Medical Microbiology Illustrated

Dedicated to Janet, Peter and David

Medical Microbiology Illustrated

S. H. Gillespie MB, BCh, BAO, MRCP(UK), MRCPath

Senior Lecturer in Medical Microbiology,
Division of Communicable Diseases,
Royal Free Hospital School of Medicine, London

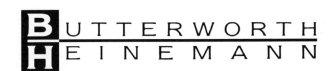

Butterworth-Heinemann Ltd
Linacre House, Jordan Hill, Oxford OX2 8DP

A member of the Reed Elsevier plc group

OXFORD   LONDON   BOSTON
MUNICH   NEW DELHI   SINGAPORE   SYDNEY
TOKYO   TORONTO   WELLINGTON

First published 1994

British Library Cataloguing in Publication Data
Gillespie, Stephen H.
  Medical Microbiology Illustrated
  I. Title
  616.01

ISBN 0 7506 0187 6

13/3/95

Composition by Scribe Design, Gillingham, Kent
Printed in France by Pollina,
85400 Luçon - n° 65293

Contents

Preface

Medical microbiology performs a vital role in the management of patients with infection. The successful microbiologist must master a diverse spectrum of knowledge which encompasses facts about micro-organisms, their classification, the diseases they cause, the way in which they harm the human host together with laboratory methods of isolation and identification. This book is intended for those coming to clinical microbiology for the first time from either a scientific or medical background. It should prove valuable to medical microbiologists in training, and public health and infectious diseases physicians who seek an introduction to laboratory-based microbiology. It should also help the medical laboratory scientist by putting laboratory practice into its proper clinical context.

In an age when textbooks are measured by the kilogram this text is not intended to be comprehensive but to provide an introduction to the laboratory–clinical interface so important in the management of patients with infections.

Acknowledgements

I am grateful to colleagues for the following figures:

Figure 2.8a and 2.8b Dr Marples, Division of Hospital Infection, Central Public Health Laboratory, Colindale, London. Figure 6.9 Mr McMillan, Central Veterinary Laboratory, Weybridge. Figure 7.11 Dr David Dance, Department of Clinical Sciences, London School of Hygiene and Tropical Medicine, London. Figures 10.2 and 10.3 Dr C.C. Kibbler, Royal Free Hospital School of Medicine, London. Figures 11.12, 11.13, 11.26, 11.27 Dr Mark Taylor, London Hospital Medical College, London. Figure 11.18 Dr T. McHugh, Department of Microbiology, St Georges Hospital, London. Figures 8.8 and 22.5 were kindly provided by Don Whitely Ltd, Figures 13.2–13.4 by MDH Ltd, Figure 14.2 by Unipath.

Tables 4.4, 4.6 and 4.7 were based on Collins, Grange and Yates (see Further reading).

I am grateful to Dr R. Gargan for his assistance in preparing many of the preparations for photography. I also gratefully acknowledge the assistance of Mrs A. Smyth, Mr A. Ramsay, and Miss L. Tilling and the staff of the Medical Illustration Department, Royal Free Hospital, in preparing and photographing material for this book.

1

Introduction to clinical microbiology

Introduction

A detailed understanding of epidemiology, and the biology of micro-organisms is required if patients with infectious diseases are to be adequately treated. Knowledge of the normal resident microbial flora facilitates the evaluation of the significance of individual organisms isolated from clinical specimens. An understanding of the pathogenicity and virulence will assist in predicting the likely behaviour of potential pathogens. In the same way, knowledge of intrinsic susceptibility or resistance to antimicrobial agents will be valuable in planning effective antimicrobial chemotherapy. This introductory chapter discusses the process of microbiological diagnosis from the initial clinical encounter to the completion of the diagnostic and therapeutic process.

The process of microbiological diagnosis

The process of making a microbiological diagnosis has many component steps. All of these must be understood and optimized if the laboratory is to collaborate fully with the clinician in achieving the best outcome for the patient.

The process begins when the clinician meets the patient, takes a history and performs a clinical examination. The clinician forms a hypothesis about the cause of the patient's complaint: the differential diagnosis. With this hypothesis a diagnostic plan must be constructed which will include laboratory, radiological and other investigations. At this point the clinical microbiologist may be contacted and discussions may lead to the development of the differential diagnosis. The clinical microbiologist can also advise on the most appropriate investigations, how the specimens should be sent and may also give advice on empirical therapy.

Relevant specimens are obtained and transported to the laboratory. It is essential that this process is closely controlled as most microbiological specimens are highly perishable. When they are received in the laboratory the specimens should be carefully documented and urgent specimens identified for rapid processing. They should then be investigated according to the standard laboratory procedures. A report is drawn up which may indicate the presence or absence of human pathogens and, where relevant, their susceptibility to antimicrobial agents. These results are communicated to the clinician, together with further advice from the clinical microbiologist, who may request further specimens, modifications to the treatment regimen or clinical and laboratory follow up. This is summarized in Figure 1.1.

Specimens

The quality of microbiological specimens is crucial to the value of the results obtained. For example the possibility of isolating an organism is much reduced if antibiotics are given before a specimen is obtained.

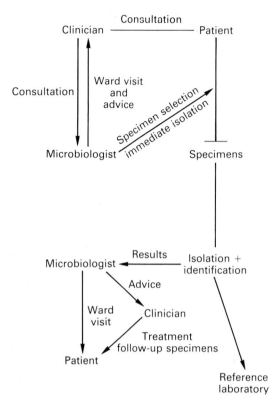

Figure 1.1 Role and function of a clinical microbiology service

The isolation of an organism from a site which is normally sterile is likely to be clinically important. Organisms may be present as a result of contamination during the clinical procedure required to collect it or during laboratory processing. Before an organism is dismissed as a contaminant, careful evaluation must be made of the clinical details usually by a visit to the patient.

In many instances, the interpretation of bacterial isolates is made more complex when important pathogenic organisms form part of the normal flora in asymptomatic subjects. *Streptococcus pneumoniae* may be found in the nasopharynx of up to 30% of healthy adults. Sputum specimens are contaminated with pharyngeal secretions which may therefore contain this organism. To overcome this problem quantitative techniques have been evolved which assume that potential pathogens are present in smaller numbers when they are acting as commensals than when they are acting as pathogens (see p. 181).

Specimen types

Specimens may be divided into two groups: those from normally sterile sites, and those containing normal bacterial flora. It is important to classify them in this way as it affects the way in which they are processed, culture results are evaluated and reports issued.

Specimens from sites which are normally sterile are inoculated into enrichment media. This protects fastidious pathogens that may be present in small numbers, provides all essential nutrients, and allows rapid multiplication so that enough organisms will be available for identification and susceptibility testing. By contrast, in specimens from a site with a normal flora, selective agents must be used to suppress the growth of commensal organisms which would obscure any pathogens. Thus for specimens from sterile sites *amplification* is the aim whereas for sites with a normal flora *selection* is the aim.

Specimen choice

Advice must be given to clinical colleagues on the most appropriate specimens for the investigation of each infective condition: for example in gonorrhoea in females an endocervical swab should be sent rather than a high vaginal swab as the former has a much higher diagnostic yield.

In the investigation of acute lower respiratory tract infection where the patient is unable to produce a satisfactory sputum specimen, more invasive techniques such as bronchoalveolar lavage may be necessary. When an abscess is drained surgically, specimens of pus should be sent in a sterile container or a sterile syringe rather than on a bacteriological swab. Pathological material may dry rapidly causing fastidious organisms to die. Swabs maximize the exposure of bacteria to drying and atmospheric oxygen resulting in a reduction in diagnostic yield; some organisms are inhibited by materials in the swab itself.

Containers

Labelled, sterile containers should be available for collection of microbiological specimens.

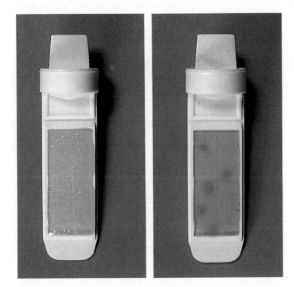

Figure 1.2 (*a* and *b*) The dipslide has two types of media on alternate sides of the paddle, MacConkey and CLED in this case. By comparing the number of colonies with a diagram the approximate number of organisms can be estimated

These should be of different sizes, depending on the specimen (i.e. a screw-capped container for cerebrospinal fluid (CSF), a wide-mouth container for mid-stream specimens of urine (MSU)). Stool pots may have a scoop incorporated in the lid to make specimen collection more aesthetic. Bottles should have a label which prompt the clinician to record essential information (i.e. name, hospital number, sex, date of birth) so that they can be reliably identified. Sodium borate can be added to urine containers to inhibit bacterial multiplication. A 'dip slide container' may be provided in which there is a paddle coated on both sides with an agar medium (usually MacConkey and cysteine lactose electrolyte deficient (CLED) agars). The paddle is dipped in the urine which is then discarded and the paddle replaced in the container. Organisms survive well on these media at ambient temperature while in transit to the laboratory where they are subsequently incubated at 37°C. Colony counts will be available on the following day and identification and susceptibility tests can be performed by subculture (Fig. 1.2).

Some perishable specimens are collected directly into a transport or culture medium and these require careful stock control to ensure that these media are kept in an optimum condition. Some workers consider that blood cultures collected into blood culture medium which is held at 37°C produces a higher diagnostic yield as this is thought to prevent 'cold shock' which retards growth. If this strategy is adopted, the microbiologist must provide blood culture bottles maintained at 37°C convenient to clinical areas and control the stock of bottles so that all media are in date.

Transport

Many bacteria, especially anaerobic species such as *Bacteroides fragilis* or aerobes such as *Neisseria gonorrhoeae,* are highly sensitive to environmental conditions. Oxygen is toxic to many anaerobic species (see p. 92), and *N. gonorrhoeae* is susceptible to drying (see p. 60). Specialized transport medium for delicate organisms and methods to generate an anaerobic atmosphere in transit are available. In both these cases delay in transport results in a significant fall in the number of viable organisms which makes it more difficult to obtain a positive result.

In specimens which are contaminated by normal bacterial flora delay in transit may allow commensal organisms to grow more rapidly than the pathogen and obscure its presence. The growth of the commensal organisms may result in the production of bacteriocins or toxic metabolites which inhibit the growth of pathogens.

When specimens cannot be processed immediately appropriate facilities for their storage should be provided. Specimens containing a normal flora should be refrigerated or discarded and repeated. For others, such as blood cultures, a small incubator outside the laboratory could be provided so that they may be incubated overnight.

Specimen quality control

The laboratory must apply a system of quality control on specimens as the results can only be as good as the quality of the specimens received. Those which are inadequately taken, delayed in transport or incorrectly stored may yield misleading results and therefore lead to inappropriate or inadequate therapy. Results generated from unsatisfactory specimens often make clinical decisions more difficult and rarely benefit the patient.

Specimens can be selected on the basis of time criteria, for example an MSU more than four hours old might not be processed. False-negative leucocyte counts may be obtained as a result of cell lysis in acid urine, and contaminating organisms initially present in low numbers will multiply and yield 'significant' counts.

Specimens may also be selected on the basis of result of direct microscopy. A poorly taken sputum heavily contaminated with saliva may yield an organism which is part of the normal oral flora. If this result is accepted and reported uncritically inappropriate antibiotics may be prescribed.

Unsatisfactory specimens must be identified quickly and the clinician requested to send another of appropriate quality. Selection of specimens in this way not only helps to optimize the use of resources, it focuses diagnostic effort into those specimens that are most likely to provide clinically relevant results.

Laboratory examination

Direct examination

Urine specimens can be examined macroscopically for cloudiness, the presence of frank pus, blood staining or xanthochromia. The characteristic offensive odour of anaerobes may be detected in abscess material.

Microscopy

Direct microscopical examination provides much useful information and it has the advantage that in some instances it provides a rapid presumptive diagnosis, which is of particular value in life-threatening infections such as acute pyogenic meningitis. For many human pathogens which are not easily cultured in artificial media (e.g. malarial parasites), microscopical examination is the only means of diagnosis available.

Unstained preparations may be examined with a light microscope. Saline-wet preparations of stool and colonic ulcers scrapings can be examined for faecal parasites (see Chapter 17). Additional information may be obtained, however, when the specimens are stained. Direct microscopy with simple stains, such as Gram's stain, are most valuable for specimens from sites that are normally sterile; thus the presence of Gram-negative diplococci in CSF enables a rapid presumptive diagnosis of meningococcal meningitis to be made. Even in specimens with a normal flora where pathogens and commensals have similar morphological appearances such as sputum, the overwhelming presence of one morphological type, e.g. Gram-positive diplococci, might indicate pneumococcal pneumonia.

Staining a micro-organism is in fact a simple biochemical reaction. Gentian violet or methyl violet in Gram's stain bind to the Gram-positive bacterial cell wall and resist decolorization with methanol or acetone. Neutral red counter stain is applied to demonstrate the organisms which have failed to take up and retain the violet dye. Thus, this process is more accurately described as Gram's reaction.

Other stains, such as the Ziehl-Neelsen (ZN), may be used in the rapid diagnosis of mycobacterial diseases. ZN stained preparations of sputum are, in some ways, more valuable than culture as a culture result can be delayed for up to eight weeks. Most clinical decisions are based on review of the clinical presentation, X-ray appearances and results of direct microscopy. Smear-positive patients are those who are most likely to transmit tuberculosis, thus ZN staining not only provides rapid presumptive diagnosis but also identifies patients to whom measures to control the transmission of infection should be applied (see Chapter 4).

Giemsa stain is used for blood and tissue parasites such as malaria and leishmania (see Chapter 11). Silver methenamine stains are employed in staining fungal cell walls and *Pneumocystis* (see Chapter 10).

The specificity and sensitivity of antibody–antigen interaction is utilized in direct immunofluorescence microscopy. Patients' specimens are air dried, fixed on a glass slide and specific antibodies are applied. After washing, fluorescence-labelled antiglobulin is added and the presence of specific antigen is demonstrated by bright apple-green fluorescence seen under ultraviolet illumination (Chapter 21).

Culture

Modern trends in diagnosis are leading to rapid diagnosis with the use of antigen detection enzyme-linked immunosorbent assay (ELISA), DNA probes and the polymerase chain reaction (PCR). However, cultural techniques will remain central to the practice of clinical microbiology. Culture enables an amplification in the number of pathogens which are initially present in very low numbers. The use of selective media will enable the discrimination between pathogens and non-pathogens which are found in the same site.

Culture on solid media is essential to produce isolated colonies for identification and susceptibility testing. Species identification is clinically beneficial as the presence of an organism of known characteristics will imply the likely pathological processes going on in the patient. Identification of *Corynebacterium diphtheriae* from a patient with a sore throat will lead to markedly different clinical and public health interventions than will the isolation of Group A β-haemolytic streptococcus.

Typing micro-organisms facilitates epidemiological studies. Some organisms have individual types which are more pathogenic than the species as a whole. For example, *Clostridium perfringens* serotype A is most frequently associated with gas gangrene, whereas serotype C is associated with clostridial food poisoning. Typing also enables the study of cross-infection within the hospital environment. Phage typing of *Staphylococcus aureus* may be used to plot the transmission of highly virulent epidemic strains, or to monitor the transmission of those staphylococci which are methicillin resistant. This is discussed in more detail in Chapter 2.

Conditions of culture

Nutrients

For successful culture, a medium must be capable of supporting the growth of the micro-organism sought. To do this, it must provide an adequate carbon and nitrogen source in a form which the organism can utilize. In addition, it must provide essential co-factors: for example *Haemophilus influenzae* requires haematin

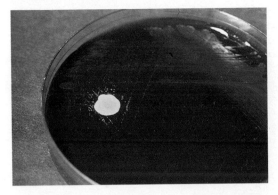

Figure 1.3 This streptococcus grows poorly on ordinary medium but forms large colonies around the *S. aureus* culture which supply essential nutrients such as pyridoxine

and nicotinamide adenine dinucleotide (NAD) for growth. Some streptococci are nutritionally fastidious, being dependent on pyridoxine. These organisms will not grow unless the medium contains pyridoxine or a *Staphylococcus* is streaked across the culture to provide this nutrient (Fig. 1.3).

Temperature

Cultures must be incubated at the temperature which is optimal for the organism sought. For most human pathogens this is 37°C but other organisms are able to multiply at higher (*Campylobacter*) and lower (*Listeria*) temperatures. *Listeria monocytogenes* can multiply at low temperatures and this can be used to select the organism from heavily contaminated sources by incubating cultures in a refrigerator. The growth of most organisms is inhibited but listerias are able to outgrow the competition.

Atmosphere

Some bacteria have strict atmospheric requirements for their growth. Some are obligate aerobes (e.g. *Bordetella*), requiring molecular oxygen as the terminal electron acceptor in their metabolic pathway. Others, such as *Pseudomonas aeruginosa*, usually utilize molecular oxygen but are able to use nitrates if they are incubated anaerobically. Anaerobes are either facultative – growing under both aerobic and anaerobic conditions – or obligate. Some members of the latter group may be aerotolerant: i.e. survive in the presence of small amounts of oxygen, or are strict anaerobes to which oxygen is toxic. Micro-aerophilic organisms use oxygen as the terminal electron acceptor but grow better if the oxygen concentration is reduced. Methods for culture of anaerobic species are noted in Chapter 8. Capnophilic organisms are those whose growth is enhanced by increasing the concentration of CO_2 to 5–10%.

Humidity

Adequate humidity is requires to prevent desiccation of the cultures. This is especially important in long-term cultures required to isolate mycobacteria, fungi or slow-growing anaerobic species. Humidification can be provided by incubating plates in a plastic bag containing a few millilitres of water, by bubbling air through a reservoir of water inside the incubator, by sealing cultures with tape, or using universal containers for culture.

Media for bacterial culture

There are three forms of bacteriological media: solid, semi-solid and liquid. Each of these has a different role to play. Bacteriological media may be solidified by the addition of agar, gelatin, alginate or silica gel. The unique melting characteristics of agar have many advantages for bacteriologists: agar melts at 95°C and solidifies at approximately 50°C so that after melting the agar it remains liquid at much lower temperatures allowing the addition of heat-labile constituents such as blood and serum.

There are basic requirements for culture medium. There must be a source of nitrogen in the form of NH_2 groups. This is provided by adding proteins which may have been partly broken down by acid hydrolysis, enzyme activity, or heat. A source of energy and carbon is also required. The proteins and peptides can be used for this purpose by many species but sugars (e.g. glucose), complex carbohydrates (e.g. starch) or alcohols can be supplied.

The metabolism of bacteria may alter pH to such a degree that growth is inhibited. In most media buffering capacity is provided by the zwitterionic effect of peptides but when fermentable sugars are available a buffer is usually required. The addition of buffer salts may adversely affect the performance of the medium as some of these salts can chelate essential metal ions. In many media mineral salt and metal ion supplements are required for optimum growth. Anaerobic organisms require a low redox potential for growth and thioglycollate and cysteine and other -SH containing substances can be added to maintain this. Some organisms require special factors for growth, e.g. NAD and haemin (X and V factors) for *H. influenzae* and others require the removal of toxic metabolites (see below). The selection of individual species for further study requires the addition of selective agents and these are discussed in more detail below.

Semi-solid media are useful for demonstrating bacterial motility or for preserving those organisms which are susceptible to desiccation. Fluid media are used in enrichment cultures and as indicator media. Bacteriological media can also be classified in three ways: enrichment, selective or indicator (Table 1.1).

Table 1.1 Examples of different types of media employed in clinical microbiology

Medium	Type	Selective agent/ indicator/enrichment
Hoyle's medium	Selective/enrichment	Potassium tellurite, lysed blood
Chocolate agar	Enrichment	Heated blood
MacConkey agar	Selective/indicator	Bile salts/lactose neutral red
Cary-Blair	Semi-solid transport	
Selenite F	Selective broth	Sodium selenite
Robertson's cooked meat	Enrichment broth	Meat/brain heart infusion
Peptone water sugars	Indicator broth	Monosaccharide and Andrade's indicator

Enrichment media

Enrichment media are used in the isolation of organisms that have fastidious growth requirements which include many human pathogens. Media may be enriched by the addition of animal products, such as blood, brain and heart infusions, meat digests, and yeast extracts. Each of these products supplies essential nutrients which the bacteria are unable to synthesize by themselves (e.g. nucleotides are richly found in yeast extract). Each of these media types can be solid, semi-solid or fluid by the addition of varying concentrations of agar. Fluid enrichment media are particularly valuable for the isolation of small numbers of pathogens from fluid specimens or tissues which are normally sterile as a single organism will multiply to sufficient numbers for subculture and identification.

It may be necessary to remove bacterial toxic metabolic products. *Bordetella pertussis* is inhibited by the products of its own metabolism and this effect is overcome by absorbents in the form of potato starch (in Bordet-Gegnou medium), or charcoal in charcoal yeast extract agar. A similar effect is also seen on *Haemophilus ducreyi* for the culture of which charcoal is added to standard media such as Meuller-Hinton.

Selective media

Selective media are essential in the microbiological investigation of specimens which contain a normal flora. Media can be made selective by the addition of antimicrobial agents or compounds which will inhibit the growth of unwanted species. Compounds used for this purpose include dyes such as crystal violet and natural components such as bile salts, which select for bile-tolerant organisms. Selective agents, however, have their disadvantages: selection is only relative and the target organism may also be inhibited. Selective media, therefore, should be used in parallel with enrichment media to ensure maximum diagnostic yield. Many organisms are inherently resistant to some antimicrobial agents and this property can be used in selecting them: for example *Bacteroides* spp. are naturally resistant to aminoglycosides and vancomycin and thus a combination of kanamycin and vancomycin is used in selective media for their isolation.

Indicator media

Indicator media include a compound which alters in its physical characteristic in response to growth of a micro-organism. This usually takes the form of a colour change to indicate utilization of a particular substrate. Indicator media may be solid, semi-solid or liquid. Solid media containing potassium tellurite are used in the diagnosis of diphtheria. Some corynebacterium reduce tellurite to an insoluble black compound, making the colonies easily distinguishable from the normal flora. The oxidative/fermentative test of Hugh and Liefson consists of a basal medium containing a single carbohydrate and an indicator in a semi-solid agar. A stab inoculum is made in two similar tubes, but air is excluded in one of them by layering mineral oil on top. Oxidation or fermentation of the carbohydrate is indicated by a change in the colour of the indicator dye. The semi-solid nature of the indicator also enables bacterial motility to be detected.

This description of bacterial culture media is, of course, a simplification as many of the media in use in the microbiology laboratory fall into more than one category. Many media used in primary bacterial culture are both selective and enrichment (see Table 1.1). MacConkey's agar or thiosulphate citrate bile sucrose (TCBS) agar are examples of selective indicator media. MacConkey's agar includes sodium taurocholate, lactose and neutral red. It selects for bile-tolerant organisms and indicates the presence of lactose fermenters which grow as pink coloured colonies. *Vibrio cholerae* may be isolated on TCBS, which is selective for vibrios on the basis of its high pH and the presence of bile salts. Selenite F is an example of a selective enrichment broth. The use and preparation of individual media are described in the relevant chapters.

Sensitivity testing

Methods of sensitivity testing are described in detail in Chapter 20.

Clinical correlation

The value of antibiotic susceptibility testing, whether qualitative or quantitative, is limited as it is unable to take account of the contribution of the patient's immune system or the negative effect of derangement in other body systems caused by infection. For example, it has been clearly shown in pneumococcal bacteraemia that patients fail to survive despite optimal chemotherapy once a 'point of no return' has been passed. Also, many patients recover from serious bacterial infection when treated with antibiotics to which the organisms are resistant. In other infections, such as atypical mycobacterioses and nocardiasis, there is a poor correlation between the results of susceptibility testing and clinical outcome.

Susceptibility results are usually obtained 48 hours after the receipt of specimens, often when the patient has already been on therapy for some time. When the clinical microbiologist, therefore, advises on antimicrobial agents, he will select the regimen on the basis of his knowledge of the likely pathogens and their usual susceptibility pattern. Bacterial culture and susceptibility testing can, however, take account of unusual pathogens or indicate unusual sensitivity patterns.

Susceptibility testing can be used as an 'intelligence network', enabling the clinical microbiologist to predict accurately the susceptibility of organisms isolated from his patients. This information can also be used to monitor the transmission of organisms within the hospital and identify patients where precautions to contain the transmission of multiresistant organisms are required.

Serology and antigen detection

The most valuable microbiological results are those which are obtained rapidly. This is especially true among immunocompromised patients, whose response to infection is poor, and those suffering from acute pyogenic infections, where rapid deterioration may occur. Antigen detection and other serological methods may also be used when organisms are difficult or impossible to culture (e.g. *Pneumocystis carinii*). Detailed methods of serological and antigen detection techniques are found in Chapter 21.

Reporting

The function of the clinical microbiologist is to transmit relevant microbiological information to clinicians as rapidly as possible, to interpret it and advise on appropriate therapy and procedures to control transmission.

Strategy

We can divide the reporting process into several stages. A preliminary report may be made, usually by telephone, when results of direct microscopical examination or primary isolation become available. As well as communicating results rapidly, the additional clinical information obtained will guide further laboratory work. The preliminary report of Gram-negative intracellular diplococci in the CSF of a child will direct antimicrobial chemotherapy towards agents active against the meningococcus and set in train control of infection measures such as source isolation and antibiotic prophylaxis to close contacts. After primary isolation and simple identification testing (e.g. Gram stain, oxidase, and catalase), a presumptive identification can be made. For example, a Gram-positive catalase-negative coccus on primary culture from CSF is likely to be *S. pneumoniae*, although final identification must await the result of bile solubility and optochin sensitivity tests. These preliminary reports, although issued by telephone or ward visit, should be carefully documented in the patient's notes and in laboratory records. Some laboratories will issue written preliminary reports. In general, most laboratories will issue a written report when the organism has been identified to an appropriate level, and susceptibility tests have been performed. In some instances, this will be at species level (e.g. *S. pneumoniae*), but in others identification to genus level will be sufficient (e.g. *Campylobacter* spp.).

Content

The content of the final written report must be carefully considered. It should include details of the macroscopic examination of the specimen and the results of any microscopical examination, including white cell count, cell type, and Gram morphology of bacteria present. The reporting of isolates will vary, depending on whether the specimen contains a normal flora. In specimens which are normally

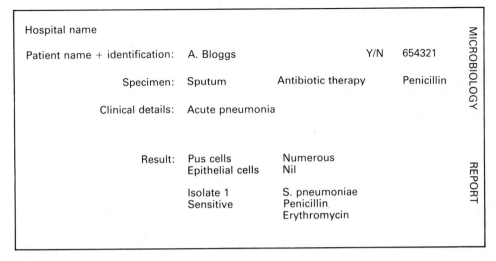

Hospital name			
Patient name + identification:	A. Bloggs	Y/N	654321
Specimen:	Sputum	Antibiotic therapy	Penicillin
Clinical details:	Acute pneumonia		
Result:	Pus cells	Numerous	
	Epithelial cells	Nil	
	Isolate 1	S. pneumoniae	
	Sensitive	Penicillin	
		Erythromycin	

MICROBIOLOGY

REPORT

Figure 1.4   Diagram of a typical report form

sterile, the presence of any bacterial isolate must be explained.

Selective reporting

In specimens with a normal flora selection of the content of report is more difficult as isolation of primary pathogens may not necessarily indicate disease. Contaminated sites may also contain several organisms of varying pathogenic potential. Difficulties such as this can be resolved only by reporting in the light of clinical symptoms and signs, and using accessory details such as white cell counts and contaminating epithelial cells seen on microscopy. Reports therefore, should guide the clinician to the organism which may be implicated in the disease process.

When a report is based on culture-selective media it should be precise; thus 'no pathogens found' is not as useful as 'no Salmonella, Shigella, Campylobacter found' as a clinician is left in no doubt as to which diarrhoea-causing organisms have been sought.

Additional comments should be applied to the report, requesting further specimens or indicating doubts about the significance of a particular isolate. Such comments are of limited value, however, in comparison with a ward visit where the patient's clinical details may be fully evaluated and a record of inter-

pretation and advice entered in the patient's case record.

Unselective reporting

Some microbiologists include a list of all organisms isolated. Such reporting is usually confusing to clinicians who may lack the detailed knowledge of normal bacterial flora and the pathogenic potential of organisms which would enable them to interpret such reports fully. In any case, reporting normal flora is in no sense more complete as artificial culture only yields organisms capable of multiplying on the medium selected.

Quantitation

Many cultures are quantified, i.e. 'heavy growth of'. This practice is illogical as the number of colonies found on primary isolation is under the influence of so many confounding variables as to make such a comment uninterpretable. In specimens left at high ambient temperature a small number of organisms could multiply before inoculation, similarly, a specimen transported under adverse circumstances could allow the numbers of a more delicate organism to fall, resulting in a scanty growth. Isolates should, therefore, only be reported in a format such as '*Staphylococcus aureus* isolated'. Where significance can be established by reference to viable count or quality of the specimen ('A significant isolate of *Staphylococcus aureus*'), or where there is doubt of the clinical relevance ('*Staphylococcus epidermidis* isolated: of doubtful significance').

Reporting susceptibilities

Selective reporting of susceptibility results should be adopted as this will help to limit unnecessary antimicrobial therapy and guide the clinician towards agents with higher activity, better safety records, or which are less expensive. Consequently, significant isolates should be accompanied with the results of antimicrobial susceptibilities, giving a choice of agents to treat that infection taking into account common problems, e.g. pregnancy or penicillin allergy. It is important also to list resistances so that antibiotics likely to be ineffective are clearly shown. This is illustrated with a report (Fig. 1.4).

Reference laboratories

When an organism cannot be fully identified in the laboratory where it was first isolated but is thought to be clinically relevant, it should be sent to a reference laboratory. Many countries have a national network of laboratories (see Further reading). A report should be issued with a comment stating that the organism isolated has been so referred.

Typing

Indications for typing

Typing is the natural extension of the process of isolation and identification and the indications for typing are similar. In simplistic terms typing can be used to show that a group of organisms are the same. By showing that a group of organisms are the same one can predict their biological behaviour, i.e. these organisms are more virulent, or they have come from a common source.

Typing bacteria can be a drain on laboratory resources unless these simple principles are adhered to. Bacteria should only be typed if there is a clear objective, in other words they should not be typed because a typing method exists.

Requirements of a typing system

A successful typing system should be simple to perform and reproducible. It should differentiate organisms into enough groups so that it is useful for distinguishing organisms that are similar but not identical. Bacteria isolated from clinical material should be found in many of the typing groups. A typing scheme is of little value if all clinical isolates are found in one or two groups no matter how many types can be differentiated. The typing method should be of proven value for the epidemiological question which is being addressed. Naturally every laboratory would wish that its typing methods were cheap.

Methods

Antibiograms

This method is based on the determination of the pattern of resistance to a range of antibiotics. For most routine purposes an antibiogram is adequate to distinguish two isolates. It has little application, however, for organisms whose resistance pattern is predictable and stable. It is clearly of value in monitoring multi-drug-resistant organisms such as methicillin-resistant staphylococci, or gentamicin-resistant Enterobacteriaceae.

Biotyping

Biotyping utilizes a group of phenotypic characteristics to separate strains. This may be useful when a common organism causing an outbreak has unusual phenotypic characteristics. Biotyping methods for *H. influenzae* have been described but have found little clinical application (see Chapter 6). Auxanograms which determine an organism's requirements for essential nutrients are a form of biotyping which is useful in the typing of *Candida albicans* and other yeasts.

Serotyping

Serotyping uses bacterial agglutination with different antibodies to distinguish isolates. This has proved useful for typing several Gram-negative pathogens notably the salmonellas, *Pseudomonas*, shigellas, and *Legionella pneumophila*. Most laboratories would expect to perform some serological typing on salmonella and shigella isolates (see Chapter 17).

Bacteriocin typing

Bacteriocins are protein antibiotics produced by bacteria to inhibit organisms which inhabit the same ecological niche including those of the same species. The activity of a test isolates bacteriocin is tested against a panel of indicator strains and the pattern of inhibition used to determine the bacteriocin type. Bacteriocin typing has found application in typing *Shigella sonnei* and *P. aeruginosa*.

Phage typing

In phage typing a panel of lytic phages is inoculated on a lawn inoculum of the isolate under investigation. Phages which are able to set up a lytic infection in that isolate produce a clear zone. The pattern of lysis is used to determine the phage type. Staphylococci can be typed by phage typing and many hospitals developed such a system when some types of organisms were causing life-threatening infections. Staphylococci are typed to determine whether the isolates belonged to the more virulent phage types so that the appropriate control of infection methods could be instituted.

Plasmid analysis

Plasmid analysis is one example of the growing use of molecular biological methods for typing. Plasmid DNA is extracted and treated by endonuclease digestion with one or more restriction endonucleases. The digested DNA is then run on a horizontal agarose gel, and the DNA is visualized by staining with ethidium bromide and examined under u.v. illumination. A permanent record can be obtained by photographing the gel. A major disadvantage of this technique is its variability and the cost of some restriction enzymes.

For bacteria which do not possess plasmids digestion of chromosomal DNA can be used. This technique can be developed further by probing the restriction fragments with DNA sequences which are found in more than one copy in the genome. A method based on this method using an insertion sequence probe is proving valuable for the typing of *M. tuberculosis*.

Computerized records

Many laboratories are now using computers to generate report forms. These systems utilize a large database programme and have a number of advantages. Printed reports are always legible and will follow a strict reporting protocol. Individual sensitivity results may be suppressed and, when necessary, further reports generated. The power of these systems, however, comes in their ability to access the database and process results in a number of ways. Multi-drug-resistant organisms such as methicillin-resistant *S. aureus* (MRSA) or virulent organisms such as *Salmonella typhi* can be flagged and cumulative reports can be generated. All the positive blood culture isolates could be collected, numbers and species of pathogens counted, and the percentage of contaminated cultures evaluated. Daily printouts of positive isolates can be used to act as a focus for clinical case review, and weekly/monthly reports can be used to identify cross-infection problems by identifying clusters of similar isolates in individual ward areas. By counting the number and type of specimens processed, the computer can be used to study work flow and assist in costing services and allocation of resources.

2

Gram-positive cocci

Introduction

Gram-positive cocci are included among some of the most significant human bacterial pathogens: primary pathogens such as *Staphylococcus aureus*, *Streptococcus pyogenes*, and *Strep. pneumoniae*, along with species of lower virulence such as *Staph. epidermidis*, *Staph. saprophyticus* and *Enterococcus faecalis*. Isolation and identification of these organisms is one of the most important but also routine tasks performed in clinical microbiology.

The Gram-positive cocci are divided into the Streptococcaceae and the Micrococcaceae; this is summarized in Table 2.1. This is an important clinical as well as taxonomic division and one which is made simply on the basis of colonial morphology, Gram morphology and the catalase test (Figs 2.1–2.3).

Staphylococcus

Introduction

The genus *Staphylococcus* belongs to the family Micrococcaceae (see Table 2.1). (The other major genus in the family, *Micrococcus*, is found as a commensal in human specimens and in the environment. It rarely causes disease.) Staphylococci are Gram positive and occur characteristically in irregular grape-like clusters, tetrads or short chains. They are catalase-positive, facultative anaerobes, non-motile, non-spore-forming and usually

Table 2.1 Differentiation of Gram-positive cocci

	O/F	*Catalase*	*Gram*
Micrococcaceae			
Micrococcus spp.	O	+	Clusters
Staphylococcus	F	+	Clusters
Streptococcaceae			
Aerococcus	F	weak	Clusters
Streptococcus	F	–	Chains
Enterococcus	F	–	Chains

O/F: Oxidative/Fermentative

unencapsulated. They may be differentiated from micrococci by their susceptibility to lysostaphin, resistance to lysozyme, fermentative reaction in the Hugh and Leifson test and their ability to ferment glycerol in a medium containing 0.4 mg/l erythromycin.

Habitat

Staphylococci are found on the skin and mucus membranes and in the gastrointestinal tract of humans, other mammals and birds. Some species have a preferred host, e.g. *S. hyicus*, pigs; *S. caprae*, goats; *S. equorum*, horses. Many are found on the human host as commensals, and can be found preferentially in some parts of the body (Table 2.2). Staphylococci survive well in the environment on skin squames and in dust and are readily transmitted in hospitals on the hands of medical and nursing staff and by the airborne route. Measures must, therefore, be taken to prevent the spread of strains of *Staph. aureus*

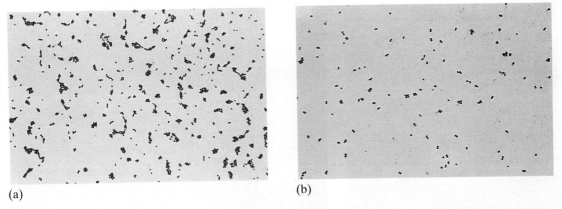

(a)   (b)

Figure 2.1 (*a*) The Gram stain shows the characteristic 'bunch of grapes' appearance which gave staphylococci their name. (*b*) Coagulase-negative staphylococci like this strain of *S. epidermidis* may be seen in tetrads. They cannot be distinguished from *S. aureus* on this characteristic alone

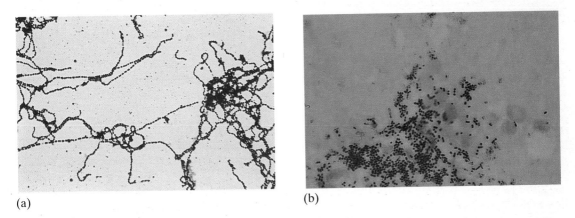

(a)   (b)

Figure 2.2 (*a*) Streptococci form long chains of cocci as in this preparation of *S. pyogenes*. (*b*) Enterococci and some other species of streptococci may apparently cluster and form short chains

that have enhanced virulence or which carry antibiotic resistance genes.

Clinical importance

Staphylococcus aureus is a common cause of primary human skin infections including impetigo, pustules, boils, carbuncles, and cellulitis. It is also frequently implicated in postoperative sepsis, in wound infections, abscesses, and in colonizing intravascular prosthetic devices and the sites of burns. Septicaemia may develop when organisms invade from any of these sites or can occur when introduced by intravenous catheters or by the unhygienic techniques employed by i.v. drug abusers. Serious localized infections may arise as a result of haematogenous spread from the site of a trivial skin infection or as part of the septicaemic process resulting in an acute endocarditis, osteomyelitis, or septic arthritis. Staphylococcal pneumonia may follow severe influenza virus infection or aspiration.

Staphylococcus aureus elaborates a number of potent toxins, including six enterotoxins which withstand heating at 100°C for 30 minutes. Foods typically implicated include ham, cream and custard. Symptoms of vomiting and diarrhoea develop after a short incubation period (4–6 hours) and are typically of short duration.

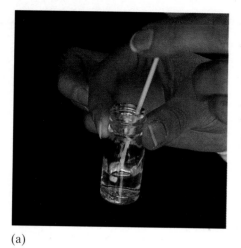
(a)

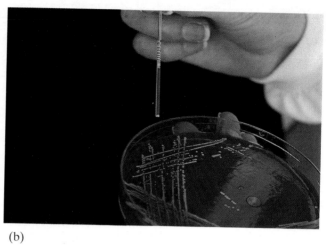
(b)

Figure 2.3 (*a* and *b*) The catalyse test is an important test for differentiating streptococci from staphylococci. Hydrogen peroxide drawn into a capillary tube is touched onto a colony: catalase-positive strains will be demonstrated by a column of bubbles rising in the tube. Alternatively a colony can be picked up with a wooden applicator and placed into a bijoux of hydrogen peroxide

Strains which elaborate exfoliatin toxin are capable of inducing the staphylococcal scalded skin syndrome (Lyell's syndrome) where the bacterial toxin causes lysis in the layers of the skin with widespread superficial skin loss. The patient appears to have multiple scalds.

Toxic shock syndrome (TSS) is a community-acquired toxaemia associated with the use of tampons or with skin sepsis where there is a localized *S. aureus* infection, with an organism which produces the toxic shock syndrome toxin-1 (TSST-1). This results in an acute life-threatening toxaemia characterized by hypotension, scarletiniform rash followed by desquamation, and multi-organ failure.

In the past staphylococci were classified on the basis of the coagulase test into *S. aureus* and '*S. albus*', the latter usually being dismissed as a non-pathogen. '*S. albus*' has now been subdivided into many species (at least 27), some of which are human pathogens.

As a result of changes in medical practice *S. epidermidis* infection is now considered to be an important clinical problem. *S. epidermidis* is a frequent cause of hospital-acquired bacter-aemia (up to 75% of positive blood cultures) often related to indwelling intravascular prosthetic devices, including prosthetic heart

Table 2.2   Examples of staphylococci found in the human host with preferred site of colonization

Species	Site
S. aureus	Anterior nares
S. epidermidis	Skin
S. saprophyticus	Genitourinary tract
S. haemolyticus	Apocrine skin
S. hominis	Apocrine skin
S. capitis	Scalp

valves, central venous cannulae and pacemak-ers. The organisms are usually introduced at the time of insertion. In these circumstances staphylococci may cause recurring episodes of bacteraemia necessitating the removal of the prosthetic device.

Staphylococcus epidermidis is responsible for approximately 40% of prosthetic joint infection and is involved in bacterial peritonitis in patients treated with ambulatory peritoneal dialysis. Patients with ventriculo-peritoneal shunts may also be infected by *S. epidermidis* and this may be accompanied by a bacter-aemia. *S. saprophyticus* is the second common-est cause of urinary tract infection in young, sexually active females. *S. haemolyticus* is the third most commonly pathogenic coagulase-negative staphylococcus and is found in prosthetic valve endocarditis, peritonitis, septicaemia and urinary tract infection. It is also important as it shows natural resistance to the glycopeptide antibiotic, teicoplanin.

Pathogenicity

Staphylococcal enzymes

Coagulase is the enzyme which catalyses the conversion of fibrinogen to fibrin. It is most closely associated with pathogenicity, having previously been used in the microbiology laboratory to separate pathogens from non-pathogens. Two types of enzyme are produced: 'bound' associated with the cell surface and 'free'. They are detected by different methods (see below). Strains of *S. aureus* lacking this enzyme are rare and other staphylococci possessing this enzyme (*S. intermedius* and *S. hyicus*) are rarely found in man.

More than 99% of *S. aureus* elaborate a deoxyribonuclease, and demonstration of this enzyme is useful in confirming the identification. Many strains of *S. aureus* produce one or more haemolytic toxins, of which there are four. These are antigenically distinct (α, β, γ, and δ) and differ in their activity against red cells of animal species. In addition, Panton-Valentine leukocidin, which is toxic to polymorphs, several lipases, hyaluronidase, and fibrinolysin are produced. Each of these enzymes may assist in establishing and disseminating infection.

Staphylococcal toxins

Staphylococcus aureus may produce exfoliation, of which there are at least two antigenically distinct types: exfoliation A, coded by a chromosomal gene, and exfoliation B, coded on a plasmid. This toxin splits the desmosomes in the stratum granulosum which link individual skin cells leading to a scalded skin appearance.

Two antigenically distinct proteins (A and B) are made by staphylococci and share many biological and clinical characteristics with streptococcal erythrotoxins. They are thought to be involved in the staphylococcal scarlet fever syndrome.

Six antigenically distinct glycopeptide enterotoxins are produced by *S. aureus*. Up to 50% of strains isolated from human sources are toxin producers and these are usually from phage group III organisms. Unlike shigella enterotoxins, these act by stimulating the vomiting centre via the vagus and sympathetic nervous system in the gut, and may also release cytokines.

TSST-1 toxin is produced by up to 20% of staphylococcal strains *in vitro*. The toxin is a polypeptide antigenically distinct from the other staphylococcal toxins. TSST-1 strains are more often found in phage group I and among untypable strains. The toxin acts by stimulating the release of cytokines such as interleukin 1 (IL-1), tumour necrosis factor (TNF) and interferon (IFN) and their consequent biological effects.

Surface factors

Most *S. aureus* express protein A on their surface. Protein A binds the Fc portion of immunoglobulin thus interfering with its antibacterial function. Many strains of *S. aureus* express receptors for the protein fibronectin which is found in the serum and on cell surfaces. These receptors may aid in attachment of the organism at the site of invasion.

Some strains of *S. aureus* are capsulate, and this enhances their virulence. In addition, strains may exhibit a pseudocapsule formation only when cultivated *in vivo*. This has been shown to be the principal pathogenicity determinant of sheep mastitis.

Staphylococcal adhesion to plastic is important in the pathogenesis of catheter-related sepsis. This adhesion is thought to be mediated through extracellular slime production. The pathogenicity determinants are illustrated in Figure 2.4.

Antibiotic susceptibility

As an important community-acquired and hospital pathogen, antibiotic resistance is a significant problem. *S. aureus* is usually sensitive to erythromycin, clindamycin, tetracycline, chloramphenicol, fucidin and gentamicin.

Originally almost all strains of *S. aureus* were penicillin sensitive, but with the clinical

(a)

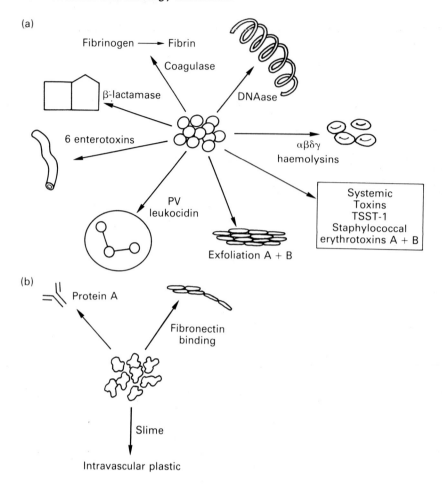

(b)

Figure 2.4   Summary of pathogenicity determinants of *S. aureus*

use of this antibiotic, almost all hospital strains and 60–70% of community strains are resistant by virtue of extracellular penicillinase production. Penicillinase stable agents such as methicillin and flucloxacillin have solved this clinical problem. More recently, however, strains which are resistant to methicillin due to chromosomally encoded mechanism have become important nosocomial pathogens, especially where other antibiotic-resistant genes are expressed.

More than half of known strains of coagulase-negative staphylococci are resistant to methicillin, and this is often combined with other resistances.

Susceptibility to methicillin is unreliable if tested at 37°C on normal media and read after 24 hours. More reliable results can be obtained if the incubation period is extended to 48 hours or testing is performed on nutrient agar containing 6% NaCl. The simplest way of obtaining reliable results is to incubate conventional sensitivity tests at 32–34°C overnight. This enables other antibiotics to be tested at the same time.

Specimens

Staphylococci are relatively easy to isolate from infected clinical material. Specimens of pus should be sent whenever these can be obtained, especially from those patients with abscess formation, accompanied by a blood

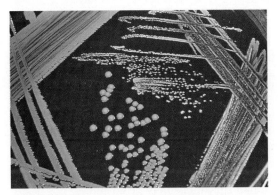

Figure 2.5 Golden-yellow colonies of *S. aureus* are seen beside the white colonies of *S. epidermidis*

optimum of 37°C at an optimum pH of 7.5. After 24 hours, colonies are 1–3 mm in diameter with a smooth glistening surface, an entire edge, and a soft butyrous consistency. They are opaque and may be pigmented. *S. aureus* may have a golden-yellow hue, whereas other staphylococci are white, hence the old name '*S. albus*'. This contrasts with the largely non-pathogenic *Micrococcus* spp. which are often a lemon yellow (Fig. 2.5). On blood agar the colonies may be surrounded with a zone of beta haemolysis and on MacConkey's agar smaller colonies are formed which are pink due to lactose fermentation.

Selective media

Selective media are used in the examination of specimens which are likely to be heavily contaminated with large numbers of other bacteria in examination of faeces or food or in searching for staphylococci from screening specimens during an outbreak.

Staphylococci tolerate high sodium chloride concentration and cooked meat broth with 10% NaCl may be used for selection and enrichment. Mannitol salt agar incorporates 7.5% NaCl, 1% mannitol and 0.0025% phenol red in a nutrient agar base. This is both a selective and an indicator medium. Many strains of *S. aureus* ferment mannitol producing colonies surrounded by a yellow zone which facilitates screening. However, it has the disadvantage that some mannitol non-fermenting organisms could be missed.

A nutrient agar which incorporates phenolphthalein can be used as an indicator medium. *S. aureus* produces a phosphatase which will liberate phenolphthalein from the medium. When the plate is exposed to ammonia vapour, the colonies will become a pink colour.

culture. Staphylococci survive well in transit and can easily be isolated from swabs from superficial sites. Multiple swabs may be sent from patients suspected of carrying multiresistant or virulent staphylococci. Sputum and other respiratory secretions may also yield staphylococci (see Chapter 16). Portions of intravenous devices may be cultured but care must be taken to ensure that only the interior of the lumen is sampled as the exterior may be contaminated when the device is removed through the skin. When outbreaks of food poisoning have occurred food may be cultured (see Chapter 22). Staphylococci can be isolated from air samples as part of hospital infection control strategies.

Direct examination

Staphylococci may easily be demonstrated by direct Gram staining of clinical specimens. They appear as spherical cocci varying between 0.8 and 1 mm in diameter, in grape-like clusters (*Staphyloi*, Greek – grapes) although they may appear singly, paired or in tetrads. Similar morphology is seen in broth culture, although occasionally short chains made up of less than five cocci may be seen (see Fig. 2.2).

Culture

Staphylococci grow readily on laboratory media growing between 12°C and 44°C with an

Identification

Staphylococcus aureus can be differentiated from the other members of the genus by the demonstration of coagulase as almost all strains produce this enzyme. *S. aureus* produces two forms of coagulase enzyme, bound and free. The bound coagulase or clumping factor is detected by a slide aggluti-

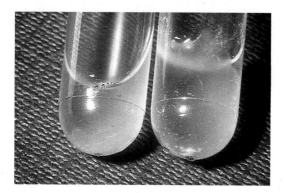

Figure 2.6   The coagulase activity of *S. aureus* (on the right) makes a solid clot whereas the *S. epidermidis* (on the left) remains liquid which is demonstrated when the two tubes are tipped

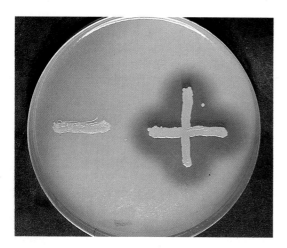

Figure 2.7   Deoxyribonuclease is a characteristic enzyme of most strains of *S. aureus*. DNAase positive strains destroy the DNA in the medium. After culture acid is placed on the plate where DNA remains a cloudiness develops leaving a clear zone around DNAase producing strains

nation test, whereas free coagulase is detected by the tube coagulase test (Fig. 2.6). As a small number of *S. aureus* strains are coagulase negative, a DNAase test should be set up in parallel. Many laboratories adopt a policy of screening suspected *S. aureus* strains with a slide agglutination technique and a DNAase test. Discrepant results are confirmed with the tube coagulase test.

The deoxyribonuclease plate test uses an agar which incorporates deoxyribonucleic acid. The suspect colony is inoculated along with positive and negative controls and incubated aerobically overnight at 37°C. After incubation, the plate is flooded with 1M HCl which causes precipitation of the DNA. After a few moments, the plates will become cloudy, except where colonies producing DNAase have destroyed DNA, producing a clear zone (Fig. 2.7). *S. intermedius* and *S. hyicus* which are animal pathogens and rarely isolated from human specimens may be coagulase positive.

Staphylococci can be further differentiated by sugar fermentation tests. Filter-sterilized carbohydrate solutions are added to a medium containing bromocresol purple to make a final concentration of 1% of the test carbohydrate.

Novobiocin resistance is found in *S. saprophyticus*, *S. cohnii*, *S. xylosus*, *S. sciuri*, *S. lentus*, and *S. gallinarum*. Only *S. saprophyticus* is a frequent human pathogen and thus this test can be used presumptively to identify this organism in clinical specimens.

All strains of *S. aureus* produce acetoin and this test may be used to distinguish *S. aureus* from *S. intermedius* and *S. hyicus*, which are occasionally coagulase positive.

The conventional biochemical methods for identification of staphylococcus species are unsuitable for use in a busy routine diagnostic laboratory. A number of commercially produced identification kits for staphylococcus species have been marketed. Identification of staphylococcus species other than coagulase-positive strains is thus a potentially expensive process. Only those isolates which are thought to be clinically significant should be identified.

Identification of coagulase-negative staphylococci may be valuable in establishing their origin in patients with intravenous prosthetic devices. Biochemical tests and antibiograms can be valuable in differentiating isolates from different blood culture bottles.

Typing

Sophisticated typing methods have been developed for staphylococcus species because of their propensity to develop significant antibiotic resistance, produce invasive infectious infections in hospitalized patients, and to be readily transmitted within the hospital

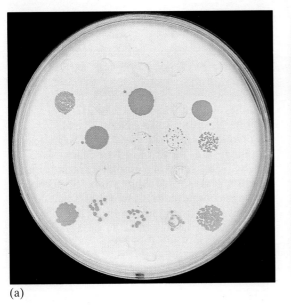
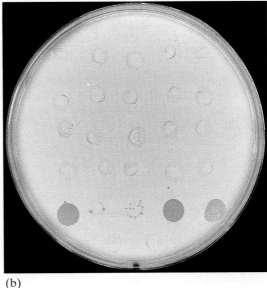

(a)   (b)

Figure 2.8   (*a* and *b*) The strain of *S. aureus* for typing is grown as a lawn on a plate. Phage is inoculated onto the lawn and where individual phage strains may infect the test strain lysis occurs

environment. These methods were initially developed to deal with the outbreaks of penicillinase-producing *S. aureus*. The development of methicillin reduced the seriousness of this problem. The advent of methicillin-resistant staphylococci which have caused invasive infections in hospital outbreaks has meant that typing strains has again become important.

Serological typing methods have been developed and more than a hundred serotypes can be distinguished. The serotype scheme has been shown to be valuable in epidemiological investigations of outbreaks. This method has not been widely utilized, however, because of the difficulties in standardization and production of antiserum.

Phage typing is the most widely accepted means of epidemiologically typing staphylococci and internationally established techniques and a standardized set of phages have been developed. In this method, a lawn inoculum of the test organism is made. Phage preparations are inoculated individually in microlitre amounts according to a preset grid pattern. After overnight incubation at 37°C,

the plates are inspected for areas of confluent lysis. The number of phages in the typing set which cause lysis are noted (Fig. 2.8). Staphylococci show continuing variation in the phages by which they can be lysed. Consequently, the international phage typing set is upgraded regularly to keep abreast of these changes.

Plasmid profiles, agar gel electrophoresis and endonuclease digestion of staphylococcal chromosomal or plasmid DNA have also been utilized for epidemiological purposes in typing both coagulase-positive and -negative species.

Stomatococcus mucilaginosis

This is also part of the family Micrococcaceae and is found in the normal oral flora. It is a slime producing Gram-positive coccus which can be seen in small clumps. It is catalase variable and is biochemically similar to the staphylococci but fails to grow on media containing a high salt content. It is an organism of low virulence but has recently been associated with infection in neutropenic patients.

Streptococcus

Introduction

The family Streptococcaceae include Gram-positive spherical bacteria growing in chains or pairs. They are typically non-motile, non-spore forming facultative anaerobes and oxidase negative. They attack carbohydrates fermentatively and are catalase negative. The Streptococcaceae are distinguished from the Micrococcaceae in that the former are catalase negative and the latter are catalase positive. In the Streptococcaceae family, only streptococci and aerococci are regularly isolated from specimens of human origin (see Table 2.1).

There have been recent taxonomic changes in the family Streptococcaceae. Several species which carry the Lancefield group D antigen have been allocated to a new genus *Enterococcus* (see below).

Classification and clinical significance

The streptococci can be classified by their phenotypic, serologic and biochemical characteristics, e.g. on the basis of haemolysis on blood agar, the group-specific carbohydrate

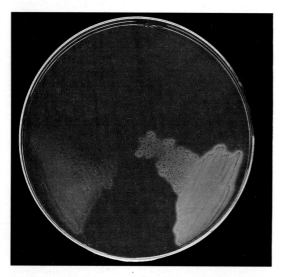

Figure 2.9 Blood agar plate showing complete 'β', partial 'α' and non haemolysis 'γ'

(Lancefield) antigen in the bacterial cell wall, and fermentation and other biochemical tests. These classification systems overlap and to some extent cause confusion as individual isolates within a species may be classified in different ways, e.g. *S. milleri* which shows variable haemolysis on blood agar, and exhibits different Lancefield antigens.

For clinical microbiologists the most useful groupings are those based on haemolysis as this helps in selecting colonies from primary isolation plates for further study. Streptococci produce complete (β) haemolysis, partial (α) haemolysis or no (γ) haemolysis (Fig. 2.9). The species which is classified as beta-haemolytic are summarized in Table 2.3.

Streptococcus pyogenes (group A streptococcus)

Clinical importance

Streptococcus pyogenes is a beta-haemolytic streptococcus frequently implicated in human infection. *Streptococcus pyogenes* can be found in the pharynx of up to 10% of healthy adults and children. The organism can be transmitted by droplet spread or direct contact, and may survive in a dry, dusty environment for prolonged periods. It causes acute pharyngitis, tonsillitis, sinusitis, otitis media and lymphadenitis. Some cases of tonsillitis may be complicated by a peritonsillar abscess (quinsy). It may infect the skin, causing erysipelas, a spreading infection often on the face which is characterized by a superficial red rash with sharp margins. Streptococcal skin infection may also take the form of a spreading cellulitis, of impetigo, or of pyoderma.

Bacteraemia is relatively common and has a significant mortality. Other suppurative complications include septic arthritis, osteomyelitis, and, more rarely, endocarditis, meningitis, and pneumonia. *S. pyogenes* spreads readily in the hospital environment and is an important pathogen of surgical wounds and in the past was a major cause of mortality through puerperal fever.

Streptococcus pyogenes can also induce post-infective complications as a consequence of immunological cross-reaction between streptococcal and host antigens. Rheumatic fever is characterized by pancarditis, arthritis, skin

Table 2.3 Summary of β-haemolytic streptococcus species and clinical significance

Species	Group antigen	Clinical syndrome
S. pyogenes *Lancefield Ag T, S protein*	A	Pharyngitis/tonsillitis/quinsy septicaemia, puerperal sepsis, cellulitis, erisypilas, impetigo, scarlet fever, rheumatic fever, glomerulonephritis
S. agalactiae	B	Neonatal septicaemia, meningitis
S. equisimilis	C	Pharyngitis, cellulitis
S. zooepidemicus	C	Septicaemia, endocarditis
S. equi	C	Rarely associated with human disease
S. dysgalactiae	C	Rarely associated with human disease
Enterococcus spp.	D	Urinary infections, abscesses, endocarditis
S. milleri	A, F, G (minute colonies)	Metastatic abscesses

rashes, and nodules and occurs four to six weeks after acute pharyngeal infection with *S. pyogenes* of any M-type (see below). Acute post-streptococcal glomerulonephritis may follow pharyngeal or cutaneous infection. A small number of individual M-types are responsible for the majority of glomerulonephritis episodes (12, 4, and 1). Post-streptococcal glomerulonephritis occurs between 10–20 days after infection.

Major antigens and pathogenicity determinants

Streptococcus pyogenes produce four main cellular antigens. A group-specific carbohydrate antigen (Lancefield antigen) is a major component of the bacterial cell wall and is used to speciate streptococci (see below). T-protein is a surface antigen which may be used as an epidemiological marker. R-protein is found in some strains of *S. pyogenes* and its biological function, like that of T-protein, is unknown.

The M-protein is a specific pathogenicity determinant. It is a surface exposed fibular protein antigen which inhibits phagocytosis by binding plasma fibrinogen and inhibiting opsonization by the alternative complement pathway. More than 80 different M-protein

types have been described, and it is this antigen to which the host's humoral immune response is mainly directed. Organisms expressing M-protein are resistant to phagocytosis in the absence of specific anti-M antibodies.

Phagocytosis may also be inhibited by a surface expressed C5a peptidase which interferes with the deposition of C3b on the surface. Some group A streptococci possess a small capsule of hyaluronic acid.

Attachment to mucosal surfaces may be facilitated by cell-surface lipotechoic acid and a fibronectin binding protein. Like other mucosal pathogens *S. pyogenes* may express IgA and IgG binding proteins.

Streptococcus pyogenes can express exotoxins, the erythrogenic toxins, and protein whose production is encoded by lysogenic bacteriophage. Three antigenically distinct toxins have been described: types A, B, and C. These toxins produce erythematous skin reactions, are pyrogenic, are cardiotoxic and are specific and non-specific T-cell mitogens. They are thought to exert their pathogenic effect by disrupting the regulation of cytokine release. Infections with organisms elaborating these toxins are complicated by an erythematous rash and are clinically described as scarlet fever. They may follow a more severe course

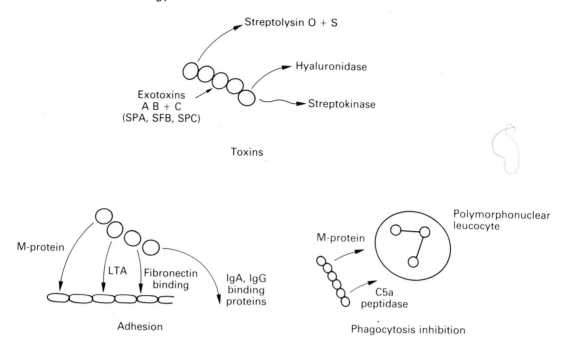

Figure 2.10   Summary of pathogenicity determinants of *S. pyogenes*

and in the past a high mortality was associated with scarlet fever.

The organism also produces two haemolysins: streptolysin O, which is oxygen labile and strongly antigenic, and streptolysin S, which is oxygen stable but poorly antigenic. Streptolysin O is one of the 'thiol activated' family of toxins found in Gram-positive organisms (see pneumolysin, cereolysin, tetanolysin). Immune response to this antigen is used in diagnosis in the anti-streptolysin O (ASO) antibody test.

Group A streptococci produce enzymes which may assist invasion: hyaluronidase, a phage encoded enzyme and streptokinase which activates plasminogen by forming an enzymic complex with plasminogen and plasmin. The pathogenicity determinants of *S. pyogenes* are illustrated in Figure 2.10.

Streptococcus agalactia (group B streptococcus)

This species was first recognized as a pathogen of cattle, causing mastitis. It is a significant cause of serious sepsis during the neonatal period, however, resulting in either septicaemia and pneumonia in the immediate perinatal period or, later, pyogenic meningitis. The organism is part of the normal flora of the gastrointestinal and female genital tracts and can be transmitted to the neonate after premature rupture of the membranes, contamination during birth, or by nosocomial transmission from other mothers, babies, or health care workers. Invasive infection is especially common in low-birthweight babies and following obstetric complications (e.g. amnionitis, operative delivery). Five main serotypes (Ia, Ib, II, III and IV) are defined on the basis of the capsular polysaccharide antigens. The majority of infections are caused by serotype III. The principal pathogenicity determinant is the antiphagocytic capsule which contains sialic acid and appears to function by inhibiting complement deposition on the bacterial surface. Neonates without maternally acquired antibody to type III are highly susceptible to infection.

Group C beta-haemolytic streptococci

There are four species of group C beta-haemolytic streptococci and they are all veterinary pathogens. The four species are *S.*

equisimilis, S. zooepidemicus, S. equi and *S. dysgalactiae*. Of these, *S. equisimilis* is the species most commonly implicated in human infection. *S. zooepidemicus* is also associated with human infection, whereas the others are less frequently isolated. A wide range of infections has been reported, including pharyngitis, cellulitis, puerperal sepsis, endocarditis, and abscess. Rheumatic fever has not been described following group C streptococcal infection, but nephritis has been documented after a group C skin infection.

Group D streptococci

The group D antigen differs from the other Lancefield group antigens in that it is a lipotechoic acid. Several species carrying this antigen have been reallocated to the genus *Enterococcus* (see below). Group D streptococci now include only two species: *S. bovis* and *S. equinus. S. bovis* is associated with infective endocarditis. *S. bovis* bacteraemia may point to underlying bowel carcinoma as *S. bovis* infection is more common in patients with gastrointestinal malignancy and inflammatory bowel disease.

Group F beta-haemolytic streptococci

Group F beta-haemolytic streptococci along with groups A and C beta-haemolytic streptococci (which form minute colonies), non-haemolytic groups A, C and G streptococci, and Streptococcus MG are all classified together under the names *S. milleri,* among European taxonomists, and *S. anginosis,* according to the Centers for Disease Control scheme. More recent DNA hybridization studies suggest that this group may be differentiated into at least three distinct species: *S. anginosis, S. constellatus* and *S. intermedius.* They form part of the normal flora at a number of body sites, being found on the hard surfaces within the mouth, in the upper respiratory tract, in the gastrointestinal tract and in the urogenital system. These organisms are responsible for odontogenic abscesses, paranasal sinusitis and are the most frequent streptococcus isolated from intracranial abscess. Endocarditis is uncommon, although bacteraemia transiently occurs following manipula-

tion of the dentition. The isolation organisms of the '*S. milleri*' group from the blood of a febrile patient should prompt a search for an occult abscess, pleural empyema, peritoneal sepsis, and hepatic abscesses which are often associated with *S. milleri* bacteraemia.

Pathogenicity determinants

The pathogenicity factors of this organism are not clearly determined. However, fine fibrillae analogous to group A streptococcal M-protein have been demonstrated as have several surface proteins which may be anti-phagocytic. A 90 kD protein has been characterized which produces T-cell suppression and B-cell activation. The organism also produces hyaluronidase, RNAase, DNAase, and proteolytic enzymes.

Alpha-haemolytic streptococci

The term viridans streptococci is used to describe organisms which characteristically produce a partial haemolysis on blood agar, although some organisms within this group may be non-haemolytic.

Classification and clinical importance

The classification of the remaining streptococci has been clarified by molecular studies. These organisms can be classified into three main groups: *S. mutans, S. oralis* and *S. salivarius* on the basis of ribosomal RNA cataloguing and DNA hybridization studies.

S. mutans

The *S. mutans* group consists of seven distinct species: *S. mutans, S. cricetus, S. downeri, S. ferus, S. rattus* and *S. macacae.*

S. salivarius

This group contains three species: *S. salivarius, S. vestibularis* and *S. thermophilus.*

S. oralis

This group can be subdivided into three subgroups which include the *S. milleri* subgroup (see above), *S. sanguis* subgroup and *S. oralis* subgroup.

The sanguis group can be subdivided into four species of *S. sanguis*, *S. gordoni*, *S. parasanguis* and *S. crista*.

The oralis subgroup contains *S. oralis*, *S. mitis* and *S. pneumoniae*. In addition to these species are the nutritionally variant streptococci *S. adjaceus* and *S. defectus* which require the addition of cysteine or adenosine to the growth of medium for isolation.

S. mutans is found in dental plaque, is associated with infective endocarditis and is thought to be important in the causation of dental caries.

S. salivarius and *S. vestibularis* are only rarely associated with human disease. *S. mitis* and *S. oralis* are normally resident in the mouth and are found in patients with infective endocarditis and more recently have been associated with severe invasive disease in patients with haematological malignancy undergoing the induction of remission or bone-marrow transplantation.

S. sanguis and *S. gordoni* are associated with dental plaque and are frequently found in patients with infective endocarditis.

Streptococcus pneumoniae (the pneumococcus)

The most significant of the alpha-haemolytic streptococci is *S. pneumoniae*, which is responsible for acute lower respiratory tract infection, septicaemia and meningitis. The pneumococcus can also be found in patients with septic arthritis, osteomyelitis, empyema, pericarditis, primary peritonitis and endocarditis. It is also an important cause of sepsis in the upper respiratory tract in patients with sinusitis and acute otitis media.

The principal virulence determinant is the anti-phagocytic polysaccharide capsule, of which there are 83 serotypes. It possesses a cell wall techoic acid antigen, the species-specific C-polysaccharide, which activates the alternative pathway of complement and stimulates inflammation in the lungs and CSF. Pneumolysin is a membrane cytotoxin analogous to streptolysin-O. Other potential pathogenicity determinants are pneumococcal surface protein A, IgA_2 protease, and neuraminidase.

With the clarification of speciation among this group of streptococci, more consistent

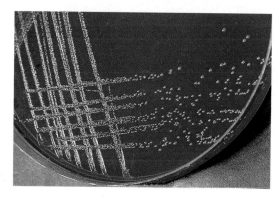

Figure 2.11 Enterococci tolerate bile and ferment lactose resulting in small pink colonies are shown here on MacConkey agar

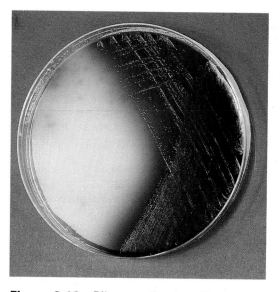

Figure 2.12 Bile aesculin plate. Enterococci can hydrolyse aesculin in the presence of 40% bile resulting in black colonies and discoloration of the medium

understanding of clinico-pathological correlation of these organisms can be expected.

Enterococcus

Classification and clinical significance

Enterococcus spp. have recently been allocated to a separate genus. They are bile salt tolerant

(Fig. 2.11) and have the ability to grow in the presence of 6.5% NaCl at 10°C, 45°C and at pH 9.6. They hydrolyse aesculin in the presence of 40% bile (Fig. 2.12). Twelve species have been defined, but *E. faecalis* is that most commonly isolated from clinical specimens. It is a normal resident of the human gastrointestinal tract and causes up to 25% of urinary tract infections. It may cause endocarditis, particularly after the instrumentation of the urinary tract. It participates in mixed infections of wounds and in abdominal abscesses. These organisms, especially *E. faecium*, are of increasing importance in the hospital environment as they are naturally resistant to many antimicrobial agents. They are therefore important colonizers and cause severe sepsis following super-infection in patients on broad spectrum antibiotics such as cephalosporins, to which enterococci are naturally resistant. The three main human species are *E. faecalis*, *E. faecium* and *E. durans*. Of these, *E. faecium* is likely to be resistant to many antibiotic agents and organisms resistant to vancomycin have caused serious infections in some hospitals.

Specimens

Streptococci may be isolated from blood, the throat, abscess pus, nasal and skin swabs, and sterile body fluids. The correct means of taking throat swabs is important for maximum isolation rates. A dry cotton wool swab should be rolled over the pharynx and tonsil, and any exudate should be swabbed. Nasal swabs should be gently moistened with sterile distilled water. Cultures from skin lesions should be obtained by firmly rubbing the sterile swab on the base of the lesion after the crusts or vesicles have been removed.

Streptococci survive well in a dry environment, but if culture is to be delayed for more than 24 hours, a transport medium such as Stuart's or Amie's medium should be used.

The isolation of *S. pneumoniae* from the respiratory tract is discussed in more detail in Chapter 16, and from the CSF in Chapter 15.

Direct examination

The direct examination of specimens from the throat, nose, or vagina is of little value as pathogenic streptococci resemble the organisms of the normal flora. However, Gram-stained smears of body fluids which are normally sterile should be examined after centrifugation.

Isolation

Streptococci are fastidious organisms which require rich media such as tryptic soy, heart infusion or proteose peptone broths. Agar containing 5–10% blood should be used for isolation on solid media. The pattern of haemolysis may vary, depending on the species of animal blood employed. Sheep blood agar is recommended for the study of haemolysis. If human blood is used the absence of inhibitors should be demonstrated by the growth of beta-haemolytic streptococci with control cultures.

Selective media

Media can be made selective for streptococci by the addition of a number of agents. Sodium azide may be used to inhibit Gram-negative rods and crystal violet to inhibit staphylococci. Combinations of antibiotics have also been used, including oxolinic acid, gentamicin, and polymyxin. Plates should be incubated at 37°C. Many streptococcal species fail to grow in an aerobic atmosphere but will grow in an increased concentration of CO_2. Streptococci grow well in an anaerobic atmosphere and beta-haemolysis is enhanced. Some strains are nutritionally demanding, requiring cysteine or pyridoxine for growth.

Identification

Identification of streptococcus species is complex, but commercial kits for biochemical testing have brought the full identification of many streptococcal species within the reach of routine diagnostic laboratories. However, to provide a useful clinical result, a simple scheme for presumptive identification of most pathogenic species should be adopted. Such a scheme is illustrated in Figure 2.13.

Suspect colonies are stained by Gram's method to determine the characteristic chains of streptococci, and the colonies are shown to be catalase negative. The first stage of

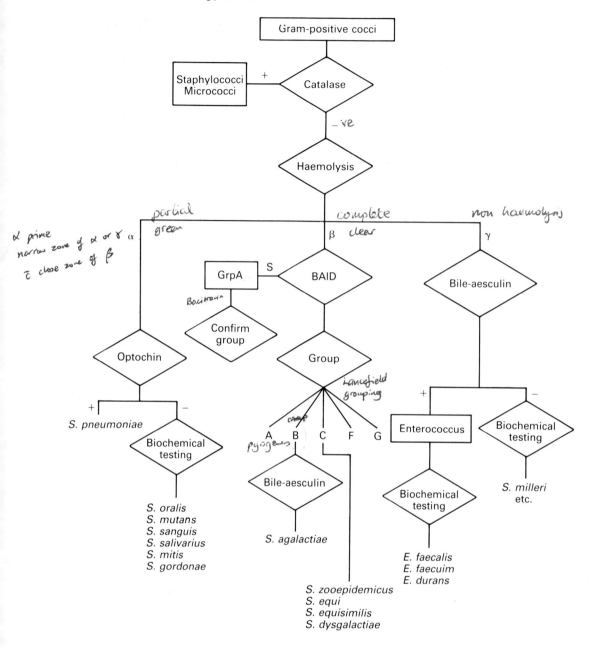

Figure 2.13   Identification scheme for Streptococci

identification of streptococci is then the description of haemolysis on blood agar. Four forms of haemolysis are described: alpha-haemolysis (a zone of partial haemolysis giving a green discoloration of a medium), beta-haemolysis (a clear zone where red blood cells have been completely destroyed), gamma-haemolysis (where no haemolytic activity has occurred), and alpha-prime haemolysis (where there is a narrow zone of partial or no haemolysis close to the bacterial colony with a zone of complete haemolysis beyond).

After incubation for 24 hours, *S. pyogenes* colonies are between 0.5 and 1 mm in diameter. They are transparent, domed with a smooth, dullish surface and an entire edge. Group B colonies may be somewhat larger than those of group A with a wider zone of haemolysis. 'Minute' colonies of groups A, C, G, and F may indicate '*S. milleri*' (see above). Among the viridans, streptococci colonial size varies from 0.1 to 2 mm. Pneumococcal colonies are 1–2 mm in diameter, round with entire edges, and may be mucoid. Older colonies may collapse in the centre, giving a draughtsman-like appearance.

Beta-haemolytic streptococci

Beta-haemolytic streptococci may be identified with a combination of disc identification tests, by serological grouping, pigment production and simple biochemical tests. Colonies should be subcultured on blood agar to provide material for the determination of the carbohydrate antigen (Lancefield group). The Lancefield group antigen is extracted and a slide agglutination test using sensitized latex beads or a coagglutination technique. Streptococcal group antigens may be extracted by the original Lancefield hot hydrochloric acid method, the autoclave, hot formamide, nitrous acid, enzymic extraction or pronase B extraction methods. The Lancefield hot acid technique is capable of extracting both the protein type-specific antigens and carbohydrate group antigen and is superior to other methods in extracting the group D (teichoic acid) antigen. Enzymic methods extract the group D antigen poorly. However, if a mixture of staphylococcal enzyme and lysozyme is used, groups A, B, C, D, F, and G antigens can be successfully extracted. In practice, most laboratories use commercial enzyme extraction kits for convenience. Results obtained by grouping can be confirmed with the other simple tests below.

Group A streptococci

Bacitracin test

Filter paper discs impregnated with 0.04 units of bacitracin are used to differentiate group A beta-haemolytic streptococci from non-group A species. A zone of inhibition is counted as a positive test but a heavy inoculum of a pure culture should be used if false-positive results

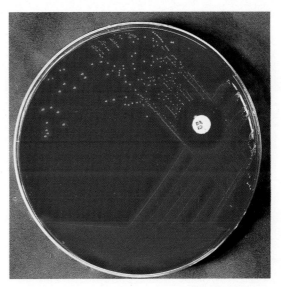

Figure 2.14   *Streptococcus pyogenes* is typically sensitive to bacitracin and exhibits beta-haemolysis

are to be minimized (Fig. 2.14). Alpha-haemolytic streptococci tested in error will also give false-positive results. In primary cultures on non-selective media, false-negative results are common but are less important if a streptococcal selective medium is used. Bacitracin sensitivity testing provides a presumptive identification and cannot replace Lancefield grouping.

PYR (L-pyrrolidonyl-beta-naphthylamide) test

The PYR reagent (N,N-dimethylaminocinnamaldehyde) is hydrolysed by all *S. pyogenes* and *Enterococcus spp.* Suspect colonies are inoculated into broth test medium and incubated for four hours. A drop of PYR reagent is added and a positive test is reported if a red colour develops after one minute.

Group B streptococci

CAMP test

The Christie Atkinson Munch-Peterson (CAMP) test may be used for the presumptive identification of *S. agalactiae* (group B β-haemolytic streptococcus). Group B streptococci produce a CAMP factor which enlarges the zone of haemolysis of *S. aureus* possessing a β-haemolysin. The suspect strain and control

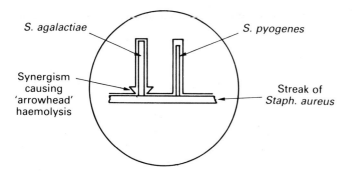

Figure 2.15 The CAMP test. Group B streptococci produce a substance which acts synergistically with staphylococcal beta toxin. *S. pyogenes* lacks this factor

Group A and B strains are streaked at right angles to the staphylococcal streak and incubated aerobically. A positive result is reported if the characteristic arrowhead is seen (Fig. 2.15). Some group A streptococci are also CAMP positive.

Hippurate test
Almost all group B β-haemolytic streptococci are hippurate positive. Some group D and α-haemolytic streptococci occasionally give a positive reaction. Hippurate medium is inoculated and incubated overnight. Ferric chloride reagent is added and, if positive, a heavy precipitate forms and remains for more than 10 minutes.

Pigment
Group B β-haemolytic streptococci produce an orange pigment when cultured on a starch/serum medium such as that of Islam.

Viridans streptococci

Optochin test
This is similar in principle to the bacitracin test. A 5 µg impregnated disc is used. A heavy inoculum should be plated on blood agar and incubated at 37°C with 5% CO_2. A positive result is reported if a zone radius (on a 6 mm disc) is >8 mm. Optochin sensitivity can be used in primary plates from specimens (e.g. sputum) likely to be contaminated by oral flora to differentiate suspected pneumococci from other alpha-haemolytic streptococci.

Bile solubility test
The bile solubility test is used to distinguish *S. pneumoniae* from other alpha-haemolytic streptococci. Suspect colonies are cultured overnight in Todd-Hewitt broth and then mixed with an equal volume of 10% sodium desoxycholate. The tubes are incubated at 30°C and a positive result is reported if clearing of turbidity occurs. Control *S. pneumoniae* and *E. faecalis* cultures should be used.

Group D streptococci and enterococci

Bile aesculin test
Suspect colonies are inoculated on a medium containing bile and aesculin. All group D streptococci, enterococci and some oral streptococci are bile-aesculin positive. After overnight incubation, positive cultures produce a blackening of the medium (see Fig. 2.12), although positive results can be observed within a few hours.

Sugar fermentation tests form an essential part of the identification process for α-haemolytic, non-haemolytic streptococci and enterococci.

Conventional biochemical techniques or commercial kits (e.g. API Strep) may be used for additional tests such as urease, arginine hydrolysis, and H_2O_2 production. The production of specific glycosidic enzyme activities can be detected with 4-methylumbelliferyl-linked substrates. Bacteria grown anaerobically are used for the test. They are mixed with the substrate and incubated for three hours. A positive result is indicated by an increase in fluorescence, signalling degradation of the substrate.

Antigen detection

Group A streptococcal antigen can be detected in throat swabs with a coagglutination or latex agglutination technique. The carbohydrate streptococcal group antigen is extracted by enzymatic means or coated with antibodies to group antigens and this is mixed with Cowan type 1 *S. aureus* in a slide agglutination test. This technique has only a moderate sensitivity (75%) but is highly specific. Several commercial kits based on this technique are available. Similar techniques can be applied to group B streptococcal antigen extracted from swabs taken from the female genital tract. A rapid diagnosis in blood culture can be obtained by antigen detection techniques. Suspect positive blood cultures which have been shown to have Gram-positive cocci in chains by direct microscopy may be examined by streptococcal antigen detection techniques of the broth.

Antibiotic susceptibility

Streptococcus pyogenes and other beta-haemolytic streptococci are sensitive to penicillins and cephalosporins, and also to erythromycin. They are naturally resistant to aminoglycosides.

The pneumococcus was previously fully sensitive to penicillin but resistant strains emerged first in South Africa and Papua New Guinea, and are now found worldwide. Penicillin resistance can be accompanied by resistance to other potentially useful agents such as erythromycin and chloramphenicol. The other viridans streptococci can also show reduced susceptibility to penicillin.

The enterococci are sensitive to ampicillin, but are naturally resistant to cephalosporins. Vancomycin may be used to treat serious enterococcal infection, but vancomycin-resistant strains have been isolated.

Serological techniques

Anti-streptolysin-O (ASO) titre

Streptolysin-O in patient serum causes lysis of red blood cells (RBCs) which can be inhibited by specific antibodies. The ASO test measures the neutralization activity of patient serum for streptolysin-O. All results are measured against a serum standardized by the World Health Organization with a value of 20 000 Todd or international units/ml. A fourfold rise in titre between acute and convalescent sera is considered significant. Commercial reagent kits for this technique are available.

Titres begin to rise one week after the infection reaching a peak four to six weeks later and remaining elevated for a number of months. False-positive results can be obtained due to bacterial multiplication in the serum, oxidation of the streptolysin-O reagent or in patients with liver disease. False-negative results can be obtained in patients with superficial infections.

An alternative technique is the measurement of anti-DNAase B antibody, which is more sensitive than the ASO titre, and may therefore be positive in streptococcal skin infection.

Aerococcus viridans

This is a rare cause of infection in man and is usually associated with infective endocarditis and infections in immunocompromised patients. It is a Gram-positive coccus growing in pairs and chains which is catalase negative but which will grow on 6.5% NaCl containing medium.

3

Gram-positive bacilli

Introduction

Aerobic Gram-positive bacilli are a taxonomically diverse group of organisms, most of which are found in the environment and rarely cause human disease. Many of them are used in industry for the production of enzymes, antibiotics, and some are important food spoilage organisms (Table 3.1). This chapter focuses on species of medical importance encountered in the microbiology laboratory. It will not refer to anaerobic species which will be discussed in Chapter 8. A simple guide to their microbiological diagnosis is found in Figure 3.1.

Corynebacterium

Classification

The genus *Corynebacterium* includes important human pathogens such as *Corynebacterium diphtheriae*, commensal organisms such as *C. hofmanii* which are pathogenic only in compromised patients, and animal pathogens. The corynebacteria are taxonomically related to the mycobacteria and nocardia. Their cell walls contain meso-diaminopimelic acid, mycolic acids and arabinogalactan polymer.

The corynebacteria are pleomorphic Gram-positive rods which are sometimes club-shaped and grow and divide in a manner which gives them a characteristic palisade or Chinese lettering morphology on Gram's stain (Fig. 3.2). They are facultative anaerobes and are catalase

Table 3.1 Examples of commercial uses of *Bacillus* spp.

Antibiotic production
bacitracin
gramicidin
polymixin
peptides
aminoglycosides
Chemical production
Enzyme production
Insecticide production

positive, oxidase negative, non-motile, non-acid-fast and non-capsulate. They break down sugars by both fermentation and oxidation.

Corynebacteria are often found as human commensals and, in this circumstance, are given the epithet 'diphtheroid' by clinical bacteriologists anxious to distinguish them from *C. diphtheriae*.

Some of the organisms previously found in the genus *Corynebacterium* have now been assigned to other genera. *Corynebacterium haemolyticum* is proposed as the only species in a new genus *Arcanobacterium*. *Corynebacterium pyogenes* will be transferred to the genus *Actinomyces* and *C. equii* to the genus *Rhodococcus*.

Corynebacterium diphtheriae

Clinical importance

Diphtheria is an acute infectious disease caused by toxigenic strains of *C. diphtheriae*.

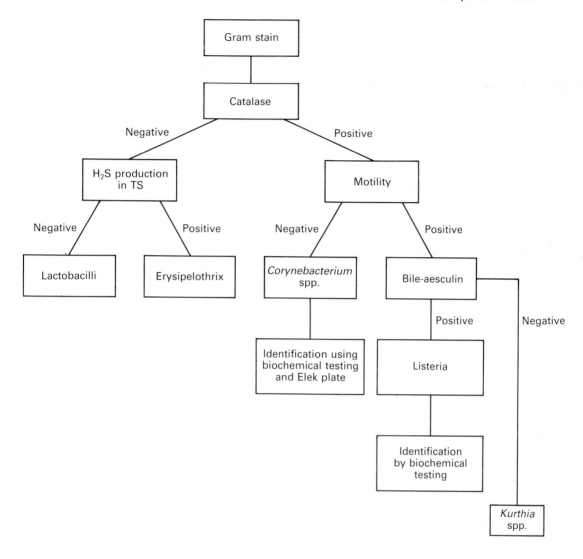

Figure 3.1 Schematic diagram of a simplified approach to the differentiation of Gram-positive bacilli

Its incidence has declined in developed countries over the last 50 years due to improvements in social conditions and the introduction of vaccination. It is still endemic, however, in many countries and may be imported by travellers and refugees.

Infection is usually localized to the respiratory tract and is characterized by an exudate which is initially white but develops into a foul, green-black necrotic membrane, with bleeding at its advancing edge. There is marked lymphadenopathy and localized oedema in the neck which give the classical appearances of 'bull neck'. The pathological consequences of diphtheria are predominantly due to the production of toxin (see below) and several clinical syndromes are recognized: nasal, laryngeal, pharyngeal, tonsillar, and cutaneous diphtheria. The severity of disease is related to the degree of toxaemia and, thus, localized forms, such as nasal, tonsillar and cutaneous infection, rarely give rise to complications.

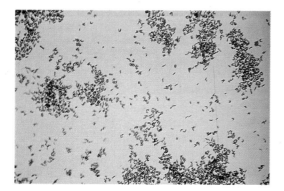

Figure 3.2 Corynebacteria are characteristically small, Gram-positive bacilli lying at irregular angles. This is sometimes known as the 'Chinese letter' pattern

They may be very important, however, in the epidemiology and transmission of infection. In the same way, laryngeal diphtheria is rarely associated with severe toxaemia, but because of the obstruction caused by the diphtheritic membrane in the larynx, death may occur.

Diphtheria toxin is toxic to all cells but severe complications affect the heart, the central and peripheral nervous systems. Myocarditis arises two weeks into the illness, usually while the oropharyngeal infection is resolving, and this may cause cardiac failure or heart block. Cranial nerve palsies develop in the acute phase of the infection but peripheral neuropathy may be delayed for up to three months.

Pathogenesis

Strains of this organism which produce toxin do so because of a lysogenic infection with a betaphage. The phage carries the full sequence for the diphtheria toxin. Diphtheria is the archetypal exotoxin disease in which a localized infection with *C. diphtheriae* produces toxin which is absorbed into the circulation and fixed to the tissues (Fig. 3.3).

The toxin consists of three portions, a receptor which mediates binding to the target cell, a hydrophobic portion which dissolves in the cell membrane enabling the third portion which contains the active portion to traverse the membrane and deregulate the cell. Diphtheria toxin acts by ribosylating diphthamide, a novel amino acid present on elongation factor 2, which is essential for protein synthesis. The toxin halts protein synthesis and cell death occurs.

Laboratory diagnosis

This organism is now rarely isolated in UK laboratories. It is important, however, that each laboratory maintains its skill in isolation, identification, and toxicity testing so when occasional isolates arise they may be rapidly identified and the appropriate public health measures taken.

It is debatable whether throat swabs should be routinely screened for presence of *C. diphtheriae*. It is argued that those who look frequently will not miss a single case when it arises. Routine screening for *C. diphtheriae* is expensive in time and materials. There is no evidence to suggest that laboratories adopting this strategy have a higher detection rate than those which culture specimens from patients with a relevant history (e.g. recent travel from an endemic country).

Specimens

Swabs from nasopharynx, fauces, nasal discharge or skin should be taken from cases as appropriate. Throat and nasal swabs are used for the investigation of suspected carriers or contacts of cases. Specimens should be sent to the laboratory directly or placed in Amie's transport medium if delay is unavoidable. The laboratory must be informed that diphtheria is suspected clinically so that appropriate isolation media can be inoculated. Microscopy of Gram-stained smears is of no value as the pathogenic organisms are morphologically similar to those found in the normal flora.

Isolation

Specimens should be inoculated on blood agar containing potassium tellurite for selection and on Loeffler's medium. The latter should be incubated for six to eight hours and growth examined by microscopy of an Albert's stained preparation. This stain is valuable for the detection of storage (volutin) granules found

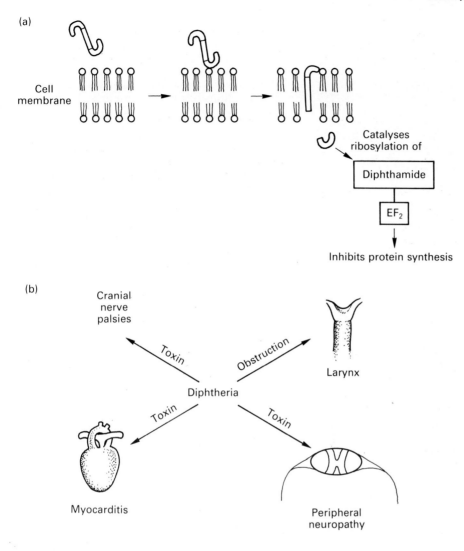

Figure 3.3 Diphtheria toxin traverses the membrane and stops protein synthesis by catalysing the ribosylation of diphthamide, a novel amino acid on elongation factor$_2$. The toxin acts on the heart and the cranial and peripheral nerves. Growth of the organism in the larynx may cause severe respiratory embarrassment

in some species of *Corynebacterium* (Fig. 3.4). Experienced workers are able presumptively to identify *C. diphtheriae* by this method but this expertise is unlikely to exist in most microbiology laboratories. When growth is detected on Loeffler's medium a subculture should be made on another plate of tellurite blood agar.

Hoyle's medium contains lysed horse blood, potassium tellurite together with a meat extract and peptone. This is the simplest medium for most laboratories. After overnight incubation colonies of corynebacteria are black and shining or grey, usually 1–2 mm in diameter (Fig. 3.5). The characteristic morphology of the biotypes of *C. diphtheriae* can be demonstrated. The colonies should be examined with a plate microscope or hand lens. It should be remembered, however, that these characteristic

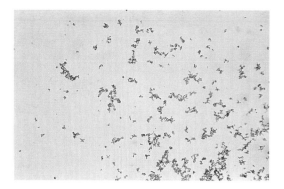

Figure 3.4 *Corynebacterium diphtheriae* and some commensal corynebacteria contain storage granules known as volutin granules which can be visualized by staining with Albert's stain

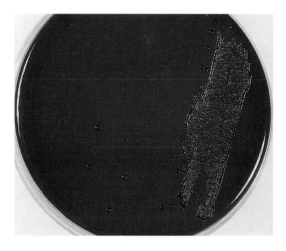

Figure 3.5 Hoyle's medium contains potassium tellurite which is reduced by corynebacteria. *Corynebacterium diphtheriae* grows well on this medium to produce shining colonies

features may be absent in some strains or can be seen in some non-diphtheria corynebacteria. If there is no growth after 24 hours' incubation, the plates should be re-incubated for a further 24 hours before being discarded as negative. All suspect colonies should be examined by Gram's stain and subcultured with a heavy inoculum. Four to six hours later there may be sufficient growth to initiate toxigenicity and biochemical testing.

Tinsdale medium (serum cystine thiosulphite tellurite agar) may be used to distinguish between *C. diphtheriae* and other respiratory tract bacteria, as *C. diphtheriae* produces a brown/black/yellow halo around the colony. This medium has been recommended for use by inexperienced staff since, as well as selecting corynebacteria, it also indicates the organisms which should be identified further. The medium is rather difficult to prepare: it may be too inhibitory and has a short shelf-life. This makes it less suitable for use as a primary isolation medium where relatively few specimens are examined. It may be valuable, however, as a rapid check for suspicious colonies found on other tellurite media.

Identification

The most important microbiological examination is demonstration of toxin production. It must be noted, however, that the decision to give antitoxin to a patient must be made clinically, as a delay in awaiting microbiological conformation will diminish the efficacy of this treatment.

Three subtypes are described and these are reflected in the colonial morphology. 'Gravis' colonies are 1–2 mm in diameter, with an entire edge convex with a matt, frosted glass appearance. 'Mitis' colonies are of a similar size, grey in colour, with a smooth consistency. They show well-defined haemolysis on whole blood media in contrast to gravis strains, which may only show a faint zone. 'Intermedius' colonies are 0.5–1 mm in diameter, circular, flat, grey-black in colour, with a smooth and finely granular surface.

Suspect colonies should be checked for the characteristic coryneform morphology on Gram's stain. Albert's stain should not be used for colonies isolated on tellurite-containing medium as this medium inhibits the formation of volutin granules.

Toxigenicity can be tested by Elek's method. A rich, clear agar containing horse serum is freshly prepared for each test, and a filter paper strip, soaked in specific antitoxin, is placed on the surface of the agar before it is finally solidified, so that it sinks into the medium. Test isolates, together with positive and negative controls, are inoculated at right angles and the plate is incubated overnight.

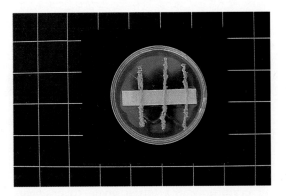

Figure 3.6 The Elek test. A strip of filter paper soaked in antiserum is placed into the medium as it solidifies. Test and control strains are streaked at right angles and after growth toxin diffuses from the streaks to form a precipitin line with the antitoxin diffusing from the strip. A line of identity with the positive control confirms the diagnosis of toxigenic *C. diphtheriae*

Precipitation will take place between antitoxin diffused from the strip and toxin produced by the organism (Fig. 3.6).

Biochemical testing

Corynebacterium diphtheriae is unable to grow sufficiently well in conventional media such as Andrade's medium, for biochemical testing serum must be added. Conventionally, Hiss's serum water sugars are used. These consist of fetal calf serum, peptone, with 0.5% acid fuchsin as indicator, together with the test carbohydrate. Alternatively, Andrade's sugars, used in the identification of Enterobacteriaceae, may be employed with the addition of one or two drops of fetal calf or horse serum.

Isolates should be tested against glucose, maltose, starch, and sucrose. In addition, nitrate reduction should be tested, together with urease hydrolysis in Christensen's medium. The usual characteristics of corynebacteria are noted in Table 3.2.

Rapid fermentation tests similar to those used for the identification of *Neisseria* may be used. These do not require the growth of *C. diphtheriae* and avoid the need for serum in the medium. In addition it is a rapid test giving results within one hour whereas serum sugars require 24 hours' incubation.

Typing

Corynebacterium diphtheriae may be typed by phage and bacteriocin typing methods. Serological methods have also been described.

Other corynebacteria

Other corynebacteria are capable of producing diphtheria toxin. These include *C. ulcerans* and *C. tuberculosis*. In addition, a dermatonecrotic toxin may be produced by *C. tuberculosis*, *C. ulcerans* and *C. haemolyticum*.

Corynebacterium ulcerans

It causes mastitis in cattle and may infect animal bite wounds. In human infections, it causes mild to severe pharyngitis, and, on rare

Table 3.2 Biochemical identification of *Corynebacterium*

Species	Glucose	Maltose	Starch	Sucrose	Urease	Nitrate
C. diphtheriae						
gravis	+	+	+	−	−	+
intermedius	+	+	−	−	−	+
mitis	+	+	−	−	−	+
C. ulcerans	+	+	+	−	+	−
C. pseudotuberculosis	+	+	−	−	+	v
C. xerosis	+	+	−	+	−	+
C. hofmanii	−	−	−	−	+	+
Rhodococcus equi	−	−	−	−	v	v
C. jeikeium	+	v	−	−	−	−

occasions, a diphtheria-like illness. It grows on tellurite medium with a similar morphology to *C. diphtheriae* and is haemolytic on blood agar.

Corynebacterium pseudotuberculosis (C. ovis)

This organism causes lymphadenitis in sheep; human infections are rare and are typically sub-acute or chronic relapsing lymphadenitis. Most patients have a close occupational exposure to sheep. The organism grows poorly on nutrient media, but grows well on Loeffler's serum slopes. After 48 hours on blood agar, colonies are 1–2 mm, dry, yellowish, with a narrow zone of beta haemolysis.

Corynebacterium pseudodiphtheriae (hofmanii)

This organism forms part of the normal flora of the human nasopharynx. It has little pathogenic potential but has been isolated from cases of endocarditis.

Corynebacterium xerosis

This organism was originally thought to be the cause of conjunctivitis, but is a part of the normal conjunctival flora. It grows well on conventional media with small non-haemolytic colonies less than 1 mm in diameter after 24 hours' incubation. Infections have been reported in severely immunocompromised patients and it has been reported as a cause of endocarditis.

Corynebacterium jeikeium

Over the last 10 years these organisms have been isolated from systemic infections in neutropenic patients. They are typically associated with the colonization of intravenous prosthetic devices, with prosthetic valve endocarditis, and there are anecdotal reports of pneumonitis. Cutaneous infection and peritonitis in chronic ambulatory peritoneal dialysis (CAPD) patients have been described.

Corynebacterium jeikeium show coccobacillary or coccal forms. They are slow growing, and form smooth, translucent, white colonies, 0.5 mm after 24 hours' incubation. They have few biochemical reactions and are more easily identified as they are naturally resistant to many antibiotics with the exception of vancomycin.

Antibiotic susceptibility

Corynebacterium diphtheriae is susceptible to penicillin, erythromycin, clindamycin and vancomycin. There is no evidence to suggest that antibiotics alter the course of the disease, but erythromycin is often given to eradicate carriage in the index case and contacts.

Rhodococcus equii (C. equii)

Rhodococcus equii is a pathogen of horses, swine, and cattle and may be found in soil. It is an intracellular organism which may cause pulmonary infections in immunocompromised human patients and has recently been associated with pneumonia in patients with the acquired immune deficiency syndrome (AIDS).

It grows easily on ordinary media, where it produces large, mucoid, salmon-pink colonies. It is non-fermentative. Gram's stain shows rods of varying lengths, which may be curved or have club forms. The cell wall is related to that of mycobacteria and some acid-fast strains have been reported.

Listeria

Classification

The genus *Listeria* contains seven species (some of which are listed in Table 3.3), of which *Listeria monocytogenes* is a human pathogen. Listerias are motile Gram-positive bacilli and catalase positive. They are facultatively anaerobic and capable of growing over a wide temperature range on simple media.

Listeria monocytogenes

Habitat

Listeria monocytogenes is widespread in nature, present in soil, plants, and as a

Table 3.3 Examples of some biochemical tests useful in differentiation of *Listeria* spp.

Species	β haemolysis	CAMP S. aureus	CAMP R. equi	Hippurate	Mannitol
L. monocytogenes	+	+	−	−	−
L. grayi	−	−	−	+	+
L. murrayi	−	−	−	+	+
L. innocua	−	−	−	−	−
L. ivanovii	+	−	+	−	−

commensal in animals and humans. It is found in meat, milk, and milk products and human infection occurs as a result of eating contaminated food or as a result of occupational exposure to animals. Changes in the way in which food is prepared, stored, and marketed (most notably refrigerated ready-cooked meals) has meant that infection with *Listeria* has become more common. The organism is able to multiply at low temperatures and may cause infection if the meal is not reheated to a high enough temperature to kill it.

Pathogenicity

It is important to remember that listeria are not predominantly human or animal pathogens. They are environmental organisms which are transmitted to man through the food chain. *Listeria monocytogenes* is able to cause human disease because of its ability to survive inside the macrophage. It achieves this by escaping from the phago-lysosome into the cytoplasm. The organism expresses a number of enzymes and toxins, including catalase which may be important in surviving the initial contact with the phagocyte. A phospholipase is elaborated which may assist in breaking down host membranes and *Listeria* along with other Gram-positive organisms possesses a cholesterol binding ('thiol activated') toxin listerio-lysin, analogous to streptolysin-O and pneumolysin.

Clinical importance

Listeriosis may give rise to a number of different clinical syndromes. These include acute meningoencephalitis, especially in immunocompromised and elderly patients. Neonatal infection takes two forms: the early-onset disease (characterized by pneumonia and septicaemia) and the rarer late-onset form (characterized by granulomatous meningitis). *Listeria* may also cause a low-grade septicaemia or an infectious mononucleosis-like syndrome which may go unrecognized by the patient or his medical attendant. Pneumonia, endocarditis, conjunctivitis, and urethritis have been reported.

Laboratory diagnosis

Specimens

Listeria are readily isolated from clinical specimens, such as blood, cerebrospinal fluid (CSF), amniotic fluid, genital tract secretions, or biopsies. Heavily contaminated specimens, such as soil or faeces, may be processed by cold enrichment techniques (see below).

Direct examination

Direct examination of normally sterile fluids, such as CSF or amniotic fluid, may be valuable for rapid diagnosis. However, specimens which may be contaminated by other organisms are not suitable for microscopy.

Isolation

Listeria monocytogenes is easily cultured on conventional media incorporating horse, sheep or rabbit blood. *Listeria monocytogenes* produces round, smooth, translucent colonies with a narrow zone of beta-haemolysis (Fig. 3.7). Colonies are small (0.5–1.5 mm in diameter). Under reflective light they have a blue-green colour.

Cold enrichment should be used for specimens from heavily contaminated sources. The specimen is inoculated into a nutrient broth

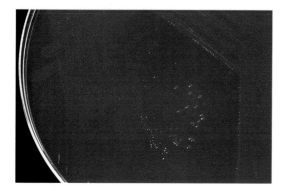

Figure 3.7 *Listeria monocytogenes* characteristically exhibit a narrow band of beta-haemolysis on blood agar

and incubated at 4°C for one month and subcultured weekly. This technique uses the ability of *L. monocytogenes* to multiply at low temperatures overgrowing other organisms which grow more slowly if at all.

Identification

Listeria monocytogenes is most frequently confused with enterococci or diphtheroids. Simple techniques can be used to differentiate these genera. Listeria are catalase positive (like diphtheroids) and bile aesculin positive (like the enterococci) (see Fig. 3.1). They exhibit characteristic tumbling motility when examined by the hanging drop method. Other biochemical tests which are useful include acetoin, H_2S production, and fermentation reactions. The CAMP test used in the identification of *Strep. agalactiae* may be modified for *Listeria* spp. (see Fig. 2.15). The typical reactions of listeria are set out in Table 3.3.

Typing

Variation in the lipotechoic acid antigens gives rise to more than 17 antigenic variants in the somatic O antigens. Flagellar H antigens may also be used for serological typing. Organisms can be typed using the O and H antigens for the investigation of food-borne outbreaks and cross-infection. Most listeriosis in man is caused by serovar 4B.

A system of bacteriophage typing has been described and is available as a reference technique.

Antibiotic susceptibility

Listerias are sensitive to ampicillin, rifampicin, chloramphenicol, erythromycin and aminoglycosides and resistant to cephalosporins. Ampicillin and gentamicin may be used in combination when treating serious listeria infections. Chloramphenicol is a useful alternative therapy.

Erysipelothrix rhusiopathiae

Classification and clinical importance

Erysipelothrix rhusiopathiae is a facultative anaerobic, Gram-positive bacillus. It is non-motile, catalase negative, and produces H_2S. It is the only species in the genus.

This organism is an animal pathogen causing an erysipelas-like syndrome in pigs. Erysipeloid is the infection which occurs in man and is characterized by a red lesion with a raised edge with central discoloration. Systemic invasion is uncommon but endocarditis can occur. Patients usually acquire *E. rhusiopathiae* through contact with infected animals or their products.

Laboratory diagnosis

Isolation

Specimens for the isolation of *E. rhusiopathiae* from erysipeloid lesions may be obtained by pinch graft biopsy. The organism is isolated by placing specimens in an infusion broth, supplemented with 1% glucose. Cultures should be incubated at 37°C and subcultured daily onto blood agar. After 24 hours' incubation, convex colonies up to 1 mm in diameter, circular, transparent, associated with the green discoloration of blood may be found.

Identification

Erysipelothrix rhusiopathiae may be presumptively identified by catalase and oxidase testing (both of which are negative) and H_2S production which can be demonstrated with Kligler's iron agar or triple sugar iron (TSI) agar. The clinical lesions are sufficiently distinctive to enable a presumptive diagnosis to be made in patients with an appropriate clinical syndrome.

Antibiotic susceptibility

Isolates of *E. rhusiopathiae* are susceptible to penicillin, chloramphenicol, tetracycline and erythromycin and are resistant to aminoglycosides and vancomycin.

Bacillus

Classification

The genus *Bacillus* consists of Gram-positive bacilli which form spores, are aerobic, or facultatively anaerobic, are usually catalase positive and motile. They characteristically form large, irregular rhizoid colonies.

More than 20 species are recognized, but of these, only *Bacillus anthracis* and *B. cereus* are pathogens of man. The remaining *Bacillus* species may be isolated from the environment. They can be found in water, plant material, soil and dust and these species rarely cause human disease. Infections, when they arise, are usually in the severely immunocompromised host or colonization of long-standing intravenous prosthetic devices.

Clinical importance

Bacillus anthracis

Anthrax is a zoonotic disease, primarily of wild or domestic herbivores, in which a fatal septicaemic infection takes place. Human infection can occur when man comes in contact with infected animals or their products (e.g. infected bone meal, animal hides or wool).

Bacillus anthracis is responsible for three clinical syndromes in man: cutaneous, inhalational and intestinal disease.

Cutaneous anthrax ('hide porters disease') follows the inoculation of anthrax spores into the skin, usually the result of occupational exposure. Lesions begin as small papules which slowly darken forming a brown eschar and blacken over the next few days. The lesion

is approximately 2.5 cm in diameter, with surrounding oedema and regional lymphadenitis.

Pulmonary anthrax arises as the result of inhalation of anthrax spores. This disease is now uncommon in developed countries, but still occurs in the developing world. Its old name, 'woolsorters disease', relates to occupational exposure. During the sorting of wool from contaminated fleeces large numbers of spores were dispersed and inhaled. The disease is characterized by an acute pneumonia followed rapidly by septicaemia. Death occurs two to three days after onset.

Intestinal anthrax may occur as a result of ingestion of spores. This is the least common form of anthrax but has a high mortality as septicaemia usually develops.

Pathogenicity

The pathogenicity of *B. anthracis* is dependent on the expression of a capsule and a toxin complex. Both of these characteristics are coded by genes found on a plasmid. The capsule is antiphagocytic and is composed of poly-D-glutamic acid. The toxin consists of three components, the protective factor, the oedema factor and the lethal factor.

Laboratory diagnosis

Specimens
Bacillus anthracis can be readily isolated from clinical specimens of blood or sputum in cases of septicaemic or pulmonary anthrax. The best specimen from cutaneous anthrax is to inoculate material aspirated from one of the vesicles onto nutrient agar (Fig. 3.8).

Direct microscopy
Direct smears and stains with polychrome methylene blue using McFadyen's method will stain the bacilli purple, with the capsule showing red (Fig. 3.9). Spores are, of course, unstained.

Isolation and identification
After 24 hours colonies of *B. anthracis* are 2–3 mm in diameter with an irregular surface and wrinkled edge giving the 'medusa head' appearance.

This organism is a category 3 pathogen according to the Advisory Committee for

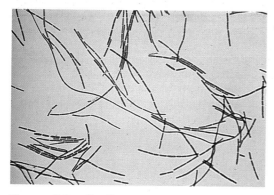

Figure 3.8 *Bacillus anthracis (Gram stain)*

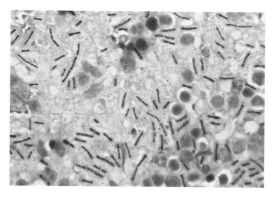

Figure 3.9 Pathogenic *Bacillus anthracis* release potent toxins and possess a capsule. Bacteria in specimens of pus from anthrax will stain pink and the capsule blue when stained with polychrome methylene blue

Dangerous Pathogens (ACDP) and suspect isolates should be referred to a reference laboratory for identification. The other organisms of this genus can be identified by the use of simple biochemical tests. The tests used include lecithinase production, anaerobic growth, citrate utilization, oxidation of ammonium salt, oxidation of sugars, acetoin production, salt tolerance, urease activity, and hydrolysis of starch and gelatin. For details of *Bacillus* identification, see Further reading.

For isolation of *Bacillus* species from heavily contaminated specimens, such as soil or faeces, a selective medium such as Knisely's (heart infusion agar with polymixin, lysozyme, EDTA and thallous acetate) can be used.

Bacillus cereus

Bacillus cereus is an important cause of toxin-mediated food poisoning. The commonest vehicle of transmission is parboiled rice which is subsequently stir-fried. During the period of storage between boiling and stir frying spores germinate and a heat stable toxin is produced. Nausea and vomiting develop one to six hours later. *Bacillus cereus* also elaborates a heat labile toxin which causes a diarrhoeal syndrome 18 hours after ingestion. The usual vehicles for this form of food poisoning are foods which are not reheated after cooling such as gravies and sauces. Infections with *B. cereus*, in immunocompromised patients, relate to indwelling intravenous catheters and are being increasingly recognized.

Diagnosis of *B. cereus* food poisoning is usually made on the basis of the clinical features and a detailed food history. Suspect food can be investigated and this is dealt with in Chapter 22.

Actinomycetales

Classification

Organisms of the order *Actinomycetales* are Gram positive, branching, filamentous bacteria, <1 μm in width, with pleomorphic morphology. They are non-motile, slow-growing organisms which are not acid fast. They may be microaerophilic, facultative or obligate anaerobes. They include genera as diverse as *Actinomyces*, *Proprionibacteria*, *Bifidobacteria*, *Nocardia*, *Streptomyces*, and *Rhodococcus*.

Actinomyces spp.

Habitat

They normally live as commensals in the mouth, gastrointestinal or genitourinary tracts, but when alterations in the host–parasite balance take place, invasive disease can occur. This takes the form of chronic destructive granulomatous inflammation, producing pus which may have granular particles known as 'sulphur granules' (Fig. 3.10). These consist of multiplying *Actinomyces* in a mycelium and are just visible to the naked eye. They are obligate anaerobes.

Classification

There are more than eight species in the genus, of which the type species *A. ovis* is a pathogen in cattle. *Actinomyces israelii* is the species most frequently found as a pathogen in humans but also forms part of the normal flora in the mouth and gut. It is the commonest cause of human actinomycosis which presents as chronic granulomatous lesion with discharging sinuses. Infection is usually found in the face and the neck, but infections in the female genitourinary tract may occur in those using an intrauterine contraceptive device.

When invasion occurs other bacteria such as *Bacteroides* spp. or *Actinobacillus actinomycetescomitans* are implicated in the process. Other species, such as *A. naeslundi*, *A. odontolyticus* and *A. viscosus* are commensal organisms which are rarely isolated from clinical specimens. *Corynebacterium pyogenes* has recently been transferred to the genus *Actinomyces*.

Laboratory diagnosis

Direct examination

Specimens of pus should be obtained, where possible, and if sulphur granules are seen, they should be separated for direct examination. Any granules found should be placed on a slide and a coverslip applied. Direct examination with the ×40 objective will demonstrate branching filaments with coccoid and bacillary forms. The coverslip can then be removed and the smear heat-fixed and stained by the Gram and Ziehl-Neelsen (ZN) methods. For the latter stain, two additional preparations should be made and decolorized with 20% and 1% H_2SO_4 for five minutes. Preparations showing only non-acid-fast organisms are likely to be *Actinomyces*, whereas those which are fast at 1%, but not 20%, may be *Nocardia*. Where no granules are present, a simple Gram stain should be performed and Gram-positive branching filaments sought (Fig. 3.11). An alternative method of rapid diagnosis is to

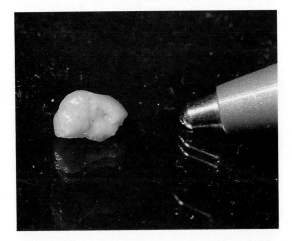

Figure 3.10 A yellow 'sulphur granule' is seen here in comparison to the head of a ball point pen

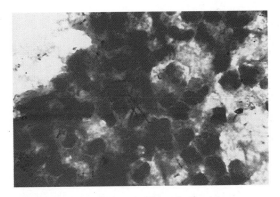

Figure 3.11 Gram-positive branching bacteria can be seen in specimens of pus from cases of actinomycosis

perform a direct immunofluorescence test on specimens of pus.

Isolation

Granules can be washed by mixing some pus with sterile saline in a universal container. The granules will settle and the supernatant fluid should be discarded. This process should be repeated several times. Finally, the granules should be crushed with the sterile glass rod and the suspension inoculated onto selective media. These should include a blood agar plate, incubated in CO_2 atmosphere and two

Table 3.4 Some characteristics of *Actinomyces* which may be utilized in differentiation

Species	Atmosphere	Nitrate	Catalase	Glucose	Mannitol	Raffinose	Xylose	Starch	Cell wall
A. israelii	O An	+	−	+	+/−	+/−	*/−	+/−	Ornithine
A. bovis	M Aer	−	−	+	−	−	+/−	+	Aspartate
A. naeslundi	Fac	+	−	+	−	+	−	+/−	Ornithine
A. viscosis	Fac	+	+	+	−	+	+/−	+/−	Ornithine
A. odontolyticus	Fac	+	−	+	−	+/−	+/−	+	Ornithine

An, obligate anaerobe; M Aer, microaerophilic; Fac, facultative anaerobe

blood agar plates incubated anaerobically. The first plate should be inspected after 48 hours and the second at seven days. A number of different agents have been described for selecting actinomyces including colistin, kanamycin, metronidazole. Enrichment media that may be inoculated include thioglycolate broth and Robertson's cooked meat medium.

Identification

Suspect colonies should be examined by Gram's method and by ZN decolorizing with 1% and 20% H_2SO_4. The colonies should also be subcultured and incubated in air, CO_2 and anaerobic atmospheres.

Definitive identification is by fermentation tests in which thioglycolate broth supplemented by yeast extract and containing a 1% solution of the sugar is used. A change in the colour of an indicator or fall in pH >0.5 can be used as an end point. Table 3.4 shows characteristic results of simple biochemical tests. Additionally the metabolic end products of organisms grown in PYG broth can be determined using gas-liquid chromatography. Successful identification using commercially produced biochemical tests can be achieved. Other identification methods which may be used are analysis of cell wall components.

Antimicrobial susceptibility

Unlike other anaerobic species *Actinomyces* are not susceptible to metronidazole. They are sensitive to penicillin, chloramphenicol, erythromycin, and tetracyclines.

Closely related to the Actinomycetaceae are the *Bifidobacteria*, of which there are more than 30 species, and *Rothia* and *Streptomyces*. These genera rarely cause human disease but form part of the normal flora of the large intestines.

Nocardia

Clinical importance

Nocardia are saprophytic inhabitants of soil. They do not occur as commensal organisms in man or animals. Mycetoma (Madura foot) is a chronic granulomatous inflammation of feet, thought to be caused by the inoculation of soil organisms through abrasions on the sole. It may be caused by a number of different *Nocardia* spp., including *N. madurae* and *N. brasiliensis*, as well as some species of *Streptomyces*. *Nocardia* spp. may also cause severe cavitating infections in the lungs in patients who are immunocompromised or have anatomical abnormalities (e.g. bronchiectasis or tuberculosis scarring). Very rarely, nocardiasis may occur as disseminated abscesses in fully immunocompetent patients.

Laboratory diagnosis

Specimens of pus or bronchial lavage may be submitted for examination and should be cultured on blood agar and Sabouraud's agar. Blood agar plates should be incubated aerobically at 37°C and another at 40–42°C. The plates should be inspected daily for up to 14 days before a negative result can be confirmed. Pigmented rhizoid colonies should be considered suspect.

Table 3.5 Some characteristics of *Nocardia* useful in identification

Species	Caesin	Tyrosine	Xanthine	Urea	Gelatin	Starch
N. asteroides	−	−	−	+	−	−
N. brasiliensis	+	+	−	+	+	−
Actinomadura madurae	+	+	−	−	+	+
Streptomyces sotrinaliensis	+	+	−	−	+	+

Isolation and identification

Suspect colonies should be examined by Gram's method. Nocardia are Gram-positive organisms with bacillary and coccoid forms, together with branching filaments. Such colonies should also be stained by ZN decolorized with 1% and 20% H_2SO_4. Definitive identification of *Nocardia* spp. may be made by the use of biochemical tests, including decomposition of casein, tyrosine, starch and the production of urease and gelatinase (Table 3.5).

Antibiotic susceptibility

The susceptibility of these organisms to antibiotics is highly variable, and often does not predict the response in clinical use.

4

Mycobacterial infection

Introduction

Mycobacteria are among the most important pathogenic bacteria infecting man. Although *Mycobacterium tuberculosis* (MTB) infection is uncommon in many parts of developed countries, more than 10 million people are infected world-wide, with an estimated 3 million deaths per year.

Classification

The taxonomy of the genus is complex, more than 50 species are recognized, although only a minority are human pathogens. They are, for the most part, environmental organisms being found in water and soil and as pathogens and commensals of animals.

The genus can be classified in a number of ways. Runyon separated the non-tuberculosis (or 'atypical' mycobacteria) organisms into four groups. Group I consisted of organisms which were pigmented when exposed to light, the photochromogens. Group II were organisms which were pigmented when incubated in the dark, the scotochromogens. Organisms which were not capable of pigment production were placed in Group III (non-chromogens) and the rapid growers were in Group IV. This classification has little clinical relevance and pigmentation can be variable in some organisms, notably *M. avium-intracellulare* and *M. szulgai*. A clinical classification is more practical giving five main groups as set out below (Table 4.1). This also provides a guide to laboratory examination and clinical advice.

Isolation of an obligate pathogen such as *M. tuberculosis* from sputum is diagnostic of tuberculosis, whereas isolation of *M. kansasii* or *M. fortuitum* would require at least a second isolation from that site together with perhaps evidence of susceptibility and appropriate clinical symptoms and signs before an aetiological role could be established.

Pathogenesis

The pathogenicity determinants of mycobacteria have been the subject of extensive research ever since the tubercle bacillus was

Table 4.1 Clinical classification of mycobacteria

Group	Example
1 Obligate pathogens	*M. tuberculosis, M. bovis, M. leprae*
2 Skin pathogens	*M. marinum, M. ulcerans*
3 Opportunistic pathogens	*M. kansasii, M. avium-intracellulare, M. xenopi*
4 Non- or rarely pathogenic	*M. gordonae, M. smegmatis*
5 Animal pathogens	*M. paratuberculosis, M. lepraemurium*

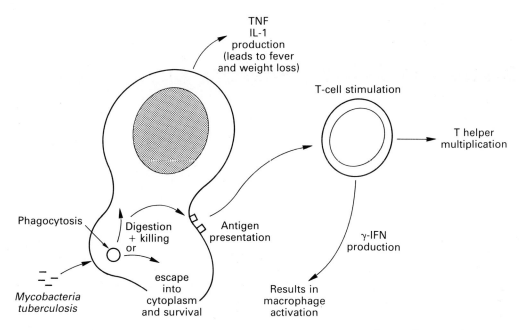

TNF
IL-1
production
(leads to fever
and weight loss)

T-cell stimulation

T helper
multiplication

Phagocytosis

Digestion
+ killing
or

Antigen
presentation

γ-IFN
production

escape
into
cytoplasm
and survival

*Mycobacteria
tuberculosis*

Results in
macrophage
activation

Figure 4.1 *Mycobacterium tuberculosis* escapes into the cytoplasm of macrophages to survive. If the organism is killed antigen is presented to T cells which proliferate and produce (gamma) interferon IFN. This cytokine activates macrophages making them more able to kill mycobacteria. Macrophages produce interleukin 1 (IL-1) and tumour necrosis factor (TNF) which are responsible for symptoms such as fever and weight loss

first identified by Koch. Central to the outcome of contact between host and pathogen is the interaction with the macrophages and T cells.

Macrophages ingest mycobacteria but they are able to survive by escaping from the phago-lysosome into the cytoplasm. Macrophages present antigens to T cells which then proliferate. Secretion of gamma interferon by T cells activates macrophages to be able to kill ingested mycobacteria. Conditions which reduce T-cell function increase susceptibility to mycobacterial disease (Fig. 4.1).

Mycobacteria differ from many other organisms in that they have a very high lipid content (up to 40% of the dry weight). A number of molecular species have been identified which may play a role in enabling the organism to survive in the human host.

Mycobacterium leprae possess a glycolipid capsular material phenolic glycolipid which has been shown to inhibit phagocyte killing by interfering with the activity of the myeloperoxide-halide system. The trehalose-containing lipo-oligosaccharides may also act in a similar manner. Lipoarabinomannan, a glycolipid, is thought to have a role in interfering with macrophage function. Protein antigens such as superoxide dismutase may play a role in protecting the organisms from the effects of oxygen and hydroxyl free radicals.

Clinical importance

Mycobacterium tuberculosis

Mycobacterium tuberculosis infection is a chronic granulomatous condition which may involve any of the tissues of the body. Three main types of disease are recognized, but this is an infection which is noted for the diversity of its modes of presentation and the symptoms it exhibits.

In countries of high endemicity primary infection occurs early in life usually in the lung with consolidation and regional lymphadenopathy. This infection may self-cure or go on to disseminated disease. Adult-type tuberculosis develops as the result of reinfection or reactivation and takes the form of a chronic progressive lung infection characterized by fever, weight loss, cough, haemoptysis and signs of pulmonary consolidation. Infection can become disseminated throughout the body and this is known as miliary disease. Miliary seeding may result in generalized infection or become dormant and allow the later development of extrapulmonary tuberculosis. Miliary tuberculosis has become more common in patients with AIDS whose failing immunity allows the reactivation of *M. tuberculosis*.

Extrapulmonary tuberculosis

Every organ in the body can be infected by MTB. In the central nervous system infection can take the form of tuberculous meningitis, a chronic progressive lymphocyte meningitis. More rarely isolated foci of infection, tuberculomas, can develop in the cerebral substance, which present with the symptoms and signs of a space-occupying lesion. On some occasions infection can be confined to the spinal cord.

The skeletal system is now rarely infected in developed countries but spinal tuberculosis and tuberculous arthritis are still common world-wide. In spinal tuberculosis collapse of the vertebrae can result in paraparesis.

Gastrointestinal tuberculosis arises from the ingestion of infected milk or swallowing infected sputum from coexistent pulmonary disease. Tuberculous peritonitis probably develops following the rupture of an abdominal lymph node. Other lymph nodes can be involved notably those in the cervical region.

Renal tuberculosis is often associated with other extra-pulmonary sites. Infection in the renal tract may present as fever, dysuria and haematuria. In long-standing or healed disease fibrosis leads to obstructive uropathy.

Mycobacterium bovis

This organism produces a tuberculosis-like syndrome in cattle and a similar disease when it infects man. It grows slowly and is encouraged by the presence of pyruvate in the medium.

Leprosy

The majority of people coming in contact with *M. leprae* are able to resist clinical disease. Leprosy was once endemic world-wide but disappeared from developed countries before the development of chemotherapy. Social, nutritional and genetic factors are thought to be responsible for the bodies' response to this challenge. *Mycobacterium leprae* mainly causes damage to the skin and the peripheral nervous system. The major complication of this disease arises as a result of cutaneous anaesthesia.

The type of disease caused by *M. leprae* differs depending on the immune response of the host. Patients who retain a degree of immunity have an illness characterized by isolated granulomas which have few bacilli within them (paucibacillary disease). As a result clinical signs in the skin and nervous system are localized. This is classified as tuberculoid leprosy.

When there is little immune response to the leprosy bacillus uncontrolled multiplication occurs and damage to the skin and nervous system is generalized. Anaesthesia of the hands and feet means that the body is unable to avoid severe progressive traumatic damage which results in the loss of fingers and toes. This form is known as lepromatous disease. Between these two poles there are three intermediate stages (borderline, borderline tuberculoid, and borderline lepromatous), although patients rarely fit into such neat classifications.

Mycobacterium leprae cannot be isolated in artificial culture but can be cultivated in the mouse foot-pad or in the nine-banded armadillo.

Cutaneous pathogens

Mycobacterium marinum

Mycobacterium marinum is found in water and is a pathogen of fish. Infection can be transmitted to man when it is inoculated into the skin, when for example tropical fish tanks are cleaned or after swimming in swimming pools. The skin lesions can take the form of a nodule which may ulcerate or it may form an abscess with local lymphatic spread.

Mycobacterium ulcerans

This is the causative organism of Buruli ulcer which is a chronic destructive ulcer usually found on the leg. It begins as a lump then ulcerates with a necrotic base which can extend into the subcutaneous fat. It is found in Africa, Australia and Mexico.

Opportunist pathogens

The opportunist mycobacteria can be divided into three clinical groups: the AIDS-related opportunists; the pulmonary group; and the rapid growers.

The development of the AIDS epidemic means that many patients with little T-cell immunity have developed generalized *M. avium-intracellulare* infection. The organism is present in the environment and infection arises late in the course of AIDS. The patient often presents with fever, weight loss, and diarrhoea. Infection is often disseminated at the time of presentation. *M. avium-intracellulare* can be isolated from many tissues including the blood. Treatment is often disappointing as this organism is naturally resistant to many of the first line agents. New therapeutic regimens using rifabutin, newer macrolides, clofazamine and the fluoroquinolones may provide some benefit.

Mycobacterium kansasii

Pulmonary infection with this organism typically arises in patients with previous or chronic lung disease, although severe disease can occur in healthy subjects. It produces a disease which is similar to pulmonary tuberculosis but is perhaps more indolent. The organism can be isolated from water supplies. *M. xenopi* occurs as commonly as *M. kansasii* and behaves in a similar manner.

The rapid growers

The organisms of the *M. fortuitum-chelonei* complex occasionally cause disease. They are environmental organisms found in the soil and water. Infection can occur when injection solutions become contaminated with these organisms and a chronic abscess develops. Infection from almost all organs has been reported, and they are being isolated more frequently from neutropenic patients.

Laboratory diagnosis

Planning mycobacterial services

All microbiological laboratories should provide diagnostic service for mycobacteria, even when mycobacterial diseases are uncommon as they form an important part of the differential diagnosis in many cases. The diagnosis of mycobacterial disease, however, requires dedicated laboratory facilities, as well as training and experience. The quality of the service is improved if there is a sufficient throughput of positive specimens for broad experience to be obtained. It is important, therefore, to plan mycobacterial diagnostic services appropriate to the needs of the institution served. Three levels of services can be planned as follows:

Level 1: direct examination

At this level laboratory specimens are examined for the presence of mycobacteria by direct microscopy using either Ziehl-Neelsen or auramine staining. Specimens are then processed and incubated with all mycobacterial isolates referred for identification.

In developing countries where tuberculosis is common, health service budgets rarely enable comprehensive TB services to be set up to provide culture facilities in district general hospitals. As a result most diagnoses are made on the basis of direct microscopic examination. This, however, provides a useful diagnostic service for TB control as only those patients who are smear positive are thought to be more infective. Thus this simple laboratory service effectively identifies the cases which it is imperative to treat to reduce TB transmission.

Level 2: identification and sensitivity

At this level the laboratory is fully equipped to culture identify organisms to species level and

Table 4.2   Examples of national schemes

USA	*American Thoracic Society*
Level I	Collect adequate specimens and forward them to laboratories at a higher level. Direct smears may be examined
Level II	As above and culture specimens on standard media, identify MTB and may perform sensitivity testing
Level III	Identify all mycobacteria, perform sensitivity tests, provide training, supervise proficiency tests and perform research

UK	*There are broadly three types of laboratory*
1	Public Health and District General Hospital laboratories where direct smears are examined and culture performed on standard media. Sensitivities are not performed
2	Public Health Laboratory Regional Reference Centres receive cultures from other laboratories, identification and sensitivity testing is performed
3	The Mycobacterium Reference Unit of the Public Health Laboratory Service provides full identification service and sensitivity testing, including rarely used drugs when indicated

test their sensitivity to a complete range of anti-tuberculosis drugs.

Level 3: national centre

The identification and sensitivity testing of mycobacteria is sometimes difficult and a national reference centre may be a useful way of pooling resources. In addition such a reference facility may provide control strains, supervise a quality control scheme and arrange national training programmes. Examples of national schemes are found in Table 4.2.

Design of mycobacteriology laboratory

The obligate pathogens are classified as Hazard Group 3 (Advisory Committee for Dangerous Pathogens) and require containment level 3 conditions. Other species are found in Hazard Group 2 and should be handled under containment level 2 conditions (see Chapter 13).

Table 4.3   Examples of specimens submitted for mycobacterial culture

Sputum (also broncho-alveolar lavages and induced sputum)
Gastric washings
Urine (an early morning urine is preferred)
Cerebrospinal fluid
Bone marrow
Pus
Tissue biopsy
Blood
Faeces

Laboratory infection with MTB is a hazard faced by those who work with this organism. Laboratory workers are about five times more likely to develop TB than the general population. Several sets of guidelines have been issued by WHO, the UK Departments of Health and the Centers for Disease Control, Atlanta. The essential requirement is for a containment laboratory in which work with any specimen suspected of containing Hazard Group 3 organisms can be contained (see Chapter 13).

Specimens

Almost any specimen may be examined for the presence of mycobacteria, some of these are summarized in Table 4.3.

Collection and transport

Specimens of sputum should be collected into sterile containers after the nature of the procedure has been explained to the patient, i.e. it is purulent sputum not saliva which is sought. Between three and six adequate specimens should be collected to maximize the chance of detecting tubercle bacilli as the organism may only be shed intermittently. Specimen collection can be improved by the assistance of a physiotherapist.

Some patients are unable to produce an adequate sputum specimen and in these circumstances alternative means of obtaining a specimen may be sought. Gastric lavage is a procedure in which the early morning stomach contents are lavaged to collect mycobacteria which have been coughed and swallowed overnight. Induced sputum is obtained when hypertonic saline is nebulized and inhaled. This induces coughing and sputum production. During broncho-alveolar lavage bronchopulmonary segments are washed via a fibreoptic bronchoscopy and the washings collected (see p. 181).

A mid-stream specimen should be collected first thing in the morning. A screw-capped bottle is satisfactory for the purpose and can easily be centrifuged without the risk of transfer of contamination to the centrifuge tubes. Twenty-four-hour urine collections frequently become contaminated during the collection process and are not recommended.

Aspirated exudate (pleural fluid) or pus should be collected into a plain sterile screw-capped bottle and another containing citrate. The citrate prevents clotting which would otherwise confound the cell count. Culture of pleural fluid is an insensitive way of making a diagnosis and where possible a pleural biopsy should also be taken and submitted for histopathological examination as well as direct microscopy and culture.

Tissue biopsy specimens should be of adequate size and should be collected into sterile screw-capped containers. It is important that such containers should be clearly marked for microbiological examination to minimize the chance of fixative being added in error.

Specimens should be transported to the laboratory with minimal delay and held at +4°C until processed. Rapid transport and processing is important to prevent the multiplication of non-mycobacterial organisms.

Direct examination

Direct examination of specimens for the presence of mycobacteria is the most important single diagnostic technique as it provides a rapid diagnosis, is cheap and specific. It identifies those patients who pose the greatest risk of dissemination of infective organisms. In the future new molecular techniques may become more widely available but must yet prove their clinical value.

Not all of these specimens, such as urine, are suitable for direct microscopic examination because of the likely presence of contaminating non-pathogenic species. Other specimens such as CSF require special handling (see below).

Preparation of specimens

Making a representative smear of sputum is very difficult because of the consistency of this material. In the preparation there is a balance to be made between thickness of the film which increases the number of mycobacteria available for detection with the problem of visualizing the organisms in the thick smear, and the risk of the material floating off during the staining process. Smears may also be made from the centrifuged deposit from the digested decontaminated specimen. This material is easier to handle, concentrates the bacteria and produces clearer films.

Direct microscopic examination may result in confusing results (see above) in specimens of urine, gastric lavage, faeces, and bone marrow. However, in patients who are HIV positive direct examination of bone marrow and buffy coat has proven valuable (sensitivity 72%, specificity 94%).

Smears from aspirated pus should be prepared as for sputum. A centrifuged deposit of pleural fluid should be used for direct examination. CSF is a precious sample, and usually only a very small volume is available. A circle should be marked in the middle of a glass slide and the centrifuge deposit dropped within the mark and dried dropwise in order to concentrate the mycobacteria for examination.

Smears should be examined systematically, and up to 300 fields should be visualized before it is reported as negative (Fig. 4.2). Microscopy can be quantified as follows:

No. of acid fast bacilli seen	*Result*
None in 300 fields	Negative
1–10 in 100 fields	+
1–10 in 10 fields	++
1–10 per field	+++
>10 per field	++++

Screening

The auramine phenol method (Fig. 4.3) is most effective when used as a screening method, but due to non-specific fluorescent material which

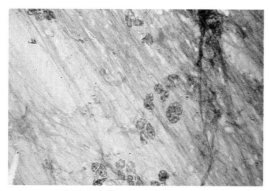

Figure 4.2 A specimen of sputum stained by Ziehl-Neelsen's method shows small pink bacilli which have resisted decolorization with the acid alcohol solution. The background is counterstained with methylene blue

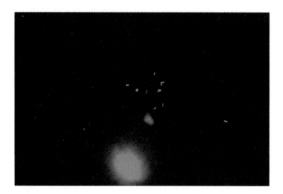

Figure 4.3 Auramine is a fluorescent dye which is retained by *Mycobacteria*. When the slide is visualized under u.v. illumination the mycobacteria can be seen fluorescing apple green

may be present in smears, all positive specimens should be over-stained with ZN. In laboratories with only a small number of specimens, ZN remains the method of choice (see Fig. 4.2).

Reporting

A positive microscopy report can have profound clinical implications, initiating a prolonged course of anti-tuberculosis chemotherapy. Care must be taken to diminish the risk of laboratory false-positive results. These may arise by transfer of acid-fast bacilli from positive specimens during the staining process (in staining jars or on re-used blotting paper), or by contamination of staining materials or rinsing water with environmental acid-fast bacilli.

New antigen detection techniques

The polymerase chain reaction (PCR) has been applied to the diagnosis of infectious diseases. A probe of known sequence with appropriate primers can now be used to detect specific sequences of mycobacterial DNA, the sequences are then multiplied using the polymerase chain reaction. This is currently under investigation, and it is yet to be seen whether it will gain a place in routine diagnosis. The technique is very sensitive but false positives may arise due to non-specific contamination. PCR is limited in scope as individual tests are specific for the sequence added, thus a probe for MTB will only detect patients with this organism. It will be many years and many technical developments later when PCR can compete realistically with a conventional culture system in routine practice.

Isolation

Decontamination of specimens

Many of the specimens submitted for mycobacterial culture are contaminated with other faster growing bacteria. In the prolonged culture period required for the isolation of mycobacteria these other organisms would overgrow and destroy the culture. Specimens of sputum and faeces should always be decontaminated, but with other materials, such as urine, which are less likely to contain other organisms, a centrifuged deposit can be examined by Gram's stain to determine whether decontamination is necessary. If organisms are seen by direct Gram smear the specimen should be decontaminated. Decontamination methods are of varying stringency, but all have one thing in common: the antibacterial effect of the method is only partly selective. 'Hard' methods (4% NaOH) are suitable for use on heavily contaminated specimen such as sputum and 'soft' methods (trisodium phosphate) for less contaminated specimens.

Culture media

There are essentially three types of culture available for the culture of mycobacteria: egg-based media, agar-based media and fluid media.

Egg-based media

These are the mainstay of tuberculosis diagnosis and include Lowenstein-Jensen (LJ), Stonebrink, and IUAT (International Union Against Tuberculosis). Lowenstein-Jensen is the most popular medium for use in primary isolation of mycobacteria. Glycerol can be added (LJG) to facilitate the growth of human type *M. tuberculosis*, whereas the addition of pyruvate (LJP) enhances the growth of *M. bovis*. Most routine isolation sets include two LJ slopes, one with glycerol and one with pyruvate. Higher concentrations of malachite green are incorporated in Petragnani medium which may be useful for the inoculation of specimens which are heavily contaminated, but the increased concentration of malachite green can inhibit some mycobacteria.

Agar-based media

These contain oleic acid, albumin, agar and are not usually used in primary culture. Their principal use is in media for identification and susceptibility test medium. A selective version of this medium has been described for the inoculation of precious biopsy material but its efficacy for primary isolation is open to question. Oleic acid is an expensive reagent and the final medium has a relatively short shelf-life (Table 4.4).

Fluid media

The principal advantage of liquid culture medium is that a larger volume of material can be cultured without inhibiting the growth of mycobacteria. A medium such as that of Kirchner is made selective by the addition of a mixture of antibiotics (polymyxin B, carbenicillin, trimethoprim and ampicillin) and is useful for isolation of mycobacteria in specimens likely to be contaminated with other bacteria (see Table 4.4).

Table 4.4 Examples of media used in culture of Mycobacteria

Name	Enrichment	Selection
Lowenstein-Jensen	Eggs, Glycerol or Pyruvate	Malachite green
Petragnani	Potato, flour, egg, milk, glycerol	Malachite green
IUAT	Egg, asparagine	Malachite green
Middlebrook	Oleic acid, albumin, dextrose catalase	Malachite green
Kirchner	Asparagine, glycerol	Polymyxin B, carbenicillin trimethoprim, ampicillin

Incubation conditions and examination of cultures

All cultures for the primary isolation of mycobacteria should be incubated aerobically at 37°C. As these cultures must be maintained for between 8 and 12 weeks, all cultivation is carried out in tightly fitting screw-top containers or, in the case of sensitivity testing, 7 ml screw-capped containers to prevent desiccation. A combination of LJG, LJP and a liquid medium provides the optimum yield of positive cultures.

Culture tubes should be examined macroscopically after 2–3 days to detect rapid growers and then weekly for 8 weeks. In cases where tuberculosis is strongly suspected cultures should be kept for a further 4 weeks (Fig. 4.4). Slopes which show evidence of contamination, i.e. growth of *Candida spp.*, should be discarded. Those with suspect colonies should be examined microscopically with a ZN stain. As well as confirming the presence of acid-fast bacilli these smears may have signs characteristic of a particular species – the serpentine cords of MTB (Fig. 4.5).

Radiometric culture techniques

The BACTEC blood culture system (see p. 164) has been modified for use in the diagnosis of mycobacterial disease. In this system the

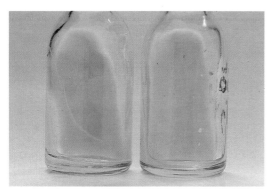

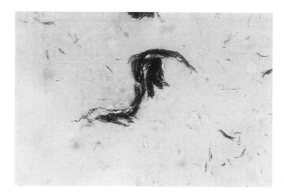

Figure 4.4 *Mycobacterium tuberculosis* has rough buff colonies on Lowenstein-Jensen medium. Other mycobacteria may be brightly pigmented on exposure to light (photochromogens), or in the dark (scotochromogens)

Figure 4.5 *Mycobacterium tuberculosis* isolated on solid medium exhibits serpentine cords. This can be an important characteristic for separating the *M. tuberculosis* complex from other species

medium used is Middlebrook 7H12 broth medium with or without an antibiotic cocktail. It contains ^{14}C-labelled palmitate. Uncontaminated specimens and the centrifuged deposit of decontaminated specimens can be inoculated to the broth.

Comparative studies show that it is as effective as a conventional three bottle culture set described above. The major advantage provided is of course that it takes a shorter time for positive growth to be detected. This system can also be modified to allow identification and sensitivity testing.

Identification techniques

Identification of mycobacteria has developed into a reference laboratory service, not because the techniques are difficult but because few microbiology laboratories have a sufficient throughput of positive specimens to develop their expertise.

Reporting

Before considering methods the sequence of reports should be set out as these will assist in the planning of the identification process. The first report is direct microscopy which provides the result, 'Acid-fast bacilli seen/not seen'. This alone does not imply that a pathogen must be present but would strongly support a diagnosis if the clinical features of the case were compatible with a mycobacterial disease. A false positive may be an opportunist, a non-pathogen or a rapid grower. A positive culture provides confirmation that the material defined on microscopy was in fact a *Mycobacterium* spp., but until further identification has been performed the report would read, '*Mycobacterium* spp., isolated, further identification to follow'. At this point the clinician has not been provided with any additional information which would cause the initiation of chemotherapy (or discontinuation). Thus the critical part of the identification process is to separate the obligate pathogens from other species. Full identification can occur later and it is important to identify all organisms fully, as some species are found as pathogens in particular clinical situations; *M. kansasii* in patients with anatomical abnormalities of lung architecture (see above). Moreover repeated isolation of a 'non-pathogen' or rapid grower from a clinical site on more than one occasion might indicate a pathogenic role for that organism. The identification of obligate pathogens will be described in detail and the principles of full species identification will be given in outline.

Screening tests

These tests are used by the Mycobacterium Reference Unit and Regional Centres for tuberculosis bacteriology but any laboratory

Table 4.5 Results of screening test for identification

Test	'Tubercle' bacilli	'Non-tubercle' bacilli
Microscopy	Cording	No cording
Growth 37°C	+	+
Growth 25°C	–	+
Pigment	–	+/–
Growth pNB	–	+/–

Based on Collins, Grange and Yates (see Further reading)

with sufficient throughput could set up screening identification with a significant increase in the speed of reporting (Table 4.5).

The following slopes should be inoculated: LJG, incubated at 37°C in a light incubator, and one at the same temperature in the dark, and LJG incubated at 25°C and a Middlebrook slope containing 500 mg/l *p*-nitrobenzoic acid (pNB). Approximately 10 µl of the suspension is inoculated on the slopes and read on days 3, 7, 14 and 21. Successful completion of this screening procedure produces a result of great practical value to the clinician (*Mycobacterium* of the tuberculosis complex isolated). *M. tuberculosis* (or *M. bovis* or *M. africanum*) is likely to be acting as a pathogen. An organism isolated several times and screening negative might prompt a search for immunosuppression in a patient with tuberculosis-like symptoms (Table 4.5).

The individual species of the *M. tuberculosis* complex can be differentiated by a small number of tests.

Identification of other mycobacteria

The principal tests which may be used to identify mycobacteria to species are as follows:

Pigment production

This is tested by incubating two LJ tubes in incubators with and without internal light at 37°C. This technique enables three groups to be defined: photochromogens (pigment production in the light only); scotochromogens (pigment production in dark or light); and non-chromogens (non-pigment producers).

Mycobacterium tuberculosis is a non-chromogen whereas *M. kansasii* is a photochromogen and *M. xenopi* is usually a scotochromogen.

Temperature of growth

Mycobacterium species differ in the temperatures at which growth can be maintained. Five tubes of LJ are inoculated and incubated at 20, 25, 37, 42 and 44°C.

Sensitivity to anti-tuberculosis drugs

Some *Mycobacterium* spp. are naturally resistant to antibiotics. This resistance is usually a stable characteristic which can be used for identification.

Enzyme production

Tests for the presence of specific enzymes are useful in speciation. These tests consist of the specific substrate and an indicator. The enzymes which can be detected by this method include catalase, nitratase, aryl sulphatase, tween hydrolase, tellurite reductase.

Examples of the usual reactions of the commonly isolated mycobacteria are illustrated in Table 4.6.

Lipid analysis

It has been shown that some mycobacteria can be identified by thin layer chromatography of cell wall lipids. Mycobacterial cell wall lipids are extracted with organic solvents and separated using a thin layer chromatogram. Comparison of the patterns obtained is then made with control strains. A method using gas-liquid chromatography has also been described and as this requires only a few organisms for a positive identification subculture may not be required.

Immunological identification

Mycobacterial antigens are divided into four groups (i–iv): group i antigens are shared with all mycobacteria, nocardia and some

Table 4.6 Examples of characteristics commonly isolated *Mycobacteria*

Species	Pigment	Growth at °C 20	25	33	42	44	Nitritase	Sulphatase (21 days)	Catalase	Tellurite reduction	Tween hydrolysis	Thiacetazone
M. kansasii	P	–	+	+	v	–	+	+	+++	–	+	s
M. marinum	P	+	+	+	–	–	–	++	++	–	+	r
M. avium-intracellulare	–/S	v	+	+	+	v	–	v	–	+	–	v
M. xenopi	–/S	–	–	–	+	+	–	+++	–	–	–	r
M. ulcerans	–/S	–	+	+	–	–	–	–	–	–	–	r
M. fortuitum	–	+	+	+	v	–	+	+++	v	+	–	r
M. chelonei	–	+	+	+	–	–	–	+++	v	+	–	r
M. malmoense	–	–	+	+	–	–	+	–	–	–	+	r

s = sensitive; r = resistant; v = variable; P = photochromogen; S = scotochromogen
Based on Collins, Grange and Yates (see Further reading)

corynebacteria; group ii antigens are found in slow-growing mycobacteria; group iii antigens occur in rapid-growing organisms; and group iv antigens are species specific. Unfortunately many species, including *M. tuberculosis* agglutinate spontaneously making a standard bacterial agglutination test impossible. This problem can be overcome by performing a gel double diffusion of bacterial cytoplasmic antigens. Species and subspecies may be identified using this technique although it is not routinely available.

New identification methods

A commercial DNA hybridization technique has recently become available for the identification of *M. tuberculosis* complex organisms and *M. avium-intracellulare*. A ^{125}I-labelled single-stranded DNA probe complementary to the rRNA of the target organism is used. Ribosomal RNA is liberated by the action of a lysing agent, heat and sonication. The probe and rRNA combine to form a stable complex which is separated from unhybridized ^{125}I-DNA with a hydroxylapatite suspension. The absorbed radioactivity is counted and calculated as a percentage of probe hybridized. Values >15% are considered positive. This system has a sensitivity and specificity in excess of 90%, is rapid but has all the disadvantages of relatively high reagent cost and of handling radiation. Non-radioactive probes are now available.

Susceptibility testing

Mycobacteria are susceptible to a wide range of agents. These are conventionally divided into first and second line partly on the basis of their activity and the frequency of their use in therapy of tuberculosis. First line agents include rifampicin, ethambutol, isoniazid, pyrazinamide, and streptomycin. Second line agents include clofazamine, para-amino salicylic (PAS) acid, cycloserine, erythromycin and ethionamide.

Therapy of mycobacterial infections is usually with a combination of antimicrobial agents. In tuberculosis this is for two main reasons: patients with pulmonary tuberculosis have a body load of approximately 10^{13} organisms. Mycobacteria spontaneously develop resistance to anti-tuberculous drugs at rates varying from 10^{-6} for ethambutol to 10^{-8} for rifampicin, consequently resistance inevitably develops if only one drug is used. When a combination is employed the possibility of two resistance mutations occurring on the one organism are reduced (to 10^{-14} for a combination of rifampicin and ethambutol). Mycobacteria are also found in four states: growing extracellularly, i.e. in cavities; growing intracellularly in macrophages; dormant with occasional bursts of metabolic activity; and completely dormant. Obviously no drug is effective against organisms which are completely dormant. Isoniazid works most effectively against extracellular organisms and has its maximum bactericidal activity early in the course of chemotherapy. Rifampicin is effective against the semi-dormant bacteria, and this is responsible for the strong sterilizing activity of this drug (the ability of the drug to render patients culture negative and to prevent relapse). Pyrazinamide is active only at acid pH conditions which are found in the macrophage and centre of caseous necrosis, thus it has its principal effect early in the course of infection since with clinical improvement the caseous foci resolve. 4-Fluoroquinolines are also concentrated in macrophages and act against mycobacterial DNA gyrase. These agents have strong early bactericidal activity and may be effective sterilizing agents. Thus in combination chemotherapy drugs perform different functions in treating the infection and preventing relapse.

Value of susceptibility testing

In countries where the prescription of antibiotics is closely controlled, resistance among wild-type *M. tuberculosis* strains is uncommon. However, in poorer countries where patients have to pay for drugs, and anti-tuberculosis agents can be purchased over the counter, inappropriate drug use is common leading to a high prevalence of multi-drug resistant strains.

The value of sensitivity testing in the management of individual cases of previously untreated tuberculosis is relatively small, if wild-type strains can be presumed sensitive.

Antibiotic sensitivities results are of particular benefit in patients who have relapsed on or after treatment where the probability of a resistant strain is high, in patients from countries where multi-drug resistance is common or in those infected with 'atypical' species. Atypical mycobacteria differ from the *M. tuberculosis* complex in that many 'wild-type' strains are resistant to first line antibiotics.

Methods of susceptibility testing

The main methods in current use include:

1   The resistance ratio method (commonly used in British laboratories)
2   The proportion method (used mainly in the USA)
3   Disc diffusion methods
4   Radiometric method.

Resistance ratio method

In this method the minimal inhibitory concentration (MIC) of a test strain is compared with the MICs of control (wild-type) strains tested on the same media at the same time. This allows for variation in the medium such as binding of drug to proteins, and thus an egg-based medium such as Lowenstein-Jensen can be used. Although an MIC method is used the results obtained are not truly quantitative as they are expressed as a resistance ratio between test and control strains.

The drug-containing medium is added in 2.5 ml volumes and inspissated 10 μl of culture suspension is added to drug-containing sets and a drug-free control tube. A set of wild-type controls are also tested in parallel. The modal values for MIC of the control strains are compared with the test strain to provide a ratio. Strains giving a ratio of 1 or 2 (i.e. the test and control values are the same or the test is one tube higher) are reported sensitive, and 4 resistant and 8 (the test is two or three tubes higher) highly resistant.

The proportion method

The proportion method is popular in the USA, and compares the number of organisms

Table 4.7   Critical concentrations for anti-tuberculous drugs for 7H10 Middlebrook agar

Drug	mg/l
Isoniazid	0.2
Rifampicin	1.0
Ethambutol	5.0
Streptomycin	2.0
Kanamycin	5.0

growing on drug-containing medium with those growing on drug-free medium. Strains are defined as sensitive or resistant on the proportion of drug-resistant organisms detected growing on critical concentrations of drug, e.g. <1% for isoniazid, PAS and rifampicin-ethambutol and <10% for the remaining agents. Middlebrook 7H10 medium is used and either quadrant plates or tubes can be used (Table 4.7).

Disc diffusion tests

In this method a high concentration of antibiotic is incorporated in a paper disc. One is placed in each quadrant of a quartered Petri dish and fresh Middlebrook 7H10 agar poured over it. When dry, test and control strains are inoculated. The quadrants are then read as in the proportion method in comparison with a quadrant containing no drug. Strains showing less than 1% of control growth are considered susceptible to the antibiotic tested. This method is very simple and produces results which correlate well with those from the standard proportion method.

Automated sensitivity testing

Using a ^{14}C-palmitate Middlebrook 7H12 medium which incorporates anti-tuberculosis agents, the BACTEC radiometric system can be adapted to perform sensitivity testing. This method produces rapid results which correlate well with standard methodology. The equipment and reagents are expensive, however, and bring the additional hazards associated with the use of radioactivity.

The advantages of the radiometric system are that rapid reporting of resistance may be especially valuable in patients infected with *M. avium-intracellulare* or where multi-drug resistance is common.

Major practical difficulties in performing the technique are in standardizing the inoculum, one which is too large results in false resistance, and if too small, false sensitivity. Problems may be encountered with bacteriostatic agents such as ethambutol which may allow growth for two to three days even in strains which are fully sensitive.

A non-radiometric alternative to this method is the use of a bioluminescence system. Bacterial ATP provides energy for the luciferin-luciferase reaction which releases light energy. (This is the same reaction which goes on in the tail of a firefly.) The light produced is directly proportional to the ATP present and thus the bacterial number. Mycobacterial sensitivity techniques using this system have been published and results are available five days after inoculation.

5

Gram-negative cocci (the Neisseriaceae)

Classification

The family Neisseriaceae contains four genera: *Neisseria*, *Moraxella*, *Kingella*, and *Acinetobacter*. The genus *Branhamella*, which had formerly been classified as a *Neisseria*, is now known to be closely related genetically with the genus *Moraxella* and has been transferred.

Acinetobacter are genetically distinct from other members of this family and it is possible that they may be included in their own family in the future.

Classification and clinical importance

All of the organisms are Gram-negative cocci or coccobacilli and all are oxidase positive with the exception of *Acinetobacter*. *Moraxella* and *Neisseria* are catalase positive and *Kingella* are catalase negative. The division of this family is illustrated in Figure 5.1.

The natural habitat of the Neisseriaceae is mucous membranes of animals including man. Although *Acinetobacter* spp. may also colonize these sites, they are more often found in the environment, living as saprophytes. There are two main pathogenic species among the Neisseriaceae: *Neisseria gonorrhoeae*, the causative organism of gonorrhoea and *N. meningitidis*, the cause of endemic and epidemic pyogenic meningitis, and acute or chronic septicaemia.

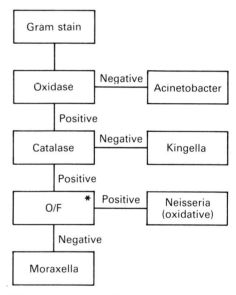

* In practice many laboratories use rapid carbohydrate utilization tests

Figure 5.1 Simplified scheme for separating genera of Gram-negative coccobacilli

Moraxellas are organisms of relatively low virulence but their role in human disease is being increasingly recognized. *Moraxella catarrhalis* colonizes the upper respiratory tract and its incidence rises in the winter months. It may cause pneumonia in patients with chronic obstructive airways disease and other chronic respiratory diseases such as bronchiectasis and pneumoconiosis. It is also associated with acute otitis media and sinusitis, and rarely with meningitis and osteomyelitis.

Moraxella lacunata is responsible for an acute angular blepharo-conjunctivitis. Of the other members of this genus *M. nonliquefaciens* has been isolated from patients with endophthalmitis and *M. osloensis*, *M. phenylpyruvica* and *M. urethralis* have been isolated in rare cases of septicaemia.

Kingella spp. are organisms of low pathogenicity. Three species are recognized: *K. kingae*, *K. indologenes*, and *K. denitrificans*. Infection usually occurs only in patients who are severely immunocompromised, and most reported infections have taken the form of septicaemia or septic arthritis.

Acinetobacter spp. are saprophytic or commensal organisms found in 7% of the normal population but more frequently in hospital patients. These organisms may be naturally resistant to many antibiotics which gives them a selective advantage in the hospital environment. When a patient is given courses of broad-spectrum antimicrobial chemotherapy and undergoes procedures which facilitate bacterial colonization such as endotracheal intubation and intravenous catheterization, colonization with acinetobacter may occur and pneumonia, septicaemia or suppuration in almost any site can develop. Acinetobacter colonize plastic prosthetic devices giving rise to soft tissue infections in i.v. cannulae sites and around intracranial shunts. Although significant bacteraemia can occur it is essential to ensure that isolates from the blood are clinically significant as blood cultures can be contaminated from the patient's skin (see p. 161).

Neisseria

Neisseria gonorrhoeae and *N. meningitidis* are the most important pathogens in this genus. Other members of the Neisseriaceae must be differentiated from these organisms as they are commensals of the human mucous membrane and may give rise to diagnostic confusion if not correctly identified. These commensal strains may be important in inducing cross-reactive immunity to *N. meningitidis*.

Neisseria gonorrhoeae

Clinical importance

In males infection with *N. gonorrhoeae* usually gives rise to acute urethritis characterized by painful micturition without frequency and a purulent discharge. Acute epididymitis periurethral abscess or infections of Cowper's glands can complicate acute infection. Asymptomatic infection can occur so the contacts of all infected patients must be traced to control the spread of the disease.

In females gonococcal infection is seated at the cervix causing a purulent discharge which may go unnoticed by the patient (up to 80% of cases of infection are asymptomatic). Ascending infection can give rise to pelvic inflammatory disease (PID). Patients complain of lower abdominal pain, nausea and vomiting and are febrile with signs of peritonitis, uterine tenderness and extreme pain on palpation of the cervix. Tubo-ovarian and pelvic abscesses may develop and fertility may be compromised if diagnosis and treatment is delayed or is inadequate. Infertility occurs in approximately 15% of patients after a single episode of PID. Patients with PID often have coexistent bacterial vaginosis.

In both males and females multiple pathogens may participate in the infective process including *Chlamydia trachomatis*, *Mycoplasma hominis*, *Ureaplasma urealyticum* or *Trichomonas vaginalis*. Mixed facultative and obligate anaerobic flora may participate in PID.

Rectal infection may also be found in approximately 40% of females, and is also common in passive homosexual males. In acute gonococcal proctitis patients complain of rectal pain, pruritus, tenesmus and a purulent discharge. Pharyngeal infection can occur after orogenital sexual intercourse. Pharyngeal infection is often asymptomatic but sore throat and local lymphadenitis can be found.

Pathogenicity

Neisseria gonorrhoeae is a mucosal pathogen with a tropism for the epithelium of the genital tract. Extensive research has revealed a number of pathogenicity determinants. Infection occurs in two phases: attachment to the epithelium followed by endocytosis and excretion into the lamina propria where the infection develops.

Pili

Gonococcal pili are hair-like projections made up of many protein subunits which are responsible for the attachment of the organism to the epithelial surface. Loss of piliation is associated with avirulence and is reflected in a change in colonial morphology. The amino acid sequence of pilus protein has a highly conserved region, which is responsible for attachment, and a variable region. This antigenic variation of this region is responsible in part failure to develop solid immunity after an infection.

Outer membrane proteins (OMP)

Outer membrane protein I makes up 60% of the outer membrane and is thought to have two functions: as a porin allowing the influx of water soluble nutrients, and as a site of attachment to membranes. Patients infected with a particular OMP I type cannot be re-infected with that type.

Outer membrane protein II enhances the attachment of gonococci to epithelial cells and expression of this protein is associated with invasiveness. With a molecular weight of 24–32 kD up to six antigenically different types of OMP II can be expressed by a single strain. Outer membrane protein II expression can be switched off and this can be seen in the colonial morphology (OMP II-negative colonies are opaque).

Like other mucosal pathogens *N. gonorrhoeae* expresses an IgA protease which may promote survival at the mucosal surface.

Laboratory diagnosis

Specimens

The specimens required for the diagnosis of gonorrhoea will vary according to the clinical circumstances, the sex and sexual practices of the patient. In females an endocervical swab should be collected together with a rectal and urethral swab. A pharyngeal swab should also be collected if there is a history of orogenital

Table 5.1 Specimens for the cultural diagnosis of *N. gonorrhoeae* infection

Males	Females
Urethral	Urethral
Rectal	Rectal
Throat[a]	Endocervical
Prostatic[b]	Throat[a]
Blood[c]	Blood[c]
Joint fluid[c]	Joint fluid[c]

a. If symptomatic or evidence of exposure
b. If symptomatic
c. In cases where disseminated infection is suspected.

contact. Urethral swabs should be collected from male heterosexuals together with rectal and pharyngeal smears in male homosexuals. Where the clinical features suggest, disseminated gonococcal infection, blood culture and culture of joint fluid and skin lesions should also be performed (Table 5.1). All specimens should be examined by direct microscopy, and inoculated on the primary isolation media immediately they are collected. This may be achieved by setting up a small laboratory as an annex of the sexually transmitted diseases clinic, and staffed by medical laboratory scientific officers (MLSOs) or nurses specially trained in these techniques.

Specimens may be collected using Dacron swabs (cotton contains unsaturated fatty acids which are inhibitory to gonococci), or with a platinum bacterial loop.

In female infection cervical swabs provide the highest diagnostic yield. To optimize results it is important that cervical mucus is wiped away and that the endocervical canal is sampled. High vaginal swabs should not be accepted as false-negative results are common. Urethral specimens should be collected at least 1 hour after micturition. Any urethral discharge should be sampled and if no discharge is present a specimen may be obtained by gently scraping the urethral mucosa with a sterile platinum loop or swab. Muco-purulent material from the anal canal can be collected with the help of a proctoscope and faecal contamination should be minimized. Conjunctival samples, pus from Bartholin's gland, and joint fluid should be obtained when clinical circumstances suggest it. Organisms can be cultured from skin biopsies or aspirated pus from skin lesions but the diagnostic yield is low.

Table 5.2 Enrichment and selective agents in media used for the isolation of *N. gonorrhoeae*

Type	Base	Selective agents	Enrichment
Thayer-Martin	Chocolate blood GC agar base	Colistin, nystatin, vancomycin	'Iso-vitalex'
Modified New York City	5% agar lysed blood	Lincomycin, colistin, amphotericin B, trimethoprim	Proteose peptone, baker's yeast

Transport

Gonococci are highly susceptible to adverse environmental conditions and are readily killed by drying. Wherever possible specimens should be examined in the clinic where they are obtained. Clinics should examine relevant Gram-stained specimens microscopically, and inoculate the specimen on appropriate media. The plates should then be incubated at 37°C in an atmosphere of 5% carbon dioxide and increased humidity and then transferred to the microbiology laboratory after overnight incubation for reading and identification.

When these facilities are not available transport media can be employed as an alternative. Gonococci survive well on transport media for up to 12 hours but are still susceptible to variation in ambient temperature. Specimens can therefore be collected on charcoal-coated swabs and sent in Amie's modification of Stuart's medium.

Direct examination

Microscopy should be performed on urethral and endocervical specimens, pus from Bartholin's abscess, and joint fluids. Direct examination of a throat swab would obviously be confusing due to the presence of commensal *Moraxella* and *Neisseria*.

In males with acute urethritis, a Gram-stained smear of urethral pus correctly identifies 95% of those subsequently shown to be culture positive. Among females endocervical swabs achieve only a 50% pick-up rate. It is important that when smears of endocervical secretions are examined, that only Gram-negative intracellular diplococci are reported as some commensal organisms can be found outside the cell. The diagnosis of gonorrhoea should be confirmed by culture wherever facilities allow.

Direct fluorescence has been used as an aid to rapid diagnosis in female subjects. Initial studies using polyclonal antibodies were disappointing but the use of monoclonal antibodies has improved the sensitivity to 80%.

An enzyme-linked immunosorbent assay (ELISA) antigen detection system which has a sensitivity of between 78 and 100% in female infection has been described. It suffers from the disadvantage of variable specificity between 70 and 100% which would lead to many false-positive results in low prevalence populations.

Culture

Neisseria gonorrhoeae is a fragile organism which is susceptible to desiccation and has fastidious growth requirements. It is usually isolated from sites which are heavily contaminated with other organisms. A nutritionally rich medium is required to isolate these organisms successfully and it must be supplemented with an antimicrobial combination to inhibit the growth of the normal flora. Because of the selective nature of the media employed, an unselective plate such as chocolate agar should be inoculated in parallel.

There are two main media for the isolation of *N. gonorrhoeae*, Thayer Martin and New York City media. Both of these media are now used in a modified form: Thayer Martin medium is chocolate blood agar supplemented with additional nutrient mixtures, e.g. Isovitalex with antibiotic agents: vancomycin, colistin, nystatin and trimethoprim (Table 5.2). In New York City medium, horse blood is completely lysed with saponin and supplemented with proteose peptone, corn starch, dextrose and yeast dialysate. The antibiotics used for selection are lincomycin, colistin, amphotericin B and trimethoprim. Lincomycin replaced vancomycin in this mixture because a

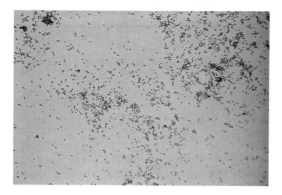

Figure 5.2   *Neisseria* are characteristically Gram-negative cocci with a peanut morphology

number of strains of *N. gonorrhoeae* are, surprisingly, susceptible to vancomycin. These strains include the fastidious arginine, hypoxanthine, uracil negative (AHU⁻) auxotypes (see below). Plates should be incubated at 37°C in 3–5% carbon dioxide with increased humidity. Candle jars may be used. Cultures should be incubated for 48–72 hours and inspected every 24 hours.

After 24 hours of incubation, colonies are 0.5–1 mm in diameter, are greyish opaque, raised and glistening with an entire edge. *N. gonorrhoeae* can be presumptively identified on the basis of demonstrating Gram-negative diplococci of typical morphology (Fig. 5.2) which are oxidase positive only if isolated from a urogenital specimen.

Definitive identification is achieved by demonstrating acid production from carbohydrates. The carbohydrates tested include glucose, maltose, sucrose, fructose, lactose (or ONPG). The conventional method of performing these tests is to use a 1 or 2% carbohydrate solution in semi-solid or solid agar (GC agar base). When media is made in-house high purity reagents must be used as contamination of maltose with small amounts of glucose has been shown to confound the results of these tests. This technique depends on bacterial growth but many laboratories now use rapid fermentation tests, which utilize a heavy bacterial inoculum in small volumes of test sugar in phosphate-buffered saline with a phenol red indicator. The heavy inoculum means that growth is not required and pre-formed

enzymes perform the carbohydrate degradation. Thus, results are available within 1–4 hours after inoculation. Several commercial versions of this technique are available. Beta-lactamases can be detected at the same time in this system in which the carbohydrate is replaced by ampicillin.

A serological identification method is also available using the coagglutination technique. Cowan type 1 *S. aureus* is coated with two monoclonal antibodies to gonococcal outer membrane proteins Pr 1A and Pr 1B. This reagent can be used with colonies from the primary culture plate, thus enabling a presumptive positive report to be made. The results of carbohydrate oxidation tests are shown in Table 5.3.

Confirmatory diagnosis can be made by detecting specific enzyme activities with chromogenic substrates. Beta-galactosidase activity is found in *N. lactima*, and gamma-glutamine aminopeptidase in *N. meningitidis*. Hydroxyprolylaminopeptidase is found in both *N. gonorrhoeae* and *N. lactima*. These tests can only be used on organisms which grow on selective media as commensal species can also give positive results.

Typing of gonococci

In auxotyping a number of different defined minimal media from which individual reagents have been omitted are inoculated. Organisms which can grow on this deficient media are described as positive and those which fail to grow negative. Strains which are arginine, hypoxanthine, and uracil negative have been associated with disseminated gonococcal infection.

Gonococci can also be typed on the basis of SDS-PAGE of outer membrane proteins. This technique is unsuitable for routine use as there is significant gel-to-gel variation.

A typing scheme has been developed based on the use of a bank of monoclonal antibodies. This is clearly able to differentiate between individual isolates but has not established itself in routine use in diagnostic laboratories.

Antimicrobial susceptibility

Neisseria gonorrhoeae was, at first, highly susceptible to sulphonamides and penicillin.

Table 5.3 Characteristic reactions of some *Neisseria* and related organisms

Species	Glucose	Maltose	Lactose	Sucrose	DNAase	Growth on nutrient agar at 35°C
N. meningitidis	+	+	−	−	−	−
N. gonorrhoeae	+	−	−	−	−	−
N. lactamica	+	+	+	−	−	+
N. subflava	+	+	−	v	−	+
N. cinerea	−	−	−	−	−	+
N. sicca	+	+	−	+	−	+
Moraxella cattarhalis	−	−	−	−	+	+

Sulphonamide resistance developed relatively quickly, but penicillin resistance arose more slowly. Because of this, therapy was possible using higher doses of penicillin and co-administration of probenecid which blocked penicillin secretion by the kidney. This form of penicillin resistance was chromosomally mediated.

In the 1970s a plasmid coding for a beta-lactamase enzyme TEM-1 was introduced into the gonococcus. This resistance gene had originally arisen among enterobacteria and disseminated to other genera by means of a transposon. These penicillinase-producing gonococci (PPNG) were also often resistant to tetracycline, one of the main alternative therapeutic agents. These organisms are sensitive to spectinomycin, an aminocyclitol antibiotic closely related to the aminoglycosides, penicillinase-stable penicillins and cephalosporins. More recently the 4-fluoro-quinolones have shown themselves to be highly active and clinically useful.

Perhaps the single most important 'susceptibility test' is the determination of beta-lactamase production. A filter paper strip may be moistened with a solution containing benzyl penicillin, and bromocresol purple and individual colonies placed on the strip which is incubated at 37°C for 30 minutes in a humidified chamber. Organisms containing beta-lactamase will produce a yellow zone due to the change in indicator colour caused by acid production secondary to the penicillin hydrolysis. A positive and negative control should be inoculated on each strip. Commercial versions of this technique are available. These may utilize a chromogenic cephalosporin (nitrocefin), which changes colour when hydrolysed by beta-lactamase.

Disc susceptibility testing

Isolates of *N. gonorrhoeae* should be tested against penicillin, spectinomycin, minocycline, a third generation cephalosporin and a 4-fluoroquinolone. A fully sensitive strain should be used as a control. When MICs are performed the agar dilution technique is reliable. A *Staphylococcus aureus* and susceptible *N. gonorrhoeae* should be tested in parallel. The inoculum should be a 1 : 100 dilution of 10^8 cfu/ml.

Neisseria meningitidis

Clinical importance

Neisseria meningitidis is a pathogen of serious public health importance. Infection can take the form of a pyogenic meningitis which may be accompanied by bacteraemia. The patient presents with fever, headache and photophobia together with neck stiffness often after a short prodromal illness. Infection may also take the form of bacteraemia in the absence of meningitis with fever, shock and a characteristic petechial skin rash. This presentation can progress to a fatal outcome in a few hours. Reactive arthritis may follow acute infection and septic arthritis may develop as part of the septicaemic process. In a small number of children bacteraemia can occur without the signs of severe sepsis and recovery follows without therapy.

Meningococcal disease is endemic with a small number of cases arising most commonly in the second winter quarter. Superimposed upon this background are periodic epidemics

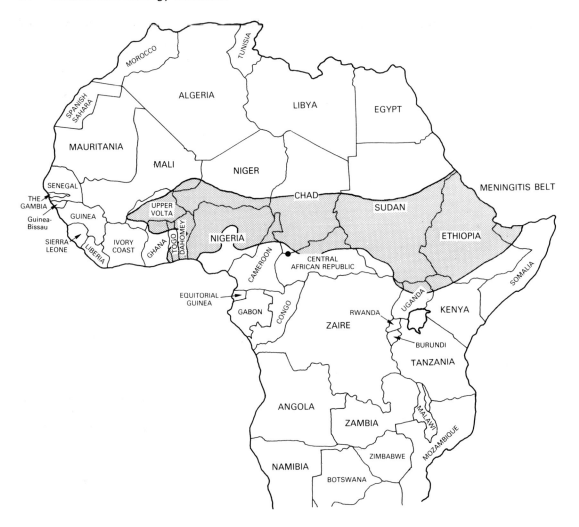

Figure 5.3   Meningitis belt

in which the number of cases may rise dramatically. Epidemic waves arise every 10–12 years. This epidemiological pattern is most graphically illustrated by the massive epidemics which develop in the 'meningitis belt' of Africa where prevalence can rise to 1000 cases per 100 000. (European 'epidemics' rarely have prevalences above 10/100 000 (Fig. 5.3).)

Classification

Neisseria meningitidis is divided, on the basis of the polysaccharide capsular antigen, into 13 serogroups. Of these the most frequent human pathogens are serogroups A, B, C and W135.

Serogroup B is usually associated with endemic disease in European countries. Group A infections are commonly found in epidemics in N. America, and C in epidemics in Africa. With increasing travel, strains of any serogroup can be introduced into the community and cause disease. Organisms can be further subdivided into serotypes on the basis of outer membrane protein typing.

Habitat

The meningococcus is most commonly isolated from the throat or nasopharynx of asymptomatic subjects. The organism circulates in the community and there is a low case-to-carrier ratio. This ratio increases during epidemics – i.e. more patients who are colonized go on to have invasive disease. Isolation of *N. meningitidis* from throat or nasopharynx is therefore not necessarily an indication for therapeutic intervention.

Pathogenicity

Capsular polysaccharide

Neisseria meningitidis possess a polysaccharide capsule of which there are at least 13 types. The capsular serotypes found most often in invasive infections are serotypes A, B, C and W135. Antibodies to capsular antigens are protective and form the basis of a successful vaccine for serotypes A, C and W135. The serogroup B capsule consists of *N*-acetylneuraminic acid which cross-reacts with the *E. coli* K1 antigen and glycoproteins in the central nervous system, liver, kidney and heart. As a result this antigen is poorly immunogenic and a vaccine based on this antigen is not practical.

Lipo-oligosaccharide (LOS)

The LOS is analogous to the lipopolysaccharide found in other Gram-negative bacteria. It is capable of stimulating macrophages to produce cytokines such as tumour necrosis factor (TNF). Tumour necrosis factor has been demonstrated in patients with meningococcal septicaemia and concentrations can be related to prognosis.

The central role of the LOS in shock opens the possibility of therapeutic intervention with anti-lipid A or anti-TNF monoclonal antibodies.

Outer membrane proteins

Endemic disease is caused by strains with a wide range of outer membrane protein 2 types whereas a single type is usually found in an epidemic. These antigens are closely bound to the LOS in the outer membrane.

Other pathogenicity determinants

Meningococci possess pili which have been shown to aid attachment to nasopharyngeal epithelium. An IgA protease is produced and may assist survival at mucosal surfaces.

Laboratory diagnosis

Methods for direct examination of CSF specimens are described in Chapter 15.

Specimens

In patients with suspected meningococcal disease specimens of CSF and blood must urgently be obtained. In cases in which a rash is present the lesions may be sampled by injecting a small amount of sterile saline and carefully aspirating it again. In practice this is rarely attempted in acute meningococcal disease, but may occasionally provide the diagnosis in the unusual chronic meningococcaemia syndrome.

Nasopharyngeal swabs can be obtained when surveys of meningococcal carriage are being performed. Cases and their contacts may also be swabbed but the results of these investigations should not alter the decision to provide prophylaxis which should be made on the basis of risk of transmission. Prophylaxis is required only for patients with intimate contact with the index case. This usually means family members or medical and nursing attendants who have performed procedures such as mouth-to-mouth respiration. Once prophylaxis has been given, nasopharyngeal swabs may prove eradication of the carriage strain.

Culture

Neisseria meningitidis are less nutritionally fastidious than *N. gonorrhoeae*, but are likely to be present in small numbers in clinical specimens. Cultures should be made on chocolate blood agar at 37°C in an atmosphere of 5% carbon dioxide and increased humidity. CSF should also be inoculated into a broth medium, e.g. Robertson's cooked meat broth. Nasopharyngeal swabs should be inoculated on chocolate blood agar and modified New York City medium, as the nasopharynx contains a large number of commensal species which will be inhibited by the selective agents contained in this medium.

Identification

After incubation for 18–24 hours colonies are usually more than 1 mm in diameter, round convex and smooth with an entire edge and a glistening surface. Mucoid colonies may occur, especially in serogroups A,C and W135. *Neisseria meningitidis* from the CSF can be presumptively identified on the basis of the characteristic Gram morphology and oxidase positivity and agglutination of specific antiserum. Confirmation of the identification is made by the techniques already described for the gonococcus.

Typing

Meningococci should be serogrouped in the laboratory of isolation. The usual method is by the slide agglutination technique using serogroup specific rabbit antiserum. This procedure must be carried out in a safety cabinet. Isolates from the nasopharynx may be difficult to serogroup. Auxotyping is of little value in typing meningococci as they are less fastidious organisms.

Typing may be performed on the basis of SDS-PAGE of outer membrane proteins. This technique enables subtypes within serogroups B, C, Y and W135 to be identified for epidemiological purposes. Several of the subtypes within group B have recently been associated with increased pathogenicity in epidemic disease.

Antimicrobial susceptibility

Neisseria meningitidis are susceptible to benzyl penicillin, and although there have been occasional reports of strains possessing the plasmid expressing TEM-1 these have not become widespread. Cefotaxime and chloramphenicol are alternatives for therapy. Sulphonamides were once the treatment of choice for meningococcal meningitis but up to 50% of strains are resistant. Isolates should be tested for rifampicin, tetracycline and 4-fluoroquinolone susceptibility as these are all useful in the eradication of carriage.

Other *Neisseria* spp.

Commensal *Neisseria* spp. are found on mucous membranes and are frequently isolated in clinical specimens *Neisseria lactamica*. They have been isolated in CSF and were once thought to be a lactose-positive variant of *N. meningitidis*. Some strains may cross-react with gonococcal and meningococcal antisera. This illustrates the importance of confirming positive isolates, both serologically and biochemically, before a definitive report is issued.

The species *Neisseria pharyngis* has been subdivided into four new species: *N. subflava*, *N. flava*, *N. perflava* and *N. sicca*. They are all nasopharyngeal commensals which produce pigmented colonies and utilize maltose, glucose, fructose and sucrose. *Neisseria sicca* has dry, tough, opaque colonies which adhere tightly to the medium in contrast to the other three species, which produce moist, pigmented colonies.

Neisseria polysaccharea resembles the meningococcus in culture. Like the meningococcus it utilizes glucose and maltose but differs in that it produces copious capsular polysaccharide material when grown in the medium containing 5% sucrose.

Neisseria cinerea can be isolated from the oropharynx and from genital sites. It is usually asaccharolytic but may occasionally utilize glucose. It does not cross-react with the gonococcus in coagglutination tests.

Neisseria flavescens was described in the 1930s as the causative organism of a group of meningitis cases in America. It produced golden yellow colonies, hence its name. Unfortunately the organism was lost in subculture and no further cases caused by this strain have been reported. *Neisseria mucosa* is a capsulate organism which produces mucoid colonies like *N. polysaccharea*, it synthesizes polysaccharide in a medium containing sucrose.

Neisseria elongata is the only rod-shaped member of the *Neisseria* genus. It also differs from the other species in that it is catalase negative.

Identification of commensal strains

There are four main techniques used to identify commensal strains: nitrate, nitrite reduction, DNAase, and polysaccharide production. Nitrate and nitrite reduction tests are performed using 0.1% solutions of potassium nitrate or nitrite in brain heart infusion broth. Polysaccharide production is determined by culture of the organism on a medium containing 5% sucrose. After culture, the fluid is flooded with Lugol's iodine and polysaccharide-producing colonies are stained deep blue in colour. DNAase is determined by a method suitable for use in Gram-negative bacteria.

Moraxella

The genus *Moraxella* includes a number of different species of which *Moraxella lacunata* is a human pathogen, causing purulent conjunctivitis presenting as an angular blepharo-conjunctivitis.

Like other members of the family Neisseriaceae, *Moraxella* spp. are part of the normal flora, but may cause opportunistic infections in immunocompromised hosts.

Moraxellas are strictly aerobic, non-capsular, non-motile, oxidase positive and catalase positive. They are asaccharolytic and susceptible to penicillin. This latter feature may be used to distinguish easily this genus from *Acinetobacter*.

Moraxella catarrhalis

Moraxella catarrhalis is a commensal of the respiratory tract. It has been associated with lower respiratory tract infections in patients who are compromised by virtue of chronic obstructive airways disease or other chronic respiratory disease. It also has a role to play in the aetiology of otitis media and sinusitis and has also been reported to cause acute pneumonia in young adults.

The organism is oval, Gram negative, and about 0.8 μm in diameter. It grows aerobically, optimally at 36°C, but may grow at 22°C. It does not require blood for growth and may be cultured on nutrient agar. After 24 hours the colonies are between 1–2 mm in diameter. They are greyish white, smooth, opaque and butyrous. The organism is strongly oxidase and catalase positive, asaccharolytic, but produces DNAase. Many strains produce beta-lactamase and are thus resistant to penicillin. They are, however, often susceptible to erythromycin, tetracycline and trimethoprim.

Kingella

Kingella spp. are short Gram-negative rods, which are oxidase positive, catalase negative and are saccharolytic. There are three recognized species, *K. kingae*, *K. denitrificans*, and *K. indologenes*. These organisms are of low pathogenicity, but are important in that they may occasionally cause opportunistic infections in immunocompromised hosts or may be mistaken for the pathogenic *Neisseria*. They are usually penicillin susceptible.

Acinetobacter

This genus has been divided into at least 17 species on the basis of DNA hybridization studies. The main species isolated in the clinical laboratory are *A. lwoffi*, *A. calcoaceticus*, *A. barmanii*, and *A. haemolyticus*. The organisms are Gram negative, bacilli or coccobacilli, are oxidase negative, catalase positive, strictly aerobic and may be capsulate. *Acinetobacter* spp. oxidizes sugars to produce acids. They are not nutritionally fastidious as they are free-living saprophytes and will, thus, grow on simple media. The colonies are white, opaque with an entire edge.

All strains are penicillin resistant and many hospital isolates of *Acinetobacter* spp. are multi-drug resistant. It is thus that they have their gained importance; colonizing patients on broad spectrum antibiotic therapy and giving rise to invasive infections in patients compromised by underlying disease, the presence of intravenous access devices, and endotracheal tubes. The resultant infections can take the form of pneumonia, urinary tract infection, abscesses, line-related bacteraemia or colonization of prostheses.

Gram-negative coccobacilli

Introduction

The small Gram-negative coccobacilli have previously been grouped together under the term Parvobacteria. This classification lacks taxonomic respectability and clinical relevance. The genera discussed in this chapter, *Haemophilus*, *Francisella*, *Pasteurella*, *Brucella*, and *Bordetella*, cause a wide range of different types of infection, from infective exacerbations of chronic obstructive airways disease (*H. influenzae*) to undulant fever (*Brucella melitensis*).

Haemophilus

Definition

Members of the genus *Haemophilus* are small Gram-negative pleomorphic bacilli which are so named because they will grow only on media containing accessory growth factors – X factor (protoporphyrin, haemin) or V factor (nicotinamide adenine deoxynucleotide NAD, or NAD phosphate, NADP) – which are found in blood. They are aerobes or facultative anaerobes and many species grow better in an atmosphere with added carbon dioxide. Carbohydrates are fermented by most species and they are mainly oxidase and catalase positive. They are non-spore-forming and may be capsulate.

Haemophilus spp. are obligate parasites, colonizing human and animal mucous membranes. They constitute approximately 10% of the bacterial flora of the respiratory tract of which *H. parainfluenzae* and non-encapsulated *H. influenzae* predominate.

Pathogenicity

The principal pathogenicity determinant of *H. influenzae* is the polysaccharide capsule. Six different capsular types (Pittman types) are produced, designated a–f, and of differing polysaccharide composition. Of these, only type b is a regular cause of invasive disease. The importance of this capsule has been shown in an elegant set of experiments with recombinant bacteria expressing different polysaccharide capsule had differing pathogenic potential in a rat meningitis model. In addition to the capsule *H. influenzae*, like other Gram-negative pathogens, possess a lipopolysaccharide which enhances the toxicity of the organism. An IgA protease is also produced.

Clinical importance

The genus contains two main pathogenic species, *H. influenzae* and *H. ducreyi*.

Haemophilus influenzae produce different forms of disease depending on the presence of a polysaccharide capsule. Those organisms which possess a capsule are genetically different from the non-encapsulate strains. They are capable of causing severe systemic infections. Of the six polysaccharide capsular types, type b is the most frequently implicated. In some countries, notably the USA, it is the most common causes of childhood meningitis. Infections are usually confined to children between the ages of six months and six years. This is because they are protected by maternal antibody in the first six months of life, and then gradually acquire immunity as a result of asymptomatic colonization by capsulate *Haemophilus* or other bacteria which express cross-reacting antigens. Another characteristic infection is acute epiglottitis which presents as croup (inspiratory stridor), fever and septicaemia. Respiratory obstruction may be rapidly progressive and complete obstruction can develop if the pharynx is examined too vigorously or swabs are taken. More rarely type b *H. influenzae* may cause severe facial cellulitis, osteomyelitis, and suppurative arthritis. Capsulate *H. influenzae* may also cause primary bacterial pneumonia and this is thought to be relatively common in children in developing countries.

A vaccine against type b *H. influenzae* consisting of protein conjugated capsular polysaccharide has been introduced and provides effective protection against this organism, and there has been a marked reduction in the incidence of cases.

Unencapsulated *H. influenzae* colonize the healthy respiratory tract. In patients with chronic obstructive airways disease, bronchiectasis or cystic fibrosis, this organism may cause lower respiratory tract infection. This arises because of damage to the mucociliary clearance mechanism which enables the organisms to colonize the lower airways. Chronic infection results in chronic inflammation and further damage to the respiratory tract.

Haemophilus aegyptius is more difficult to isolate *in vitro* than *H. influenzae* although it shares the phenotypic characteristics of *H. influenzae* bio-type 3 (see below) and is responsible for acute purulent contagious conjunctivitis, especially in the tropics. An organism of this biotype has been isolated from children with an acute haemorrhagic infection, Brazilian purpuric fever.

Haemophilus ducreyi is the causative organism of chancroid or 'soft sore', a sexually transmitted disease which is uncommon in developed countries but is an important cause of genital ulceration in sub-Saharan Africa (see Chapter 19).

The other species of this genus have a very limited pathogenic potential but have all been reported as occasional pathogens in endocarditis and as opportunistic infections.

Laboratory diagnosis

Specimens

When meningitis or septicaemia is suspected specimens of blood and CSF should be obtained for culture. Capsulate *H. influenzae* type b may also be isolated from osteomyelitis pus and aspirated joint fluid. Isolation of *H. influenzae* from the throat is of no diagnostic significance as the organism is often present as a commensal. No attempt should be made to obtain swabs of epiglottis pus in cases of suspected acute epiglottitis as any interference with the throat may result in acute obstruction and respiratory embarrassment.

Specimens of sputum should be examined for the presence of non-encapsulated *H. influenzae* in patients with acute community acquired pneumonia. As this organism is a common commensal of the upper respiratory tract, culture results must be interpreted with care. Specimens can be obtained by by-passing the nasopharynx, i.e. bronchoalveolar lavage. To help decide the significance of an isolate from expectorated sputum it is useful to quantitate the numbers of organisms cultured. It is usual to accept that more than 10^5 organisms/ml are more likely to be associated with a significant infection (see Chapter 16).

In cases of suspected chancroid the genital ulcer should be thoroughly cleaned with cotton wool swabs moistened with saline, the base of the ulcer then sampled with a swab moistened in sterile broth and inoculated directly into the appropriate medium (see p. 229). Careful clinical examination should be performed to demonstrate the presence of a suppurating lymph node from which pus could be aspirated for culture. Scrapings from the ulcer base may also be examined by direct microscopy.

Direct examination

Direct examination of CSF is of particular importance in providing a rapid diagnosis in the cases of suspected meningitis (see Chapter 15). The presence of the organism can be inferred by antigen detection technique including countercurrent immunoelectrophoresis (CIE), latex agglutination, coagglutination and enzyme-linked immunosorbent assay (ELISA) (see p. 229).

Microscopic examination of conjunctivitis and ulcer scrapings provide an important supplement to diagnosis as *H. aegyptius* and *H. ducreyi* may be difficult to cultivate. Attempts to develop a successful antigen detection assay for *H. ducreyi* have not yet proved successful.

Smears should be fixed with methanol and stained by Gram's method.

Isolation

Haemophilus influenzae requires factors X and V for growth. The organism grows poorly on fresh blood agar but if blood is added to agar at 80°C 'chocolate' agar is created. The disrupted red cells release factors X and V allowing a luxuriant growth. Clear media may be produced by adding a peptic digest of blood to nutrient agar (Fildes agar) or a filtrate of heated blood (Levinthal's agar).

Media can be made selective for *Haemophilus* by the addition of penicillin, 0.2–0.5 units/ml, and bacitracin 80 mg/l. Cloxacillin (5 mg/l) may be substituted for penicillin.

To cultivate *H. ducreyi* chocolate blood agar should be supplemented with 1% Isovitalex. Many other organisms may be present in the chancroid lesion and thus this medium should be made selective by the addition of an antibiotic supplement which should include vancomycin (5 mg/l). Optimum isolation of all species is obtained by incubating cultures in an atmosphere with 5% carbon dioxide and increased humidity, the optimum temperature is 35°C. Cultures for *H. influenzae* should be incubated for 24 hours and for *H. ducreyi* up to 7 days. It is essential that plates used for the isolation of *Haemophilus* species are as fresh as possible and should be moist as drying is inimical to their survival.

A differential selective media for *H. influenzae* has been described which consists of chocolate agar supplemented by bacitracin (80 mg/l), 1% sucrose, and neutral red as an indicator. This differentiates *H. parainfluenzae* which ferments sucrose and forms yellow colonies. *H. influenzae* which does not ferment

sucrose forms small grey semi-translucent colonies.

Identification

The most important step in identification of *Haemophilus* species is to determine X and V factor dependence. This can be achieved by demonstrating satellitism on blood agar. A lawn inoculum is made from a suspect colony on blood agar and *S. aureus* is streaked across the diameter. The plate is incubated overnight. If the organism is XV dependent, colonies will only grow close to the *S. aureus* streak (Fig. 6.1). It is essential to make a Gram stain of organisms which exhibit satellitism as nutritionally fastidious streptococci may also demonstrate this phenomenon. Although easy to perform, satellitism is not a sufficiently specific technique and most laboratories test X and V factor dependence with a disc technique. A lawn inoculum of a suspect colony is made on nutrient agar (which is deficient in both X and V), paper discs impregnated with factor X alone, V alone and a combination are placed on medium. The pattern of growth round these three paper discs determines the identification (Fig. 6.2). It has been shown that the paper disc test may be unreliable for demonstrating X requirement as misleading results may be obtained in up to 20%. The more specific porphyrin test may be used in which preformed bacterial enzymes convert delta-amino-laevulinic acid into porphyrins which fluoresce brick red in ultra violet light.

Carbohydrate utilization tests are also useful in differentiating species (Table 6.1). When sucrose and lactose fermentation reaction are performed the broths must be supplemented with X and V factors. Commercial diagnostic systems, such as API 10S or 20E systems, are capable of identifying and biotyping *H. influenzae* and *H. parainfluenzae* when adapted. Several commercial identification kits based on preformed bacterial enzyme/ substrate reactions are now available and these compare well with conventional tests (98.8% agreement).

Haemophilus influenzae may be biotyped by methods which detect indole production, urease activity and ornithine decarboxylase. Eight biotypes of both *H. influenzae* and

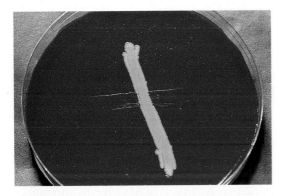

Figure 6.1 *Haemophilus influenzae* are unable to grow on blood agar except where the streak of staphylococci produce essential nutrients

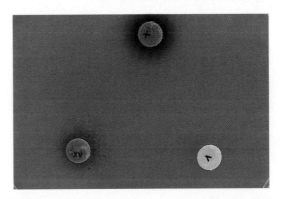

Figure 6.2 *Haemophilus influenzae* can only grow on the nutrient agar near the X and V discs as nutrient agar lacks these nutrients essential for the growth of *H. influenzae*

Table 6.1 Characteristics of *Haemophilus* spp. useful in identification

Species agglutination	X	V	Indole	Urease	ODC	β-haemolysis	Sucrose	Lactose	Glucose	CO_2
H. influenzae	+	+	+/–	+/–	+/–	–	–	–	–	–
H. aegyptius	+	+	–	+	–	–	–	–	+	–
H. haemolyticus	+	+	+/–	+	+/–	+	–	–	+	–
H. parainfluenzae	–	+	–	+/–	+/–	–	+	–	+	–
H. parahaemolyticus	–	+	–	+	+/–	+	+	–	+	v
H. aphrophilis	+	–	–	–	–	–	+	+	+	+
H. paraphrophilus	–	+	–	–	–	–	+	+	+	+
H. sequis	–	+	–	–	–	–	w	–	w	–
H. ducreyi	+	–	–	–	–	–	–	–	–	–

ODC: ornithine decarboxylase; v: variation; w: week.

H. parainfluenzae can be distinguished. This scheme is of little clinical value as many of the isolates found in human disease come from biotype III. A scheme for auxotyping *H. influenzae* has been reported.

Antibiotic susceptibility

Haemophilus influenzae is susceptible to derivatives of penicillin, to chloramphenicol, sulphonamides, trimethoprim, 4-fluoro-quinolones and tetracyclines. It is also susceptible to the later cephalosporins, but many of the oral cephalosporins with the exception of cephaclor have little activity.

In recent times *H. influenzae* has developed resistance to penicillins by the acquisition of a beta-lactamase TEM-1. In addition some strains have increased resistance due to altered affinity of the penicillin-binding proteins. The frequency of beta-lactamase producing *H. influenzae* is variable but can reach more than 50% in countries where the use of antibiotics is not closely regulated. This organism has also acquired chloramphenicol resistance due to the presence of chloramphenicol acetyl transferase enzyme.

Susceptibility testing

When disc susceptibility tests are performed by comparative methods an *H. influenzae* control NCTC 11931 should be used. Beta-lactamase production can be demonstrated by similar techniques to those employed for *Neisseria* spp. (see p. 63). Media for quantitative methods requires growth supplements, for example Fildes digest.

Bordetella

Definition

Bordetella are small Gram-negative coccobacilli which are obligate aerobes. They are characteristically catalase and oxidase positive and do not attack carbohydrates. They are non-motile, non-capsulate and non-spore-forming.

Classification and clinical importance

There are three members of this genus: *B. pertussis*, *B. parapertussis*, *B. bronchoseptica*.

Bordetella pertussis is the most important human pathogen, responsible for whooping cough. The organism infects ciliated epithelial cells of the respiratory tract. Whooping cough begins with a mild cough, fever and nasal discharge, the catarrhal phase, during which the child expresses the symptoms of an upper respiratory tract infection. This is followed by a prolonged period of cough which may last up to three months. The cough comes in paroxysms which are followed by deep inspiration. In older children the rapid inrush of air gives rise to a whooping sound which gives its name to the condition. Although a characteristic feature it is not invariably present, and is often not found in the youngest children.

Severe infection can occur in unvaccinated children and those under the age of one year. Conjunctival haemorrhages, petechial haemorrhages around the eye, and rectal prolapse are the result of the cough. The prolonged bouts of coughing can cause intracerebral haemorrhage which may lead to brain damage. Whooping cough is frequently complicated by secondary bacterial respiratory infection and otitis media.

Bordetella parapertussis also may cause whooping cough although it is much less common. *Bordetella bronchoseptica* is a respiratory pathogen of pigs, horses, sheep and dogs and may cause respiratory infections and wound infections in humans. It does not cause whooping cough syndrome.

Pathogenicity

Fears about the toxicity of the whole-cell killed pertussis vaccine have led to an attempt to develop an acellular vaccine. There has been an explosion of knowledge about the pathogenicity determinants of *B. pertussis*. Pertussigen is the major toxin which stimulates islet cells to secrete insulin, promotes the production of lymphocytes, and stimulates the coughing reflex in the respiratory tract. Several other toxins also play a role in the pathogenesis including adenylate cyclase which interferes with neutrophil function and is cytotoxic. Tracheal cytotoxin causes ciliostasis and later destruction of the respiratory epithelium. The fimbrial haemagglutinin is a fibrillar protein which is important in attachment of the organism to the respiratory tract. Heat labile toxin is a dermatonecrotic toxin originally described by Bordet. Two lipopolysaccharides are produced, one with a lipid A core which has limited toxicity and one with a lipid X core which is more toxic. More recently a 67 kD protein of unknown function has been shown to have an important role in pathogenesis: organisms lacking the antigen have diminished pathogenicity. The way in which this constellation of pathogenicity determinants interact is not known with certainty (Fig. 6.3).

Laboratory diagnosis

Specimens

To make the diagnosis of pertussis a pernasal swab should be obtained. This is a small, tightly wound swab of cotton or Dacron which is passed through the anterior nares to sample the nasopharynx (Fig. 6.4). Often the action of taking a pernasal swab will initiate a paroxysm of coughing which may assist the clinical diagnosis. Throat swabs have a very low

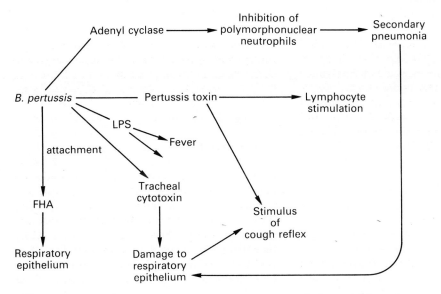

Figure 6.3 Schematic diagram illustrating some of the activities of *Bordetella pertussis* toxins and antigens

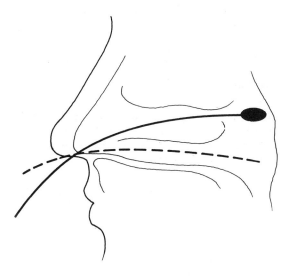

Figure 6.4 Diagram indicating the way in which a pernasal swab is taken

diagnostic yield and cough plates, where the child is encouraged to cough over a plate of Bordet-Gengou agar, are of historical interest only.

The highest diagnostic yield occurs in children during the catarrhal phase when *B. pertussis* can be isolated from up to 80% of cases. As the paroxysmal stage develops the diagnostic yield falls rapidly.

Direct examination

Gram stain of respiratory secretions is of no diagnostic value, but immunofluorescence with specific antiserum has been described. Although not routinely used, this method is more rapid and sensitive than bacterial culture.

Isolation

Bordetellas are fastidious organisms that grow slowly on specialized media. *Bordetella pertussis* is readily inhibited by many normal constituents of media and the products of its own metabolism. Protective substances such as activated charcoal or starch act to absorb these and enable these organisms to grow. The classical media for pertussis isolation is Bordet-Gengou which contains starch obtained from potatoes, but charcoal blood agar is effective. Each of these media contains a much higher concentration of blood than conventional blood agar. After repeated subculture on artificial media a number of times a phase change takes place and pertussis will then grow on normal media.

Pernasal swabs should be carefully inoculated by rolling them on charcoal blood agar and incubated in aerobic atmosphere with increased humidity for up to seven days. Charcoal blood agar is supplemented with beef extract, starch and peptone, and cefoxitin is incorporated to suppress the growth of commensal organisms. The highest diagnostic yield is probably obtained by use of Lacey's modification of Bordet-Gengou which is a rich blood agar supplemented with potato starch using diamidine and penicillin as the selective agents. This medium is difficult to make, however, and should be used only in laboratories with a high throughput. Media for the diagnosis of *Bordetella* should be preferably made up on the day of use because of its very short shelf-life.

Bordetella pertussis produces minute shiny dome-shaped colonies, 'bisected pearl or mercury drops', after 48 hours' incubation. Plates should not be discarded as negative until seven days have elapsed.

Identification

Colonies should be presumptively identified by Gram staining and direct agglutination with specific antiserum. Definitive identification of the species is not normally performed in a routine diagnostic laboratory. The characteristics which are used to differentiate the genus *Bordetella* include: growth on blood agar at primary isolation, brown soluble pigment on heart infusion agar, and nitrate production (Table 6.2).

Typing

The organisms are serotyped by use of agglutinogens of which there are 14 in the genus and six are specific to *B. pertussis*.

Serological diagnosis

Many serological methods have been described for the diagnosis of pertussis. None have gained a place in routine diagnosis but have proven valuable in epidemiological and vaccine studies. These include standard bacterial agglutination tests, indirect haemagglutination and complement fixation tests. More recently ELISAs to detect anti-whole cell or anti-LPS IgM and IgA have demonstrated a good diagnostic yield but in only half of these can the diagnosis be made on a single acute specimen. Antigen detection methods using countercurrent immunoelectrophoresis have been described and compare favourably with culture and provide a positive diagnosis on a single acute specimen.

Brucella

Definition

Brucella spp. are small Gram-negative coccobacilli which are non-motile, non-capsulate and non-spore-forming. They are catalase positive and mainly oxidase positive. Sugars are attacked by an oxidative process, and nitrate is reduced by most strains. Brucella are readily killed by pasteurization, and are sensitive to the acid found in fermented cheeses. They are sensitive to u.v. light but are able to survive in a dusty environment for several months.

Table 6.2 Some phenotypic characteristics of *Bordetella* spp.

Species	Oxidase	Urease	Browning	Growth on nutrient agar	Growth on sheep blood agar
B. pertussis	+	–	–	–	–
B. parapertussis	–	+	+	+	+
B. bronchoseptica	+	+	–		+

Classification

Modern DNA hybridization studies show that all *Brucella* spp. are closely related and may in the future be classified in a single species *B. melitensis*. The current species would then be reclassified as biovars. In the meantime there are four 'species' which regularly cause disease in the human population: *B. melitensis*, *B. abortus*, *B. suis*, and *B. canis*. There are other species such as *B. ovis* which infects sheep but is not known to cause human disease.

Pathogenicity

Brucellas are intracellular pathogens which invade the liver, spleen and bone marrow. The ability of this organism to cause disease depends on its ability to survive inside phagocytes which is thought to arise, in part, due to the production of inhibitors of the myeloperoxidase-H_2O_2-halide antibacterial system. Many of the symptoms associated with brucellosis may be due to the release of brucella lipopolysaccharide and the stimulation of macrophage-derived cytokines.

Epidemiology

Brucella spp. are predominantly pathogens of animals (Table 6.3). They have become important as causes of human disease because of transmission from domesticated animals kept for food or as pets. Brucella infection is relatively uncommon in goats in the wild, or in those able to range widely but this incidence rises steeply with herding. Herding and the use of animal products brings the human population in contact with infected animals.

Table 6.3 Species of *Brucella* associated with host animals

Species	Main animal host
B. abortus	Cattle
B. melitensis	Goats, sheep
B. suis	Pigs
B. canis	Dogs
B. ovis	Sheep
B. neotomae	Desert wood rat

The bacteria have a tropism for animal placentas and cause abortion in cattle and infertility in goats and sheep. Infection is therefore common in those who work closely with animals or their products: farmers, veterinarians, abattoir workers.

Brucellosis has been controlled in most developed countries by a policy of vaccination with the *B. abortus* strain 19 live attenuated vaccine, testing and selective slaughtering. Sporadic cases occasionally arise in these countries. Brucellosis remains an important infection in the Middle East, South America and Africa.

Clinical importance

Brucellosis has an incubation period from one week to several months. The clinical features are equally variable. Some patients present with acute illness with high remittent fevers and drenching sweats which give the infection its name 'undulant fever'. These are associated with lymphadenopathy, hepatosplenomegaly and musculoskeletal pain. Other patients have a more insidious disease with non-specific symptoms of malaise, weakness and anorexia. This may be associated with depression, anxiety, or other mental abnormality which may lead to a misdiagnosis of neurosis. This is a particular diagnostic trap when patients are likely to receive compensation as part of an industrial compensation claim.

Musculoskeletal complications are common (20–85%) and include osteomyelitis and spondylitis most often in the lumbosacral spine. Arthritis may develop in the major weight-bearing joints and may be septic or reactive. Patients with frequent exposure to brucella antigens may suffer allergic cutaneous reactions which make take a wide variety of forms, e.g. vesicular or papular rashes. Neurological complications may be acute such as meningoencephalitis or myelitis or take a more chronic and insidious form such as depression or psychosis. Epididymo-orchitis occurs in up to 10% of males, and prostatitis may also develop. Although abortion is an important complication in cattle it is not a major problem in humans. This is because human placentas do not contain erythritol present in animal placentae and which is responsible for its unusual tropism.

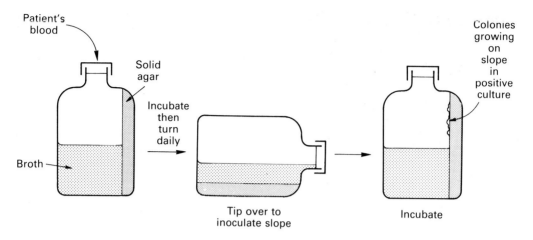

Figure 6.5   Casteñeda technique

Laboratory diagnosis

Specimens

Brucella spp. are intracellular pathogens which are preferentially found in the cells of the reticuloendothelial system. During acute infection blood cultures should be taken, but bone marrow culture has a higher diagnostic yield. Positive cultures are most likely to be obtained during the acute phase of the illness, and also more likely in *B. melitensis* infection. When osteomyelitis or arthritis is diagnosed samples of pus should be obtained. If liver biopsy or splenic aspirates are obtained as part of the diagnostic process they should be cultured.

Isolation

Brucella spp. are ACDP category 3 pathogens and must be handled in a containment level 3 laboratory. They grow slowly in artificial culture so incubation periods should be prolonged. Blood and marrow cultures should not be discarded for at least three weeks. Brucellas may be isolated on trypicase soy agar, brucella agar, which contains tryptone, peptone, dextrose and yeast extract, or serum dextrose liver infusion agar.

Blood and marrow cultures will require broth versions of the above medium. The growth of brucella is readily supported in the commercial medium supplied in the BACTEC

system. To facilitate the prolonged incubation period which is often required in conventional detection systems the Casteñeda technique may be employed. A bottle containing a vertical slope of agar and a liquid phase is inoculated (Fig. 6.5). Each day the bottle is inverted so that the slope is inoculated without the risk of contamination. The solid and liquid phases of this bottle may contain the solid and liquid versions of any of the media noted above.

Identification

Non-haemolytic colonies of Gram-negative coccobacilli which are oxidase and catalase positive and which agglutinate specific antiserum can be presumptively identified as *Brucella* spp. Most laboratories will not proceed to further identification but will refer the isolate to a reference laboratory.

Definitive identification is made on the basis of H_2S production, urease activity, growth dependence for CO_2 and dye susceptibility tests. Test and control strains are inoculated on agar incorporating two concentrations of thionine and one of basic fuchsin (Fig. 6.6). Growth on medium containing either penicillin or erythritol can be used in the same way. Three types of absorbed antiserum are used, A (abortus) and M (melitensis) and R (rough), in agglutination tests with monospecific antisera. Bacteriophages do not provide a system of typing for this genus but

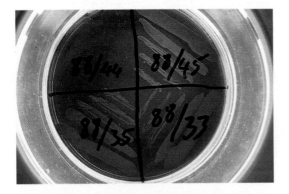

Figure 6.6 A routine dye tolerance test. Three of the strains tested here are capable of growing in the presence of the dye

may be used to differentiate species using different dilutions of the Tiblisi phage. These characteristics are used to identify the 16 species or biovars as shown in Table 6.4.

Serological diagnosis

During the acute infection IgG and IgM are produced. In relapse or chronic infection only IgG antibody concentrations rise significantly (Fig. 6.7). Most laboratories will employ the standard bacterial agglutination test. Dilutions of patient serum are mixed with killed whole bacteria which may be stained to make reading more easy. This may be performed by a slide technique, which is economical of reagents, or by a tube method. It is important that a 1 : 80 and 1 : 160 dilution are included in the screening as some patients may have very high concentrations of antibody which may cause a false-negative result due to the 'prozone' effect.

The results from this test can be used in two ways: single high values which exceed those of the local community provide support for a diagnosis of brucellosis, or rising titres in sera taken at least 10 days apart. In European populations a value of >1 : 80 in a patient without occupational exposure is suggestive of infection, whereas in a developing country a value of 1 : 160 or 1 : 320 might be employed.

Definitive serological diagnosis can only be achieved by use of specific ELISA or radio-immunoassay tests which measure IgG and IgM antibody.

Antimicrobial susceptibility

Brucella are susceptible to aminoglycosides, tetracycline, trimethoprim/sulphamethoxazole,

Table 6.4 Characteristics of *Brucella* species used in identification

| Species | | Biotype specific agglutination | | CO_2 | | Test Theonin | | Basic fuctisin | Lysis by | Lysis |
		A	*M*	*required*	*H_2S*	*a*	*b*	*20 µg*	*Tiblisi RTD*	*$10^4 \times RTD$*
B. melitensis	1	–	+	–	–	–	+	+	–	–
	2	+	–	–	–	–	+	+	–	–
	3	+	+	–	–	–	+	+	–	–
B. abortus	1	+	–	+	+	–	–	+	+	+
	2	+	–	+	+	–	–	–	+	+
	3	+	–	+	+	+	+	+	+	+
	4	–	+	+	+	–	–	+	+	+
	5	–	+	–	–	–	+	+	+	+
	6	+	–	–	–	–	+	+	+	+
	7	+	+	–	+	–	+	+	+	+
	8	–	+	+	–	–	+	+	+	+
B. suis	1	+	–	++	–	+	+	–	–	+
	2	+	–	–	–	–	+	–	–	+
	3	+	–	–	–	+	+	+	–	+
	4	+	+	–	–	+	+	–	–	+
B. canis		–	–	–	–	+	+	–	–	–

a 1:25 000; *b* 1:50 000

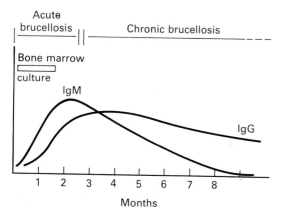

Figure 6.7   Bone marrow culture has a high diagnostic yield during the acute phase. IgM antibodies peak within three months and then fall slowly. IgG concentrations rise more slowly and remain elevated for prolonged periods

rifampicin, and fluoroquinolones. The organisms are naturally resistant to penicillins and cephalosporins. Therapy is difficult because of the intracellular location of the pathogen. Uncomplicated cases may be treated with tetracycline for six weeks, and this may be supplemented with aminoglycosides (traditionally streptomycin) for the first one or two weeks. The use of rifampicin or co-trimoxazole alone is associated with a very high relapse rate.

Francisella tularensis

Definition and classification

Francisella tularensis is a small, non-motile, bipolar staining Gram-negative coccobacillus. It is an obligate aerobe and grows poorly on ordinary culture media. Its growth is stimulated by the presence of cysteine in the medium. It expresses a small lipid-containing capsular envelope.

Francisella tularensis is the only species in the genus but there are two biovars: *F. tularensis* var. *tularensis* which is found only in North America and *F. tularensis* var. *palearctica* which is found throughout the northern

hemisphere but not in the UK. Disease initiated by the first biovar is more severe.

Clinical importance

Francisella tularensis is the causative agent of a plague-like disease of rodents and other small animals which is transmitted by ticks and biting flies between the natural hosts. The disease is widespread in North America and is found in localized areas in Northern Europe. The infection may be transmitted to man by the bite of an infected arthropod or by direct contact with the tissues of an infected mammal. The organism is readily transmitted by the aerosol route and is the third commonest laboratory infection in the USA. Natural infection is not found in the UK, but cases may arise in campers and hunters who travel to areas of mainland Europe such as Swedish Lapland.

Tularaemia is an acute febrile illness which may fall into one of five clinical syndromes: ulceroglandular, typhoidal, oculoglandular, oropharyngeal or gastrointestinal tularaemia. Ulceroglandular disease is characterized by a cutaneous ulcer at the site of inoculation which is associated with fever. Later, painful lymphadenopathy develops. Rarely there is direct inoculation into the eye with a resultant acute purulent and very painful conjunctivitis. Oropharyngeal tularaemia is characterized by a severe sore throat which may be mistaken clinically for diphtheria. In gastrointestinal infection there is severe gut ulceration. Typhoidal disease is the most serious form but is relatively rare. There is a typhoid-like illness with rapid progression and death may follow in up to 60% of cases.

Laboratory diagnosis

When tularaemia is suspected specimens from ulcers or aspirates from glands or other infected body fluids should be collected together with blood cultures. These should be stained with a polychromatic stain to demonstrate small, poorly staining coccobacilli. The specimens should be cultured on an enriched medium, for example: blood agar enriched with 0.1% cysteine, inspissated egg yolk medium, or glucose cysteine agar. Francisellas are relatively slow growing and cultures should be incubated for at least one week. *NB:* This is an important laboratory pathogen (category 3) and must be handled under ACDP containment level 3 conditions.

Pin point colonies are present after 24 hours of incubation and are 1–1.5 mm after 48 hours. *Francisella tularensis* may be identified by Gram stain which shows individual, faintly staining, minute, Gram-negative coccobacilli. Routine microbiology laboratories should not attempt to identify this organism but definitive identification can be performed by reference laboratories by using simple biochemical tests (see Table 6.5).

Serological diagnosis may be performed by standard bacterial agglutination if acute and convalescent sera are available, and this is the usual means whereby the diagnosis is made in many laboratories. Commercial kits are available in the USA and an individual acute titre of >1 : 40 is usually associated with acute infection. As *F. tularensis* shares minor cross-reacting antigens with *Brucella* species a control antigen should be set up in parallel.

Antibiotic susceptibility

Francisella spp. are susceptible to aminoglycosides, chloramphenicol and tetracycline. Streptomycin is usually used in treatment. The organism is resistant to penicillins and cephalosporins.

Pasteurella

Definition

Pasteurella spp. are small Gram-negative coccobacilli which exhibit bipolar staining. They are aerobic and facultatively anaerobic, do not form spores, and are non-motile. Almost all species are oxidase and catalase positive.

Classification

Eleven species are recognized, but most human infections are caused by *P. multocida*, *P. haemolytica*, *P. pneumotropica* and *P. ureae*.

These organisms are phenotypically similar to *Actinobacillus* and several species of the genus (*P. ureae*, *P. haemolytica*, and *P. pneumotropica*) are likely to be transferred to this genus as a result of DNA hybridization experiments.

Habitat and clinical importance

Pasteurella multocida is found in the nasopharynx or gastrointestinal tract of domestic and wild animals. It is capable of causing sporadic and epidemic pneumonia and septicaemia in animals. It is most often isolated from septic wounds following animal bites. Other infections include upper respiratory tract infection or meningitis and these infections are usually associated with intense exposure to animals.

Pasteurella multocida may be isolated from blood cultures or in pus from wounds, abdominal abscess, cerebrospinal fluid, or respiratory tract secretions.

Pasteurella haemolytica is found in the nasopharynx of animals causing episodes of pneumonia in cattle and sheep, septicaemia in lambs and cholera in chickens. Human infection is only rarely reported.

Pasteurella ureae is usually found in sputum of patients with chronic or respiratory disease, or those with acute suppurative infections.

Laboratory diagnosis

Isolation and identification

Pasteurellas are aerobic and facultatively anaerobic, growing best at 37°C. They are not fastidious and grow well on nutrient agar producing small circular colonies within 24 hours. They will not grow on MacConkey agar and are non-haemolytic on blood agar.

Pasteurellas may be identified by methods suitable for identification of Enterobacteriaceae (Table 6.5). *P. multocida* can be typed using somatic 'O' antigens.

Antibiotic susceptibility

Pasteurellas are usually susceptible to penicillin, tetracycline, chloramphenicol and aminoglycosides.

Table 6.5 Examples of characteristics useful in the identification of *Pasteurella* and *Francisella*

Species	Nutrient agar	MacConkey agar	Urease	Indole	ONPG	Glucose	Sucrose	Maltose	Oxidase	Catalase	ODC
P. multocida	+	–	–	+	–	+	+	–	+/–	+	+
P. pneumotropica	+	–	+	+	+	+	+	+	+	+	+
P. haemolytica	+	+/–	–	–	–	+	+	–	+	+/–	+
P. ureae	+	–	+	–	–	+	+	–	+	+	+
F. tularensis		–	–	–	–	+	–	+	+/–	+/–	–

Other rare Gram-negative coccobacilli

Actinobacillus

Actinobacillus spp. are commensals and pathogens of cattle and humans. Three species, *A. equuli*, *A. suis*, and *A. ligneresii,* can infect animal bites. *Actinobacillus actinomycemcomitans* is found in the mouth as part of the normal flora and is associated with chronic *Actinomyces* infections. It participates in periodontal infections and is rarely isolated in endocarditis. These organisms are susceptible to cephalosporins, aminoglycosides and chloramphenicol.

   Actinobacillus spp. grow on blood agar but may take up to seven days. They do not grow on MacConkey medium. Growth is enhanced by incubation in 5% CO_2.

Capnocytophagia

These are Gram-negative bacilli which exhibit gliding motility. They were previously known as DF-1 and DF-2 (dysgonic fermenter DF) but have been divided into five species: *C. gingivalis*, *C. ochracea*, *C. sputigena*, *C. canimorsus* and *C. cynodegmi*. They are found in the oral cavity and are associated with periodontal disease causing septicaemia in neutropenic patients, and rarely normal subjects. *Capnocytophagia canimorsus* can infect dog bite wounds which may be followed by septicaemia.

Cardiobacterium

This genus has only one species, *C. hominis*, which is part of the normal flora of the mouth. It rarely causes invasive disease but can cause endocarditis, usually in patients with previous valvular abnormalities.

Eikenella corrodens

Eikenella corrodens is a capnophilic Gram-negative bacillus which colonizes the human mucous membrane and has been isolated from patients with osteomyelitis, arthritis, septicaemia and meningitis. It forms small colonies after 24 hours on blood agar but after several days flat colonies have developed which pit the agar.

7

Gram-negative bacilli

Introduction

The Gram-negative bacilli include a diverse group of organisms in widely differing genera. Many have already been described in other chapters and will not be referred to here. This chapter will be divided into two main sections and will focus on the Enterobacteriaceae, and the genus *Pseudomonas*.

Enterobacteriaceae

Definition

The Enterobacteriaceae are Gram-negative rod-shaped bacteria which are typically motile by virtue of peritrichous flagella, are non-sporing, facultative anaerobes which will grow in the presence of bile salts. They are oxidase negative, catalase positive, reduce nitrate and almost all ferment glucose often with the formation of acid and gas.

Habitat

The Enterobacteriaceae include common human pathogens and are widely distributed in the environment, being found in the soil and water, on plants, and in the intestines of animals. They can be saprophytes, opportunist pathogens, zoonotic pathogens or primary human pathogens. Some of the species are predominantly environmental saprophytes, e.g. *Serratia* spp., but may infect patients who

are predisposed to colonization by chronic respiratory disease or immunosuppression. *Klebsiella pneumoniae* is a species typically found in the environment where it plays an important role in the biochemistry of the soil. It may also act as a primary human pathogen causing severe cavitating pneumonia. In patients in the hospital environment colonization can give rise to septicaemia, meningitis, and urinary tract infection. Some of the family are more limited in their distribution: *Shigella* spp. and *Salmonella typhi* are found only in the human host. They give rise to acute infections: acute diarrhoeal disease and typhoid respectively, or chronic asymptomatic excretion. The non-typhoid salmonellas are found in the intestines of humans and animals. Humans become infected when contaminated food which has been inadequately cooked is ingested.

Classification

The taxonomy of this family is complex and was previously based on the results of phenotypic and antigenic characteristics. DNA-DNA hybridization techniques have been applied to the genus more recently (Fig. 7.1).

Antigenic structure

The Enterobacteriaceae share the common structure of the Gram-negative cell wall with an inner plasma membrane, a peptidoglycan layer and the outer membrane (Fig. 7.2).

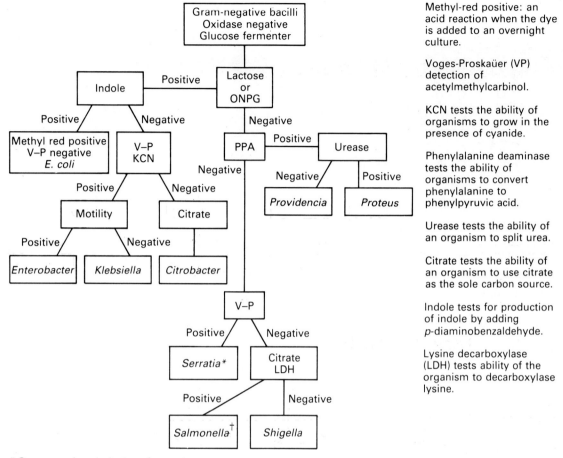

Methyl-red positive: an acid reaction when the dye is added to an overnight culture.

Voges-Proskaüer (VP) detection of acetylmethylcarbinol.

KCN tests the ability of organisms to grow in the presence of cyanide.

Phenylalanine deaminase tests the ability of organisms to convert phenylalanine to phenylpyruvic acid.

Urease tests the ability of an organism to split urea.

Citrate tests the ability of an organism to use citrate as the sole carbon source.

Indole tests for production of indole by adding *p*-diaminobenzaldehyde.

Lysine decarboxylase (LDH) tests ability of the organism to decarboxylase lysine.

* Some species are lactose fermenters.
† Some exceptions.

Figure 7.1 A simplified scheme for separating some of the genera commonly isolated in clinical laboratories

Somatic antigen

The major outer membrane antigen is the somatic O antigen, or lipopolysaccharide (LPS) (Fig. 7.3). This antigen has three main components, lipid A, the oligosaccharide core, and the repeating polysaccharide chain.

The lipid A portion is responsible for the toxicity of LPS as it is a potent activator of host macrophages inducing the release of potent cytokines such as interleukin 1 (IL-1) and tumour necrosis factor (TNF). It is these mediators which initiate the chain of pathophysiological responses associated with Gram-negative sepsis: fever, hypotension, metabolic acidosis, and platelet activation (Fig. 7.4). The core oligosaccharide contains hexoses and heptoses and a unique sugar residue 2-keto-3-deoxyoctonoic acid. The polysaccharide chain is made up of a repeating sugar motif which defines the serological reactivity of the antigen. It is also important in protecting the organism from the effects of serum and phagocytosis.

Flagellar H antigen

Most of the Enterobacteriaceae are motile as they possess flagella. The H antigen is a protein

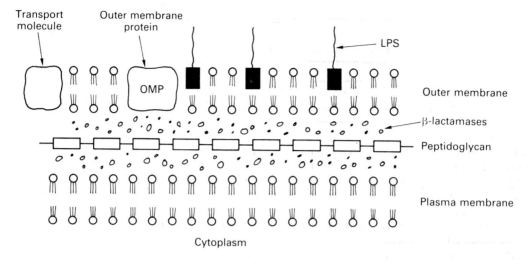

Figure 7.2   Schematic diagram of the cell wall of a Gram-negative bacterium

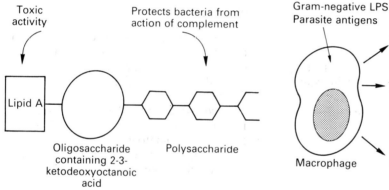

Figure 7.3   Schematic diagram of somatic antigen

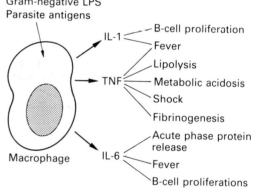

Figure 7.4 Schematic diagram of stimulation of macrophages by bacterial lipopolysaccharide and parasite antigens

and therefore heat-labile. Flagellar antigens can be used in the identification of species and serotypes. The flagella undergo phase variation in the salmonellas (see Chapter 17), and segregation (two or more probably non-reversible variants) in *Citrobacter*.

Capsular K antigens

Several species express a polysaccharide capsule, or an envelope of protein or fimbriae. These mediate adhesion and protect against phagocytosis. Important examples in human

disease are the Vi antigen of *Salmonella typhi*, the K1 antigen of *Escherichia coli* and the K88 antigen of *E. coli* (see p. 203). Capsular antigens may interfere with serological reactions with O and H antigens but can be removed by boiling for one hour.

Toxins

Toxins play an important part in the pathogenicity of these organisms especially those causing enteric disease which are discussed in Chapter 17.

Adhesins

Type 1 fimbriae are expressed by most Enterobacteriaceae and their role in pathogenesis is uncertain, but they do promote adherence to host cells and assist in colonization. Phase variation means that there is a reversible switching on and off of the expression of type 1 fimbriae. Strains of *Proteus* spp. expressing type 1 fimbriae were more pathogenic in the urinary tract than strains not expressing fimbriae. They may also aid delivery of toxins to the host cells to which they bind. The binding of the common type 1 fimbriae is specifically inhibited by mannose whereas the other types are not.

Other fimbriae have been partially characterized. The colonization factors CFA I and CFA II are important in promoting adhesion for enterotoxigenic *E. coli* (see p. 203), and P fimbriae which are found in uropathic strains.

Clinical importance

The Enterobacteriaceae contain several important pathogens of the gastrointestinal tract, *Salmonella*, *Shigella*, *Yersinia enterocolitica*, and *E. coli* and these are described in more detail in Chapter 17.

Proteus

The genus *Proteus* contains four species which are highly motile, swarming on most media, and possessing urease and phenylalanine deaminase. The four species are *P. mirabilis*, *P. vulgaris*, *P. peneri* and *P. myxofaciens*. They are closely related to *Morganella* and *Providencia* spp.

Proteus are the second most frequent Enterobacteriaceae isolated in most clinical laboratories. *Proteus* spp. colonize and infect the urinary tract, and are the second most common aetiological agent. A urea-splitting enzyme is produced which raises the pH of the urine creating conditions in which renal stones may form. This may become a nidus for further infections. Most infections are caused by *P. mirabilis*.

Proteus spp., especially the indole-positive species, are important pathogens in the hospital environment colonizing wounds and causing septicaemia in patients who are debilitated. They are found in the gastrointestinal tract of hospitalized patients where they may act as a reservoir of multi-drug-resistant organisms.

Klebsiella

Klebsiella spp. are non-motile, ornithine decarboxylase, gelatinase and indole negative. They are capsulate, ferment glucose, lactose and inositol, and are citrate, urease, and Vokes-Proskaüer positive. Seven species are recognized including *K. pneumoniae*, *K. ozaenae*, *K. oxytoca*, and *K. rhinoscleromatis*.

Klebsiellas are normally found in the soil and water and they may colonize the human gastrointestinal tract. *Klebsiella pneumoniae* is associated with a primary cavitating pneumonia which is typically found in patients predisposed by diabetes mellitus, obstructive airways disease, alcoholism or malnutrition. Klebsiellas may also act as a secondary invader in postoperative patients especially when broad spectrum antibiotics have been given. Septicaemia is a common complication in debilitated hospital patients. Klebsiellas are frequent pathogens of the urinary tract.

Klebsiella ozaenae has been associated with bronchiectasis and *K. rhinoscleromatis* with a chronic granulomatous infection of the nasopharynx, rhinoscleroma, which is usually found in tropical countries.

Enterobacter

Enterobacter spp. are closely related to *Klebsiella* but differ in that they are motile, produce ornithine decarboxylase and are usually urease and gelatinase negative. Ten species are described but *E. cloacae*, *E. aerogenes* and *E. agglomerans* are most often isolated in the clinical setting. They are found in water, soil and plants and can colonize the gastrointestinal tract. They are rarely primary pathogens but are important colonizers in hospitalized patients and may cause invasive infections and line-related sepsis in some cases.

The closely related species *Hafnia alvei* shares many of the characteristics of *Enterobacter*, but is a lactose non-fermenter. It can cause confusion in the clinical laboratory as it shares some antigens with salmonellas and will lead to false-positive reports if 'salmonellas' are reported on serological grounds before biochemical confirmation is obtained.

Serratia

Serratia spp. are closely related to *Klebsiella* and *Enterobacter*, but are motile, produce ornithine decarboxylase, gelatinase and DNAase. There are nine species of which *S. marcescens* and *S. liquifaciens* are most frequently isolated from human specimens. They are found in the soil and water. Colonization, when it occurs, is more likely to be in the urinary or respiratory tract. *Serratia* can colonize wounds and may cause urinary infection, line-related sepsis and septicaemia.

Citrobacter

There are three recognized *Citrobacter* spp., of which *C. freundii* and *C. diversus* are regularly isolated from clinical material. Citrobacters ferment lactose and produce H_2S and thus may be confused with salmonellas. Late lactose and non-lactose variants of *C. freundii* which also share some *Salmonella* antigens can be a particular problem. Citrobacters are differentiated from *E. coli* in that they are indole negative and citrate positive.

Human infection is rare and usually takes the form of colonization and septicaemia in hospitalized patients.

Yersinia

Eleven species are recognized of which three are primary human pathogens: *Y. enterocolitica*, *Y. pseudotuberculosis* and *Y. pestis*. *Yersinia enterocolitica* is an important cause of an acute enterocolitis which clinically resembles campylobacter infection and may give rise to a terminal ileitis. This, and mesenteric adenitis, may be mistaken clinically for appendicitis. Erythema nodosum and reactive arthritis may follow acute infection.

Yersinia pseudotuberculosis is a zoonotic infection transmitted through contaminated water or by direct contact with infected animals. Infection typically takes the form of mesenteric adenitis. This may develop into septicaemia in a very small number of cases.

Yersinia pestis is the agent of plague. It is a zoonotic infection transmitted to man from the rat reservoir host by the bite of a flea, *Xenopsylla cheopis*. The disease is endemic in parts of Africa, South-East Asia, South America and some southern states of the USA. Plague takes one of four forms: bubonic, septicaemic, pneumonic plague or meningitis. The characteristic lesion of bubonic plague is the bubo which is a large, intensely painful, inflamed lymph node draining the site of the bite which develops two to seven days following infection. There is local oedema and the patient is febrile and shocked, and the liver and spleen are palpable. Skin lesions may develop: pustules, vesicles or purpura which can become generalized and cause skin necrosis. Infection can be overwhelming developing from bubonic into septicaemic disease with a high mortality. Some patients may develop septicaemia without a bubo. Secondary pneumonia is a serious complication with a high mortality. It is also highly infectious by being transmitted by the respiratory route. Meningitis is rare and follows inadequately treated bubonic plague.

Laboratory diagnosis

Specimens

Enterobacteriaceae can be isolated from almost every site and specimen. These organisms survive well in transit to the laboratory and will multiply confounding the results of urine culture methods which depend on accurate quantitation of bacterial number.

Isolation

All of these bacteria grow well on simple non-selective media, and on media which contain bile salts such as MacConkey. Selection between coliforms and non-lactose fermenters plays an important part in the diagnosis of intestinal infection (see Chapter 17). Cefsulodin-irgasin-novobiocin can be used as a selective medium for *Yersinia*. Swarming of *Proteus* can obscure the growth of other pathogens and prevent quantitative counts being performed. Swarming can be prevented by increasing the concentration of agar to 2%, by using electrolyte-deficient medium, incorporating bile salts or *p*-nitrophenylglycerol.

Almost all belong to Hazard Group 2 with the exceptions of *Yersinia pestis* and *S. typhi* which are in ACDP category 3.

Identification

The tests for the identification of the Enterobacteriaceae are technically simple which in part explains the wealth of detail and species which have been described. Identification depends on biochemical reactions and serology.

Toxonomists insist that equal weight be given to individual biochemical reactions, in the clinical laboratory more emphasis is given to those tests which distinguish pathogens from closely related species found in the same environment.

Central to identification are the sugar fermentation tests where mono-, di- and polysaccharides are incorporated into a basal liquid medium together with an indicator. Fermentation is detected by the indicator and gas production with a small upturned (Durham's) tube inside the medium (Fig. 7.5).

The possession of enzyme activity is useful diagnostically. Some of these are tested in the same way as fermentation tests by detecting a pH change consequent on enzyme activity, e.g. ornithine decarboxylase. Gelatinase is detected by incorporating charcoal into a tablet of gelatin and noting release of the charcoal. Production of some chemicals can be detected in the medium as in the case of H_2S by the incorporation of iron in the medium, or by adding specific reagents after growth has taken place as in the case of indole production. A small number of tests make it possible to identify species to genus level. Full identification requires an extended battery of tests, and ideally a computer database to collate the results.

Several commercial products have been developed to identify the Enterobacteriaceae. The main advantages of these kits is the diversity of reactions which can be simply performed relieving the laboratory of the task of media preparation and quality control.

The API systems use desiccated reagents in plastic cupules to which a suspension of the test organism is added and incubated for 18 hours in the case of the API20E or six hours for the rapid tests. The Minitek system uses reagents incorporated into filter paper discs placed in the wells of a microtitre plate. Reagents can also be incorporated directly on microtitre trays or the specialized 'cards' of computer-driven automated identification and sensitivity test methods. In the Enterotube system a needle is inoculated and then drawn through pre-prepared medium in a tube (Fig. 7.6).

Additional reagents are added after incubation and the tests interpreted according to the manufacturers' instructions. The results are turned into a numeric code and the identification of the test organism can be determined by referring to manuals prepared by the manufacturers. Additional discriminative power can be obtained by entering the results into a

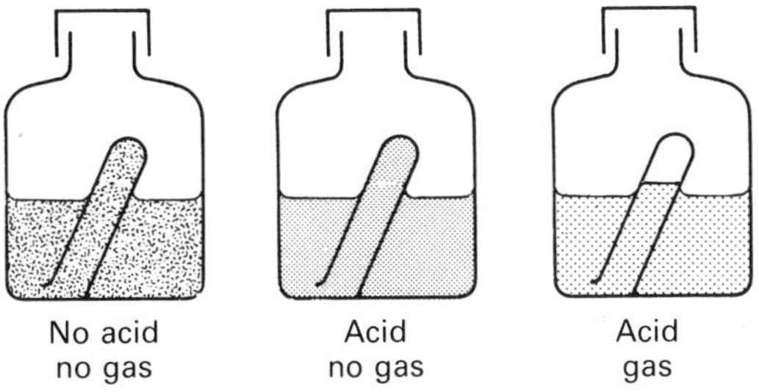

No acid   Acid   Acid
no gas   no gas   gas

Figure 7.5 The tubes contain a substrate, indicator and a small tube (Durham's tube) to detect gas production

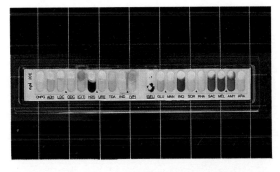

Figure 7.6 Commercial identification system: multiple wells with pre-prepared reagents enable a large number of tests to be performed rapidly

computer database where the probability of an isolate's correct identification can be calculated. The results obtained with commercial kits should not be read in conjunction with identification tables derived from conventional tests as minor differences in methodology can give different results in some organisms.

Serological identification is performed by bacterial agglutination techniques. The methods used are similar to those employed for salmonellas and shigellas and these are described in Chapter 17.

Typing

Many different typing methods have been applied to the Enterobacteriaceae. For some species serotyping is usually adequate for most purposes (e.g. *Klebsiella*), but in others additional methods are required. These include bacteriocin typing (*Sh. sonnei*) and phage typing (*Sal. typhimurium*).

Antibiotic susceptibility

Most Enterobacteriaceae are susceptible to aminoglycosides, penicillins, cephalosporins, and penem antibiotics. Resistance to other agents which were previously used such as tetracycline, chloramphenicol, trimethoprim and sulphonamides is variable.

Initially the majority of isolates of *E. coli* were sensitive to ampicillin but resistance developed in the face of general use. Indole-positive *Proteus* and *Klebsiella* spp. are intrinsically resistant to ampicillin but the later cephalosporins and penem antibiotics have been developed to which these species are susceptible. As expected with increasing use specific degradative enzymes are appearing and spreading in the bacterial population. Many of the resistances are transmitted within the Enterobacteriaceae by plasmids.

Pseudomonas spp.

Definition

These are aerobic Gram-negative bacilli which break down sugars by oxidation. They are motile (except *P. mallei*), oxidase and catalase positive. Many species produce pigments: *P. aeruginosa* produces fluorescein, pyocyanin, pyorubrin, and pyomelanin. The fluorescent *Pseudomonas* also produce fluorescein.

Classification

There are more than 100 species in the genus *Pseudomonas*. Most of these are environmental organisms and some are plant pathogens. Others colonize and infect patients made susceptible by surgery, burns, immunocompromise or other diseases. There are two primary pathogens, *P. pseudomallei* and *P. mallei*.

Pseudomonas spp. can be separated into a number of groups on the basis of phenotypic characteristics such as flagellar morphology, biochemical reactions, temperature of growth, etc., and ribosomal RNA homology. With this system *P. aeruginosa* is grouped with *P. fluorescens* and *P. putida*. *Pseudomonas pseudomallei* and *P. mallei* are classified with *P. solanacearum*, *P. cepacia*, *P. gladioli* and *P. pickettii*. Although useful for identification purposes as it groups organisms together around phenotypic characteristics it is of limited value in the clinical laboratory because it does not separate species between pathogens, opportunists, and environmental strains.

Clinical importance

Pseudomonas aeruginosa

Pseudomonas aeruginosa is a saprophytic organism which has come to be an important human pathogen, especially in the hospital environment, because of its innate resistance to many antibiotics and disinfectants. It thrives in warm, moist areas including the drains, sinks, and any place where even small amounts of water are able to collect such as humidifiers, respirators or ocular solutions. In the general population *P. aeruginosa* is carried by very few people but this can rise to over 30% after a stay in hospital. The invasive potential of this organism means that it causes disease in a wide range of hospital patients. It is a particular problem to the neutropenic patient where it can cause fulminant septicaemia and death.

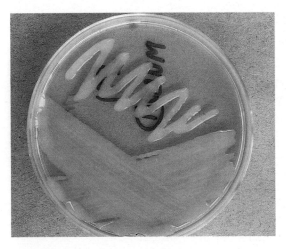
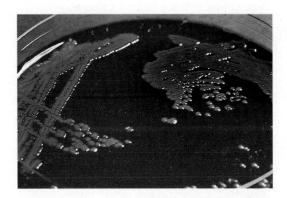

Figures 7.7 *Pseudomonas aeruginosa* may produce the characteristic blue-green pigment or none at all

Patients undergoing artificial ventilation for extended periods in intensive therapy units may become colonized with *P. aeruginosa* and secondary lower respiratory tract infection may follow. Extensive burns become colonized and septicaemia develops in a proportion of patients. Multidose optical solutions can be contaminated by *P. aeruginosa* which, when used, can produce a rapidly progressive corneal infection which ends in ocular perforation.

Pseudomonas aeruginosa is an important pathogen for patients with cystic fibrosis where colonization with this organism is inevitable. Patients suffer recurrent infections with continuing deterioration of respiratory function.

Skin infection may arise in healthy subjects exposed to high infective doses such as deep sea divers and users of contaminated hydrotherapy pools and jacuzzi.

Other *Pseudomonas* spp. can act as opportunits but generally do so less frequently. These include *P. cepacia, P. fluorescens, P. stutzeri* and *P. putida. Xanthomonas maltophilia* has recently been transferred from the *Pseudomonas* genus on the grounds of its phenotypic differences. It also acts as an nosocomial opportunist.

Pseudomonas pseudomallei

This is the causative organism of melioidosis which is found in South-East Asia, Australia and rarely in Africa. It is an environmental saprophyte found in warm, standing water such as paddy fields and it can act as a primary pathogen. In most cases infection is asymptomatic but relapse can occur years later when host immunity fails due to other diseases, typically diabetes mellitus or malignancy. Acute infection is characterized by acute or chronic pneumonia from which septicaemia may develop or arise *de novo*. Multiple abscesses may develop in skin bone and other organs including liver and brain. The septicaemic form of the disease has a high mortality.

Pseudomonas mallei

This is the causative organism of glanders, a disease of horses characterized by nasal, cutaneous and lymphatic abscesses. Human infection is rare but takes the form of an indolent glanders syndrome or fulminant septicaemia with a high mortality.

Pathogenicity

Pseudomonas aeruginosa is motile and expresses flagellar antigens. Like other Gram-negative pathogens *Pseudomonas* spp. possess a lipopolysaccharide which is capable of inducing macrophage-derived cytokines. At least two exotoxins are produced: exotoxin A and exotoxin S. Exotoxin A has been most studied and it is a potent inhibitor of protein synthesis by a mechanism similar to that of diphtheria toxin (see p. 33). Exotoxin S is also an ADP ribosyltransferase which is cytotoxic to a wide range of cell types.

In some clinical conditions, commonly found in cystic fibrosis patients, *P. aeruginosa* is able to secrete extracellular polysaccharide capsular material. Bacteria expressing this antigen grow in microcolonies in the lungs are are protected from the activity of antibiotics and host phagocytes. Alteration to mucoid phenotype is often accompanied by loss of multiple antibiotic resistances so that the organism becomes highly sensitive to penicillins and aminoglycosides. The capsular material is known to inhibit the activity of aminoglycosides.

Pseudomonas pseudomallei and *P. mallei* are both capable of surviving and multiplying inside host macrophages. Several toxins have been isolated from *P. pseudomallei* but have not been further characterized.

Laboratory diagnosis

Specimens

Pseudomonas aeruginosa is isolated from many clinical specimens, including blood pus, sputum and urine. It can be sought in environmental samples when cross-infection is a problem. *Pseudomonas pseudomallei* is usually isolated from sputum, blood or pus from abscesses. *Pseudomonas mallei* and *P. pseudomallei* are ACDP Hazard Group 3 organisms.

Isolation

Bacteria of the genus *Pseudomonas* grow readily on simple media such as nutrient or blood agar, and will also grow on the less inhibitory selective media such as MacConkey. Media can be made selective for *Pseudomonas* by the incorporation of one or more of the antibiotics or disinfectants to which it is naturally resistant such as irgasin, cetrimide or nalidixic acid. Pseudomonas isolation agar contains irgasin, peptone, magnesium chloride and potassium sulphate which as well as being selective also encourages the production of pyocyanin pigment. Specific media are used to

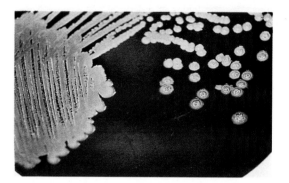

Figure 7.8   The typical dry and wrinkled colonies of *Pseudomonas pseudomallei.* (Courtesy of Dr DA Dance)

optimize production of each of the other pigments (Fig. 7.7).

Colonies of *P. aeruginosa* are morphologically diverse and dwarf, rough, mucoid, rugose, coliform-like colonies and the more commonly encountered large convex, flat, oval colonies are described (see Fig. 7.7). A culture of *P. aeruginosa* has a characteristic musty odour. The colonies of *P. pseudomallei* and *P. mallei* are slower to appear and are typically wrinkled with a faint pinkish colour developing after about five days (Fig. 7.8). A similar colonial appearance is found with *P. stutzeri.*

Identification

Pseudomonas aeruginosa is unreactive in many of the biochemical tests used to identify the Enterobacteriaceae. Hugh and Liefson recognized that bacteria which metabolized sugars poorly would preferentially utilize peptones with the result that the increase in pH produced by peptide metabolism would balance any fall in pH caused by acid production from carbohydrate. A low peptone medium was produced enabling acid production from oxidative bacteria to be detected. For each sugar tested two tubes are inoculated, one of which has a mineral oil overlay to produce anaerobic conditions. *Pseudomonas aeruginosa* will produce acid in the oxidative tube but no colour change in the fermentative tube. Other tests which are valuable in the identification of *P. aeruginosa* are lactose and fructose   oxidation,   arginine   dehydrolase,

Table 7.1 Examples of biochemical tests used in the identification of *Pseudomonas* spp.

Species	Oxidase	Lactose	ADH	ODC	Gelatin
P. aeruginosa	+	−	+	−	+
P. capacia	+	+	−	+/−	+/−
P. stutzeri	+	−	+/−	−	−
P. pseudomallei	+	+	+	−	+
Xanthomonos maltophilia	−	−	−	−	+

gelatinase and lysine decarboxylase and growth at 42°C. Typical reactions of *Pseudomonas* spp. are illustrated in Table 7.1.

Many commercial identification systems have now been adapted for the non-fermenting Gram-negative bacilli, and these successfully will identify the species of *Pseudomonas* isolated by clinical laboratory including *P. pseudomallei*. When this latter organism is suspected its identity can be confirmed rapidly by a fluorescein-labelled specific antibody.

Typing

There are seventeen somatic antigens which define the serotype of *P. aeruginosa* and can be used in epidemiological studies. Phage typing is possible but bacteriocin typing is most widely employed. It is based on pyocins of which there are four types. The method employed is similar to that described for the typing of *Sh. sonnei* (see p. 20).

Antibiotic susceptibility

Pseudomonas spp. are naturally resistant to a wide range of antibiotics. They are often susceptible to aminoglycosides, to carbenicillin, ticarcillin, the ureidopenicillins: azlocillin and piperacillin; the monobactams, penems and the third generation cephalosporin, ceftazidime. The 4-fluoroquinolones are also active and have the advantage that they can be given orally.

The mortality from acute melioidosis is high and *P. pseudomallei* is naturally resistant to aminoglycosides and penicillins. It is, however, susceptible to ceftazidime, imipenem, and the amoxycillin clavulanate combination. The 4-fluoroquinolones have no useful activity.

8

Anaerobes

Introduction

Micro-organisms can be divided into five groups on the basis of their ability to utilize oxygen as a terminal electron receptor in the processes of metabolism. Obligate aerobes require molecular oxygen in their metabolism, micro-aerophilic bacteria also require oxygen, but will not grow in an atmosphere containing 20% O_2 and will not grow under strict anaerobic conditions. Anaerobic bacteria do not require oxygen and may be described as facultative anaerobes if they are able to grow in either an aerobic or anaerobic atmosphere. Obligate anaerobes, in contrast, are unable to grow in the presence of oxygen and may be inhibited by it. Aerotolerant anaerobes grow best under anaerobic conditions, but although inhibited by oxygen may grow poorly in an aerobic atmosphere. Most obligate anaerobes (moderate) are inhibited by oxygen but are able to tolerate the oxygen concentration of up to 6%. Strict obligate anaerobes are unable to grow if exposed to greater than 0.5% oxygen.

Obligate anaerobes form an important part of the body's normal flora. They act as a non-specific defence by competing for nutrients and attachment sites with potential pathogens. The final products of their metabolism, free fatty acids, are toxic to other bacteria and inhibit colonization with new organisms. This property (colonization resistance) is very important in patients admitted to hospital who may otherwise be colonized with multi-drug-resistant organisms.

Table 8.1 Normal anaerobic flora of humans

Species	Skin	Mouth and pharynx	Large bowel	Genital tract
Prevotella melaninogenicus group		+		+
Bacteroides fragilis group			+	+
Actinomyces israelii		+		
Treponema phagedenis, etc.		+		
Clostridium perfringens			+	+
Peptostreptococcus magnus	+	+	+	+
Peptostreptococcus anaerobius	+	+	+	+
Veillonella parvula		+	+	+
Fusobacterium nucleatum		+	+	
Fusobacterium necrophorum		+		
Proprionibacterium acnes	+	+	+	+

Pathogenesis

Conditions for infection

Anaerobic bacteria are found in the larynx, mouth, gastrointestinal tract, vagina, external genitalia, and skin (Table 8.1). Anaerobic infections are either endogenous in origin or are from environmental organisms, e.g. *Clostridium tetani*.

An anaerobic infection can develop only when a sufficiently low redox potential has been established in the tissues. This may arise as a result of surgery where tissue damage may be coupled with inoculation of local anaerobic flora. Accidental trauma is an important risk factor as tissue may become devitalized or foreign bodies contaminated by *Clostridium* spp. inoculated into the wound. Ischaemia, where vascular disease has resulted in decreased blood supply to the tissues, may provide the conditions in which anaerobic pathogens may grow. Obstruction of a hollow viscus by malignancy or with a foreign body will allow anaerobic sepsis to develop. These infections are usually pyogenic and polymicrobial. The mechanisms whereby microbial synergy is achieved is not clear, but metabolism by facultative organisms may lower the redox potential creating the conditions in which obligate anaerobes may multiply. Elaboration of exotoxins by facultative organisms, e.g. hyaluronidase, may facilitate invasion. The non-sporing anaerobes may also inhibit phagocytic potential of polymorphs and macrophages, thus protecting the facultative organisms.

Once infection is initiated, anaerobes elaborate a number of potential virulence factors to maintain and extend infection. An example of this is Meleney's synergistic gangrene where facultative Gram-positive cocci combine with *Bacteroides* to produce a rapidly progressive gangrenous necrosis in the skin.

Virulence determinants

The pathogenicity determinants of *Bacteroides* and *Fusobacteria* include adhesin molecules, fimbriae and slime. *Bacteroides fragilis* possesses an anti-phagocytic capsule. Many species elaborate hydrolytic enzymes such as hyaluronidase, gelatinase, collagenase, and lecithinase. These

Table 8.2 Prevalence of anaerobic species in human infection

Species
B. fragilis group
B. melaningenicus group
Fusobacterium spp.
Peptostreptococcus spp.
Clostridium spp.
Propionibacterium acnes

Table 8.3 Specimens suitable for anaerobic culture

Blood
Bone marrow
Aspirated pus
Wound/abscess swabs
Sterile body fluids
Lung aspirates (see Chapter 16)
Aspirated urine specimens

Gram-negative bacteria have a bacterial lipopolysaccharide (LPS) which has endotoxin-like activity. It is structurally different from the LPS of other Gram-negative bacteria as it lacks 2-keto-3-deoxy octanoic acid.

Among clostridia the main pathogenicity determinants are potent exotoxins such as the neurotoxins produced by *C. botulinum* and *C. tetani*, and lecithinase C produced by *C. perfringens*. In addition to these, many other hydrolytic enzymes are secreted including haemolysins, hyaluronidase, gelatinase and collagenase.

Although there is a wide diversity of obligative anaerobic species in the environment and in the normal human flora a limited number of species are associated with human infections, principally *Bacteroides*, *Peptostreptococci*, *Clostridium*, and *Actinomyces* spp. (Table 8.2).

Laboratory diagnosis

Specimens

Collection of specimens

Obligate anaerobes not only require an anaerobic atmosphere for growth but are inhibited by oxygen. The way in which specimens are collected and transported to the bacteriological laboratory is therefore crucial if the best results are to be obtained.

Anaerobic species should be sought only in specimens which are not likely to be contaminated with normal flora (Table 8.3). An exception to this is stool which may be cultured by selective techniques for the purpose of detecting *C. difficile* or *C. perfringens* where pseudomembranous colitis or perfringens food poisoning is suspected. In the case of pseudomembranous colitis it is more important to detect the toxin as this organism can be carried asymptomatically. *Clostridium perfringens* and *C. difficile* are also part of the normal bacterial flora and only when they are present in excess is isolation significant. Anaerobes may also be cultured from the upper gastrointestinal tract in patients with suspected blind loop syndrome.

Transport

Specimens should be sent to the laboratory with a minimum of delay so that contact with atmospheric oxygen is as short as possible. For optimal results, the laboratory should be informed when operative procedures are undertaken to obtain specimens for bacteriological culture, e.g. open lung biopsy, aspiration of abdominal abscess, so that rapid transport of specimens can be arranged and the specimen processed immediately on arrival. Pus, when obtained, may be sent in the syringe in which it was collected or in a sterile screw-capped container which has been filled so that all the air has been excluded. Swabs should be avoided where possible as these permit desiccation of the specimen and the maximum exposure to atmospheric oxygen.

Transport systems for swabs have been marketed which contain semi-solid reduced transport medium such as modified Stuart's, Cary-Blair, or Amie's. Swabs which have been coated with haemoglobin and glycerol have an improved yield over uncoated swabs. Specimens could be inoculated at the bedside or in the operating room onto the appropriate media and transported to the laboratory in an anaerobic atmosphere. Commercial anaerobic bag systems are available for this purpose.

Direct examination

The appearance and smell of pus should be recorded as it may have a foul odour. Pus from cases of actinomycosis may contain 'sulphur granules'. Microscopic examination of Gram-stained specimens for the presence of anaerobes cannot be diagnostic by itself (Fig. 8.1). It can, however, provide valuable information, for example, the presence of brick-shaped Gram-positive rods without many accompanying polymorphs in a specimen of abscess pus might indicate the presence of *C. perfringens*. The pale bipolar staining of *Bacteroides* and *Fusobacterium* and their pleomorphic or fusiform morphology may be seen. The branched filamentous rods of *Actinomyces* may be demonstrated in specimens from cervicofacial

Figure 8.1 Gram-stained preparation of pus showing scanty pus cells, many organisms including a few large brick-shaped Gram-positive organisms, *C. perfringens*

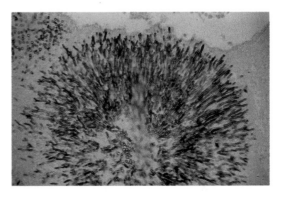

Figure 8.2 Ziehl-Neelsen preparation of an Actinomyces 'club'

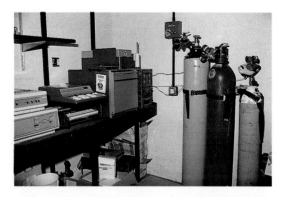

Figure 8.3 Gas-liquid chromatography. The three-fold gas supply leads to the chromatograph which contains a long column with specialized packing material and a flame ionizer. The pen recorder provides a written record of the tracing

lesions by Gram stain and the 'clubs' can be stained with modified Ziehl-Neelsen (Fig. 8.2).

In addition to alerting the microbiologist to the presence of individual pathogens the Gram-stained smear provides a degree of internal quality control as failure to grow anaerobic species when bacteria with typical morphology are seen may alert the microbiologist to failures in technique.

Smears may be examined by a direct fluorescent antibody technique. Labelled antibodies to *B. fragilis* and *Prevotella melaninogenicus* can be obtained commercially and provide a rapid diagnosis. The results obtained correlate well with culture but direct fluorescence is not suitable for routine diagnostic use due to the multiplicity of anaerobic species causing disease and the expense of individual reagents.

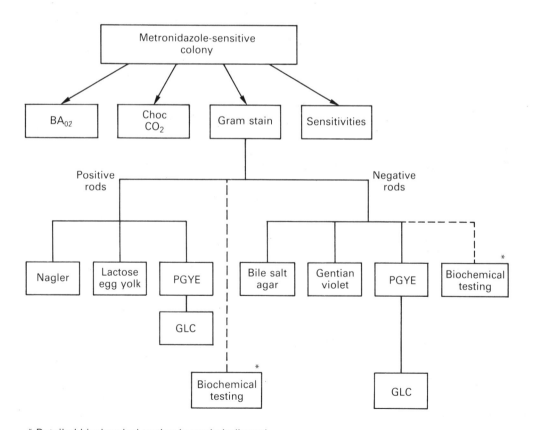

* Detailed biochemical testing is rarely indicated.

Figure 8.4 Example of a process for identification of Gram-positive or negative anaerobic bacilli

The presence of anaerobes in pus can be detected by measuring the volatile and non-volatile metabolic products of anaerobic metabolism by gas-liquid chromatography (Fig. 8.3). The cost effectiveness of this technique must be questioned as it is time-consuming to perform and irrespective of the result, patients are likely to be treated for presumptive anaerobic infection on the basis of clinical suspicion.

Isolation

For primary isolation of obligate anaerobic species, a combination of selective and an enrichment media must be used. Specimens for anaerobic culture should be inoculated on blood agar incubated aerobically, blood agar incubated anaerobically, and a selective blood agar incubated anaerobically, one of which would be inspected after 24 hours and one after 48 hours. Robinson's cooked meat broth should also be inoculated and subcultured after 24 hours if primary plates are negative. A Gram stain of all colonies isolated on incubation should be studied. This process is summarized in Figure 8.4.

Enrichment media

Enrichment (non-selective) media should be nutritionally rich, e.g. with a base media such as fastidious anaerobe agar, columbia agar, brucella or brain heart infusion agar. This should be supplemented with 5% sheep or horse blood. Haemin and vitamin K are essential supplements to all non-selective anaerobic media. Other supplements which have been recommended include yeast extract, cysteine and Tween-80, which is said to encourage the growth of anaerobic cocci. The latter compound may be inhibitory if media containing it is kept in aerobic conditions.

Selective media

Medium may be made selective for anaerobic species by the addition of antibiotics. Gram-negative anaerobes such as *Bacteroides* spp. are naturally resistant to aminoglycosides and vancomycin and these agents can be incorpo-

Table 8.4 Examples of selective isolation media for anaerobic species

Medium	Selected genera
Neomycin 75 µg/ml	Bacteroides,
Vancomycin 75 µg/ml	Fusobacteria
Neomycin 70 µg/ml	Clostridia/anaerobic cocci
Nalidixic acid 10 µg/ml	Bacteroides/pepto-
Tween 1%	streptococci
Phenylethyl alcohol 0.25%	

rated in media designed for their isolation (Table 8.4). Neomycin agar gives excellent results for the isolation of clostridia and anaerobic cocci.

Liquid media

Thioglycolate broth may be supplemented by the addition of yeast extract and Robertson's cooked meat medium may also be used as an anaerobic enrichment broth. Before the inoculation of liquid media, tubes should be held in a reducing atmosphere for 8 hours or placed in a boiling water bath for 10 minutes to drive off dissolved oxygen then cooled to 37°C before inoculating the specimen. An additional advantage of broth culture is that in the event of failure of the anaerobic atmosphere anaerobic pathogens in the specimen will survive in the anaerobic condition provided by the broth.

Generation of anaerobic atmosphere

Some of the clinically important anaerobic species are highly sensitive to the presence of oxygen. Consequently laboratory procedures should be orientated to reduce the contact between anaerobes and oxygen in the atmosphere or in microbiological media. There are a number of methods generating an anaerobic atmosphere.

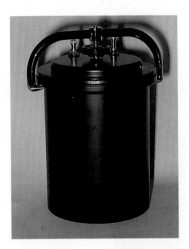

Figure 8.5 Anaerobic jars are airtight containers of metal or clear plastic within which an anaerobic atmosphere can be generated for the isolation of strict anaerobes

Anaerobic jars

Anaerobic jars are cylindrical containers made of plastic or metal and are airtight (Fig. 8.5). These jars may have vents or valves through which gases can be added or air evacuated. An anaerobic atmosphere is generated because the jar contains a catalyst consisting of palladium-coated aluminium pellets to catalyse a reaction which uses up the atmospheric oxygen by combining it with hydrogen to form water. This reaction is common to all anaerobic jar methods and takes place at room temperature over approximately 30 minutes. The catalyst is inactivated by H_2S and moisture, but can be regenerated by heating in an oven at 160°C for two hours. There are two methods:

Method 1

Air is evacuated from the anaerobic jar and replaced with a mixture of nitrogen, carbon dioxide and hydrogen. The jar is then put aside for the catalyst to allow hydrogen to react with the residual oxygen to form water, reducing the atmospheric oxygen concentration. Proof that this reaction has taken place is demonstrated by the presence of a secondary vacuum. Additional anaerobic gas mixture is then admitted and the jar incubated at 37°C.

Method 2 'Gas-pak' generating system

In this method, foil envelopes containing two tablets, one consisting of citric acid and sodium bicarbonate and the other of sodium borohydride, are placed in the jar. Water is added and carbon dioxide and hydrogen are generated and the reaction between and hydrogen and oxygen is catalysed by the palladium catalyst, thus depleting the jar of oxygen. With this method, O_2 concentration is less than 0.6% one hour after activating. If a reaction has taken place, condensed water will be visible on the inside surface of the jar.

In both of these methods the generation of anaerobic conditions should be confirmed by use of an anaerobic indicator such as methylene blue which is colourless under anaerobic conditions, or a rezaurin strip which becomes pink on exposure to oxygen. If after incubation the strip is pink, the jar should be examined for mechanical failure and broths subcultured for the recovery of pathogens.

Anaerobic cabinet

An anaerobic cabinet is an airtight box of flexible plastic or solid gastight (Fig. 8.6) construction in which cultures may be handled in an anaerobic atmosphere. An air-lock forms part of the system so that newly inoculated plates can be admitted to the anaerobic chamber and cultured plates can be removed

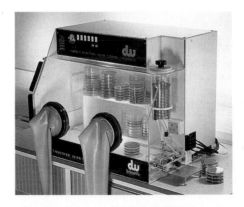

Figure 8.6 An alternative to the anaerobic jar is the anaerobic cabinet which permits the manipulation of cultures through the glove ports. Cultures and plates enter through the airlock at the side

for further work. Cultures can also be manipulated using glove-ports. The worker may have to work with gloves, but some cabinets allow 'bare hands' working.

The cabinet is supplied with a mixture of nitrogen, carbon dioxide and hydrogen which recirculates across a palladium catalyst to remove any oxygen. The air from the air-lock is evacuated by vacuum pump and replaced with nitrogen. This cycle may be repeated and anaerobic gas mixture is used on the last cycle before the inner door of the air-lock is opened and plates brought into the main part of the cabinet. Plates are incubated within the cabinet which is maintained at 37°C. Anaerobic conditions should be confirmed by a meter which measures the redox potential.

The ability of anaerobic atmosphere to suppress the growth of obligate aerobes and to support the growth of strict anaerobes should be tested by inoculating control organisms, *P. aeruginosa* and *C. tetani*, daily.

As the chamber is maintained at a slight positive pressure minor leaks will not result in loss of anaerobiosis but will cause excessive use of gas.

Holding jar technique

The holding jar technique is used in conjunction with anaerobic jars. After inoculation, plates are placed in a holding jar which is similar in construction to an anaerobic jar. It is connected to a supply of O_2-free CO_2, which is run into the jar continuously to exclude air (Fig. 8.7). When the holding jar is full, its contents are transferred to an anaerobic jar and put up in the usual way.

Incubation period

Anaerobic pathogens are often slow growing, and up to 20% of non-sporing anaerobes require five days for isolation. Some species, *Porphyromonas*, and some fusobacteria are especially sensitive to O_2 exposure during the early period of incubation. Ideally, anaerobic cultures should not be examined until after 48 hours. Reading of anaerobic plates does facilitate the interpretation of the aerobic plates and therefore where plates are

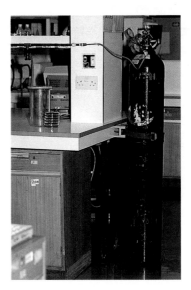

Figure 8.7 While plates are waiting to be placed in a cabinet or jar they can be placed in a holding jar which resembles an anaerobic jar but is connected to a CO_2 cylinder

examined after 24 hours, a duplicate set of cultures should be set up and incubated in a separate jar for examination after 48 hours. This problem is, of course, obviated by an anaerobic cabinet where plates can be inspected whenever required without exposure to O_2.

Identification of anaerobic species

The complete identification of anaerobic species can require complex procedures. Laboratories will vary in the degree to which they identify anaerobes depending on the clinical case mix, and interests of the laboratory. It can be argued that there is little additional clinical information to be gained from speciating Gram-negative anaerobes. In most clinical settings this is correct but without accurate speciation new pathogens such as *Fusobacterium ulcerans* would not have come to light. More detailed methods and tables of identification for the major pathogenic species are found with the relevant organism.

Differentiation of anaerobes

Feature/test	Example
Colonial morphology	u.v. fluorescence *P. melaninogenicus* Haemolysis *C. perfringens* Pitting of agar *B. ureolyticus*
Gram morphology	Classification into Gram positive and negative, characteristic morphology of, e.g. *Fusobacteria*
Spore position	In *Clostridium* spp.
Bile tolerance	Found in the *B. fragilis* group
Dye tolerance	*Bacteroides* spp., sensitive to gentian violet, *Fusobacteria* resistant
Antimicrobial resistance	*B. fragilis* group penicillin resistant
Toxin/antitoxin testing	Nagler testing for *C. perfringens*
Biochemical testing and gas-liquid chromatography	Used to identify anaerobes to species level.

The most important initial step in identification is to confirm the relationship of each suspected anaerobe to oxygen. This can be determined by plating the colony on anaerobic medium which is incubated into an anaerobic atmosphere, on chocolate agar which is incubated in 5–10% carbon dioxide, and blood agar incubated in an aerobic atmosphere. The anaerobic plate should also contain a metronidazole disc to confirm sensitivity to this antibiotic agent.

The colonial morphology of anaerobic isolates should be carefully inspected with a hand lens or plate microscope. *Prevotella melaninogenicus* produces black colonies on blood-containing medium. Cultures of *C. perfringens* exhibit a double zone haemolysis on blood agar caused by two haemolysins, the alpha and theta toxins. Several anaerobic species fluoresce when exposed to u.v. light. Brick-red fluorescence can be detected in cultures of *P. melaninogenicus* and *C. difficile*. *Fusobacterium necrophorum* fluoresces green on media containing cysteine, and *C. difficile* will show yellow fluorescence.

The Gram reaction is an important stage in identification of anaerobic species. The size and shape of the bacteria, the presence of branching and the shape and position of bacte-

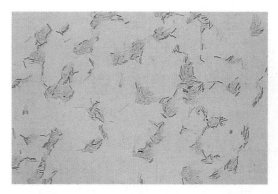

Figure 8.8 The morphology of the spores can be studied by staining them specifically

rial spore should be noted. Spores may be seen on Gram stain as they are unstained but are more clearly demonstrated by phase contrast microscopy (see Fig. 8.8). Spores are more likely to be seen on older cultures.

Dye and bile tolerance can be tested by incorporating 0.5% sodium taurcholate (or 20% bile), and 1 in 100 000 gentian violet (final concentration) into an agar base supplemented with yeast extract, vitamin K and haemin.

Antibiotic susceptibility testing

Resistance to antibiotics can be used in the identification of anaerobes. These techniques, together with bile and dye tolerance, are especially applicable to small laboratories that wish to identify anaerobic species only to genus level with the minimum of tests. The tests are performed in the same manner as susceptibility tests but use antimicrobial agents not usually used therapeutically or concentrations well in excess of that achievable in tissue. A lawn inoculum is made on blood agar and the following antibiotic-containing discs applied: vancomycin 5 µg, penicillin 2 U, metronidazole 5 µg, phosphomycin 200 µg, kanamycin 1000 µg, colistin 10 µg, novobiocin, 5 µg, sodium polyanethol sulphate (Liquoid).

Toxin/antitoxin testing

Detection of lecithinase production is useful in the identification of *Clostridium* spp. and

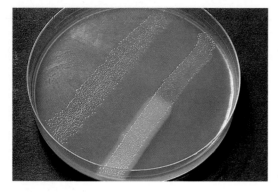

Figure 8.9 The Nagler plate is divided in two with antitoxin spread on one half. On the half without antitoxin the positive control (on the right) produces a cloudy zone caused by lecithinase activity and a pearly layer caused by lipase activity (compare with the negative control on the left)

Fusobacterium necrophorum. The test organism is streaked on a medium containing egg yolk together with the appropriate toxin and non-toxin-producing strains as controls. Elaboration of lecithinase causes an opalescence in the medium surrounding the streak. Organisms which also produce a lipase will be identified by a 'mother of pearl' sheen around the colonies. Specific antitoxin spread on one half of the plate will inhibit the homologous toxin activity allowing for the rapid identification of *C. perfringens* (Fig. 8.9). If the medium also contains lactose and neutral red, as for example in lactose egg yolk milk agar, lactose fermentation can also be demonstrated (see below).

Gas-liquid chromatography

The end products of fermentative metabolism consist of volatile (acetic propionic, iso-butyric, butyric, iso-valeric and iso-caproic) and non-volatile (lactic and succinic) fatty acids. The pattern of these fatty acids is typical of individual species. The gas-liquid chromatography (GLC) is essential for the definitive identification of many *Bacteroides*, *Porphyromonas* and *Fusobacterium* species.

A gas chromatograph consists of gas supply (N_2, H_2) an injection port, a column, and a flame ionizing detection system. Fatty acids can be detected by injecting culture supernatant fluid directly onto some columns, but the columns rapidly become contaminated and must be repacked. It is preferable, therefore, to make an ether extraction of all fatty acids.

Peptone glucose yeast extract broth (PGYE) is inoculated with the suspect colony and incubated in anaerobic conditions until adequate growth is obtained. A sample is transferred and acidified with sulphuric acid to pH 2. The bacteria are removed by centrifugation and the supernatant extracted with ether. Excess water is removed by passing over anhydrous calcium chloride and sample is injected into the gas chromatography column. Non-volatile fatty acids (lactic, succinic, and phenylacetic) must be previously methylated by mixing the culture supernatant fluid with sulphuric acid and methanol and incubating overnight at room temperature. A chloroform extract is made and injected on the GLC column.

At the start of each GLC run standard solutions of mixtures of volatile and non-volatile acids should be used and a non-inoculated PGYE medium control. Fatty acids are detected and recorded. Their identification is determined by measurement of elution time in comparison with the controls.

Biochemical testing

Biochemical identification of anaerobic species can be divided into two groups, the conventional tests and newer commercial kits.

Anaerobes may be identified by determining the pattern of sugar fermentation reactions. Conventional techniques use a solution of test carbohydrate added to proteose peptone yeast extract broth to make a final concentration of 1%. After inoculation and incubation, fermentation of the specific sugar may be detected by measuring the change in pH with an indicator (e.g. bromothymol blue) or measuring the fall in pH directly with a pH meter (>0.5 is considered positive). Urease activity is detected in a similar way and a rise in pH greater than 0.5 is considered positive.

Indole production may be detected by extracting a PGYE broth culture with toluene and adding Erlich's indole reagent. A red-

Table 8.5 Characteristic reactions of clostridia on lactose egg yolk milk agar

	Lecithinase C	Lipase	Lactose	Proteolysis	Spore
C. perfringens	+	−	+	−	OS/CNP†
C. novyi ST	+	+*	−	−	O, C or ST
C. histolyticum	−	−	−	+	O, C or ST
C. septicum	−	−	+	−	OST
C. sordelli	+	−	−	+	OC
C. botulinum					
ABF	−	+*	−	+	OSTP
CDE	−	+*	−	−	
C. tetani spherical	−	−	−	−	T
C. difficile	−	−	−	−	OST/OT

* Limited lipase activity found in *C. botulinum* (all types) and *C. novyi* (Type A).
† Does not usually sporulate in clinical material or laboratory medium containing fermentable carbohydrate specialized sporulation medium (e.g. Ellner (1956), *J. Bacteriol.* **71**, 495–6) must be used.
Adapted from Willis and Hobbs (1959). Some new media for the isolation and identification of clostridia. *J. Pathol. Bacteriol.* **77**, 511.
O, oval; ST, sub-terminal; C; central; T, terminal; P, projecting.

purple colour indicates a positive result. Nitrate reduction is also a useful test.

Aesculin hydrolysis is performed in a cooked meat broth to which aesculin has been added. Hydrolysis is detected by adding aqueous ferric ammonium citrate solution. Gelatinase activity is detected by observing the disintegration of a gelatin disc incorporating charcoal which has been placed in a tube of Robertson's cooked medium broth.

Commercial identification tests

The Minitek system consists of a multi-welled plate. Biochemical substrates are impregnated on filter paper discs added to each well and a heavy suspension of organisms is added to each well. The plates are incubated anaerobically for 48 hours and the manufacturers provide a numerical system to identify species.

The API 20A system is similar to the API 20E system consisting of a plastic strip of 20 cupules containing dehydrated biochemical substrates. The microtubules are inoculated with a heavy suspension and a strip incubated in an anaerobic atmosphere for 48 hours. Isolates are identified with a manufacturer's numerical scheme.

The API ZYM or AN-Ident use a heavy bacterial inoculum and colour changes arise due to the action of bacterial preformed enzymes. They do not depend on the growth of the anaerobe and identification may be possible within four hours. The process of identification of anaerobic species isolated is summarized in Figure 8.4. A simplified identification scheme based on Willis and Hobbs is illustrated in Table 8.5.

For the small routine laboratory such commercial identification holds the prospect of accurate identification without a major investment of time and materials. For anaerobes which are asaccharolytic, however, these techniques, which depend heavily on sugar fermentation tests (or glycolytic enzymes), may lack diagnostic power.

Gram-negative non-sporing anaerobes

Introduction

The Bacteroidaceae include anaerobic Gram-negative species found in many human infections. The genera *Bacteroides* and *Fusobacterium* are phylogenetically related to the *Flavobacterium* and *Cytophaga* genera.

The main Gram-negative anaerobic organisms isolated from human sources are found in the *Bacteroides*, *Prevotella*, *Porphyromonas* (see below), *Fusobacterium* and *Leptotrichia* species. These organisms form the major part of the bacterial flora of the gut, mouth, and female genital tract and form an important part of the non-specific defence against infection with pathogens.

Bacteroides

Classification

The genus *Bacteroides*, as previously consti-
tuted, included a very diverse range of organisms with a DNA base composition varying
between 28 and 61 mol per cent. Three main
groups were distinguished: the 'fragilis group'
which contained the bile-tolerant organisms,
the 'oralis-melaninogenicus' group which
contained non-bile tolerant saccharolytic
organisms, and the asaccharolytic group. It has
been proposed that these groups be designated
as new genera. The *B. fragilis* group will
include the other bile-tolerant anaerobes such
as *B. thetaiotamicron* and *B. disatonis*. The
oralis-melaninogenicus group has been
assigned to the genus *Prevotella*, and includes
the former *B. bivius*, *B. oralis*, *B. disiens* and
B. melaninogenicus. The asaccharolytic group
including *B. asaccharolyticus*, *B. endodontalis*
and *B. gingivalis* have been reclassified with
the new genus name *Porphyromonas*.

Bacteroides fragilis

This organism is numerically the most important
cause of serious anaerobic sepsis although not
the most numerous member of the anaerobic
flora. Together with the other members of the
group it is a small Gram-negative pleomorphic
rod with rounded ends. Organisms of the group
are non-motile, non-spore forming, obligate
anaerobes. *Bacteroides fragilis* grows well after
24 hours' anaerobic incubation with smooth,
circular, grey, non-haemolytic colonies, 1–2 mm
in diameter. They are all penicillin resistant by
virtue of beta-lactamase production.

Pathogenesis

Although not the most numerous in specimens
from healthy subjects it is most frequently
isolated in clinical specimens. The bacterial
capsule is central to *B. fragilis* pathogenicity
enabling the organism to resist phagocytosis.
In addition a direct anti-phagocytic effect is
seen inhibiting phagocytosis of other facultative organisms and this may be one of the
mechanisms of synergistic infections.
Bacteroides fragilis also produce a wide range
of lytic enzymes including protease, DNAase,

heparinase and neuraminidase; the exact
pathogenic role of these is not yet clear but
they are likely to facilitate invasion. A potent
beta-lactamase is produced.

Clinical importance

Bacteroides fragilis is typically associated with
postoperative sepsis in abdominal and gynaecological surgery. It is also found as part of the
polymicrobial flora in cerebral, hepatic and
lung abscess.

Prevotella

Classification

Prevotella melaninogenicus is the type strain of
the new genus which incorporates the old
melaninogenicus-oralis group of organisms.
They are moderately saccharolytic, and
produce acetic and succinic acids in PGYE.
Other species included in this genus are *P.
oralis*, *P. disiens*, *P. bivius* and *P. buccale*.

Isolation and identification

They are small Gram-negative pleomorphic
coccobacilli or short rods growing slowly to
produce small colonies (1 mm) after 48 hours'
incubation. Some of the species produce a
black pigment on blood-containing medium
after prolonged incubation due to the production of protoporphyrin. Colonies of *P.
melaninogenicus* will fluoresce brick red in
long wave u.v. light (365 nm). Other species in
the genus are not pigmented: *P. oralis*, *P.
bivius* and *P. disiens*.

They fail to grow on media incorporating
either bile or gentian violet, are sensitive to
neomycin and penicillin and are resistant to
kanamycin.

Clinical importance

This group of organisms is found chiefly in the
oral cavity causing endogenous infections. They
are associated with periodontal disease, gingivitis, dental abscess, sinus infection, cerebral and
lung abscesses. They are also found in association with *Borrelia* and *Fusobacteria* in cervico-

facial ulcerative diseases such as Vincent's angina and cancrum oris.

Porphyromonas

Classification

This group of organisms was formerly classified with *Bacteroides* as the pigmented asaccharolytic group. This group includes *Porphyromonas gingivalis*, *P. asaccharolyticus*, and *P. endodontalis*. Like *Prevotella* they also produce black pigmented colonies on blood-containing media. These organisms are non-motile, non-sporing, pleomorphic small Gram-negative rods. They produce a major butyric peak on GLC.

Porphyromonas spp. form an important part of the normal flora of the gastrointestinal and female genital tract. They are therefore associated with endogenous infections arising from these areas.

A large number of other species previously classified with *Bacteroides*, but differing widely in G+C content, cell wall composition and metabolic end products, are being reclassified. These include animal species found in infected bites such as *B. levii* and *B. macaccae* which closely resemble the pigmented asaccharolytic species but have yet to be renamed. *B. amylophilus* has been reassigned to *Ruminobacter*, and *B. gracilis*, a pathogen in head and neck sepsis, has been assigned to the genus *Wolinella*.

Fusobacteria

Fusobacteria are defined on the basis of their characteristic Gram morphology. All the members of this genus produce butyric acid as their major metabolic end product, differentiating this genus from *Leptotrichia* which has similar morphology but produces a lactate peak. The cell wall contains diaminopimelic acid and/or lanthionine as the dibasic amino acid in their peptidoglycan. There are more than 15 species in this genus.

Clinical importance

Fusobacteria are found in mixed infections along with spirochaetes in the destructive facial condition cancrum oris or Ludwig's angina. They also participate in mixed infection with *Borellia vincentii* to give severe mouth ulceration known as Vincent's angina. They are also found in dental and periodontal abscesses, gingivitis, liver abscesses, cerebral abscess, in anaerobic cellulitis, and necrotizing fasciitis.

Fusobacterium necrophorum is predominantly a pathogen of animals which only occasionally causes severe human infections. It may cause peritonsillar abscess, jugular vein thrombosis and metastatic abscesses. *Fusobacterium nucleatum* is associated with ulcerative gingivitis and is found only in low numbers in healthy people and in much higher numbers in patients with gingivitis.

Fusobacterium ulcerans has been identified in patients with tropical ulcer and has been implicated in the causation of this previously enigmatic condition.

Isolation and identification

After 48 hours' incubation at 37°C colonies are raised, irregular and have a crenated edge. Microscopic examination of Gram-stained organisms show very long slender rods, wider at the centre and tapering towards the end. Pleomorphism is the rule with coccobacillary and long, straight, slender rods being found.

The fusobacteria are strict anaerobes sensitive to metronidazole and tolerant of bile and gentian violet. They are non-spore-forming and are usually non-motile. Fusobacteria are sensitive to vancomycin, kanamycin and penicillin.

Leptotrichia buccalis may be isolated from human infection although its role is controversial. It is a commensal organism found in the mouth. The Gram morphology is characteristic with Gram-negative rods up to 15 μm long. The organisms are metronidazole sensitive and bile tolerant.

Anaerobic cocci

Classification

Strictly anaerobic Gram-positive cocci are found in the family Peptococcaceae which include the genera *Peptococcus*, *Peptostreptococcus*, *Ruminococcus*, and *Sarcina*. Of these only *Peptococcus* and *Peptostreptococcus* are regularly found in human specimens. Of the

Gram-negative cocci only *Veillonella* are regularly isolated from human material.

Recent re-evaluation of the G+C content, cell wall structure, fatty acid content, and SDS-PAGE of whole cell proteins has resulted in the reclassification of the 'Peptococci' *P. asaccharolyticus*, *P. indolicus*, *P. prevoti*, and *P. magnus* to *Peptostreptococcus* leaving only *P. niger* in this genus.

Veillonellas are divided into seven species: *V. parvula*, *V. atypica*, *V. criceti*, *V. caviae*, *V. dispar*, *V. ratti*, and *V. rodentium*.

Clinical importance

Anaerobic cocci are usually found in mixed infections in dental sepsis, cerebral or lung abscesses, wound and soft tissue infections. They are also associated with a severe fasciitis, 'Melany's synergistic gangrene', which is a mixed infection of anaerobic cocci, facultative streptococci, and possibly also *S. aureus*. Veillonella are rarely implicated in human infection.

Isolation and identification

Anaerobic cocci grow readily on conventional rich blood-containing media, thioglycolate and Robertson's cooked meat broth. Blood agar incorporating nalidixic acid-tween, or neomycin or gentamicin are useful selective media.

These organisms are somewhat difficult to identify in the routine diagnostic laboratory. Sensitivity testing can be useful: discs incorporating 5 µg novobiocin can differentiate *Peptococcus* from *Peptostreptococcus* but there are many exceptions (peptococci are resistant). *Peptostreptococcus anaerobius* is usually sensitive to a Liquoid-containing disc. Other valuable tests include indole production, fermentation tests, and GLC. Commercial identification systems have been shown to have low reliability.

Clostridia

Classification

The genus *Clostridium* includes all the anaerobic spore-forming bacteria. Most of the organisms are Gram-positive rods but pleomorphism occurs with coccoid and filamentous forms. They form bacterial endospores, but these may not be seen in isolates grown on artificial media (e.g. *C. perfringens*). There are 83 species described but a minority are human pathogens. Most of the organisms are obligate anaerobes, but there is wide variation in oxygen tolerance from *C. carnis* and *C. tertium* which are able to grow in aerobic conditions to strict anaerobes such as *C. haemolyticum* and *C. novyi* type B. They are motile by peritrichous flagella, the exceptions being *C. perfringens*, *C. innocuum* and *C. ramnosum*. They are catalase and oxidase negative and acetate and butyrate are produced as the end products of metabolism in PGYE broth.

Clostridia may be classified into four main groups: those which are proteolytic and saccharolytic; those which are proteolytic but non-saccharolytic; those whcih are saccharolytic but non-proteolytic strains; and those which are non-saccharolytic and non-proteolytic.

Habitat

Clostridia are widely distributed in the environment in soil, fresh water and in the sea. Several species including human pathogens form part of the normal flora of the gut in humans and other animal species.

Pathogenicity

The pathogenicity of clostridial species depends on the production of potent exotoxins. These include neurotoxins such as botulinum and tetanus toxin, cytotoxins such as hyaluronidase and collagenases and enterotoxins. These are discussed in more detail with the descriptions of the individual species.

Isolation

Clostridia grow well in ordinary media and glucose promotes the growth of the saccharolytic species. Colonial morphology is diverse with many species exhibiting swarming (e.g. *C. tetani*; Fig. 8.10) or having colonies with irregular edges and branching projections.

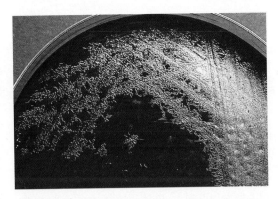

Figure 8.10 The typical spreading branching growth of *Clostridium tetani*

Many specimens from which clostridia are sought are heavily contaminated with other bacteria. Clostridia can be selected by using the survival properties of the spore by alcohol, or heat treating the specimen. A 1 ml sample of the specimen is mixed with an equal volume of absolute ethanol for one hour and then subcultured. One millilitre of specimen is added to cooked meat broth pre-heated to 80°C and incubated at this temperature for 10 minutes before subculture.

Identification

The tests which are useful in the identification of clostridia include lecithinase production (plus or minus antitoxin inhibition), lipase, urease, gelatinase production, sugar fermentation (glucose, lactose, inositol maltose), and gas-liquid chromatography.

A simple medium, lactose milk agar (anaerobic), may be used together with antitoxin inhibition to obtain much of the necessary biochemical information to identify clostridia. Those organisms which produce lecithinase (phospholipase-C) attack the glycerol-phosphorylcholine producing an insoluble complex which results in the development of an opaque halo around the colonies. On a plate on which antitoxin has been streaked, inhibition on one side is seen (see Fig. 8.9). Clostridia which have lipase activity produce opacity in the media beneath bacterial colonies and a pearly appearance on the surface which may extend a little beyond the colony, an effect which requires 48 hours' incubation. The medium also contains lactose and neutral red,

so in organisms able to ferment lactose a red halo is found in the medium around areas of growth. (NB: Colonies remain uncoloured until they are exposed to the air.) The role of gas-liquid chromatography and other biochemical tests are illustrated in Table 8.5.

Clostridium perfringens

This organism is a large Gram-positive rod which may be capsulate in tissues. It forms a part of the normal flora of animals and humans. It does not form spores in the presence of fermentable sugar (on artificial media) but spore production can be induced on medium which contains ox bile.

Colonies are large, convex and opaque and on horse blood agar are surrounded by a zone of β (complete) haemolysis and a wider zone of partial haemolysis (Fig. 8.11). Occasionally mucoid colonial forms are found.

Clostridium perfringens elaborates many exotoxins, named α to ν. These consist of the major lethal toxin α β ε ι and the minor lethal and non-lethal toxins. The combination of major lethal toxins is used to define five serotypes. A1 is associated with gas gangrene and other systemic infection and A2 with food poisoning. Type C is a cause of enteritis in sheep and other animals and is an important cause of food poisoning. Other serotypes are also animal pathogens.

The most important toxin is the alpha toxin, a cation-dependent phospholipase-C. This produces opalescence on egg-containing media which can be inhibited by specific antitoxin,

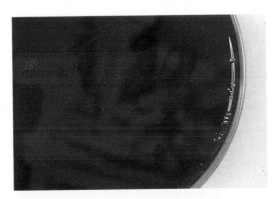

Figure 8.11 Typical wide zone of haemolysis in a culture of *C. perfringens*

the basis of the Nagler reaction (see Figure 8.9). The other toxins include collagenase, hyaluronidase, and haemolysin and lipase.

Clostridium spp. (usually *perfringens*) can also cause infections of the skin and soft tissue with muscle involvement. Gas production in the tissues occurs giving it the name crepitant cellulitis.

Food, often meat cooked in bulk, contaminated with *C. perfringens* may cause diarrhoea. The slow rise in temperature allows the organism to sporulate and survive the cooking process which also generates an anaerobic atmosphere as the dissolved oxygen is driven off. As the food cools the spores germinate and the vegetative cells multiply. The ingested vegetative cells sporulate in the gut producing an enterotoxin with a similar mode of action to cholera toxin. The illness has a short incubation period of 8–12 hours and has a high attack rate and short-lived symptoms. The diagnosis is usually made clinically.

Clostridium perfringens is the normal inhabitant of the stools and its presence does not imply disease. Similarly high spore counts can also be found in normal subjects. A causal relationship can only be deduced if *C. perfringens* is isolated from stool and the implicated food. Toxin tests using ELISA or reverse passive latex agglutination techniques may prove valuable (see Chapter 21).

Enteritis necroticans (pig bel or Darmbrand) is caused by a strain of *C. perfringens* producing a beta toxin. It occurs in Papua New Guinea at pig feasts, and in the severely malnourished world-wide. It results in necrosis of the small bowel. Alpha and beta toxins produced by *C. perfringens* are normally destroyed by proteases in the gut. Sweet potatoes eaten at the pig feasts contain a protease inhibitor which allows the toxins to survive and cause disease.

Clostridial myonecrosis (gas gangrene)

Clostridial myonecrosis is a rapidly progressive infection characterized by toxin-mediated destruction of muscle. *Clostridium perfringens* is the most frequent pathogen isolated (80%) but other clostridia are found including *C. novyii* (40%), *C. septicum* (20%), and less commonly *C. histolyticum* and *C. bifermentans*.

Predisposing factors to gas gangrene include severe tissue damage with devitalization of muscles of the limbs or buttocks, foreign bodies, e.g. shrapnel inoculated into the wound, delay in surgical debridement of a contaminated wound, and compound fractures. Conditions favouring development of gas gangrene commonly arise in war situations. Spontaneous myonecrosis has also been reported. In addition to the local destructive effects the patient suffers severe toxaemia. The diagnosis must be made clinically as early surgical and medical intervention is required for treatment to be successful.

The isolation of *C. perfringens* from a wound is not sufficient for the diagnosis of gas gangrene as this organism may colonize wounds without causing disease. On microscopic examination of a smear large brick-shaped Gram-positive rods without spores can be seen. Few intact polymorphs are seen as these have been destroyed by clostridial toxins.

Clostridium tetani

The organism is a strictly anaerobic Gram-positive rod which may show Gram-negative forms especially in older cultures (see Fig. 8.10). It is slender and long, possessing a round oval projecting spore. It is motile. Colonies have a raised ground glass centre with branching projections at the edge, a spreading growth may be seen. Ten different serotypes (flagellar H) have been described but each produces the same toxin, tetanospasmin, the principal virulence determinant. Most strains are asaccharolytic, and indole is formed by almost all strains.

Habitat and pathogenesis

The organism is distributed widely in the environment in soil, water and the faeces of humans and animals. Infection arises in contaminated wounds, puncture injuries and by inappropriate umbilical stump management. Symptoms are caused by tetanospasmin, the tetanus toxin, which is elaborated by *C. tetani* while growing under anaerobic conditions. The toxin is a protein with a molecular weight of 150 kD. Bacterial enzymes cleave the toxin to produce an extracellular form with two chains. The toxin is taken up by peripheral sensory and motor nerves and moves to the neuronal cell body, crosses the synapses to the gamma aminobutyric acid (GABA)-ergic spinal inhibitory neurones. This leads to increased muscle tone and later tonic contractions.

Clinical importance

Tetanus is caused by infection with a toxin-producing strain of *C. tetani*. The disease begins with spasm of the muscles of mastication resulting in trismus, hence the name 'lockjaw'. Progressive involvement of other muscle groups occurs with spasms being stimulated by sudden noises, movements and clinical procedures. Opisthotonos and later convulsions occur as may laryngeal spasm. Death may occur due to pneumonia, respiratory embarrassment, aspiration of food and secretions or the complications of long-term immobilization. A localized and often mild form of tetanus occurs in the partially immune, usually associated with a puncture wound in the hand or a finger.

Clostridium botulinum

Botulism is a neuroparalytic disease caused by a neurotoxin elaborated by the Gram-positive, spore-bearing rod, *C. botulinum*. It is characterized by acute descending paralysis which begins in the facial and pharyngeal muscles. Death may result from respiratory failure.

Botulism may develop after ingestion of food in which *C. botulinum* has multiplied. Cases have been associated with process failures in canned food, in home preserved meat and vegetables, or contamination of food in cans after production via a break in the surface. In the appropriate conditions surviving organisms multiply and elaborate toxin. The food, if not adequately cooked (botulinum toxin is heat-labile), will contain active botulinum toxin. It is thought that *C. botulinum* is able to multiply in the infant gut and the toxin absorbed causing a neonatal botulism. More rarely wound infection with *C. botulinum* can lead to the botulism syndrome.

Isolation and identification

The diagnosis is made by the isolation of *C. botulinum* or identification of botulinum toxin in suspect food or in the faeces of the patient. Sensitive ELISA assays can be used to detect toxin.

Clostridium botulinum is a motile Gram-positive bacillus with an oval subterminal spore. There are seven serotypes which are differentiated by antigenic differences in the botulinum toxin produced. Types A, B and E are associated with food-related disease, and types A, B and F with infant botulism.

Pseudomembranous colitis

Pseudomembranous colitis is an acute inflammatory condition of the bowel which arises when changes in the gut microflora enable overgrowth and toxin production by *C. difficile*. It typically arises after antimicrobial chemotherapy especially with agents which are active against anaerobic organisms such as clindamycin and ampicillin. It is characterized by watery diarrhoea usually with mucus which may rapidly lead to dehydration and shock. Severe colitis or megacolon can develop.

Clostridium difficile

This motile Gram-positive rod with fine subterminal non-projecting spores forms part of the faecal flora of up to 50% of neonates. It grows well on blood agar and on selective agar – cycloserine cefoxitin fructose agar – with large ground-glass colonies. Colonies fluoresce yellow green in u.v. light.

Pathogenesis

The organism produces at least three toxins, the cytotoxin toxin B and the enterotoxin toxin A in addition to a substance which is thought to alter the muscle tone in the bowel.

Diagnosis

Diagnosis is made by demonstrating toxin in the stool of suspected cases. Toxin is detected by observing the cytopathic effect of fresh stool on a tissue monolayer of Hep-2 or HeLA cells which is inhibitable by anti-*C. difficile* antitoxin (or the cross-reacting anti-*C. sordellii* antitoxin). Isolation of the organism from stool provides only supportive evidence as the organism may form part of the normal flora. *Clostridium difficile* can be detected in stool by antigen testing with a commercially produced latex agglutination technique. This has the advantage of rapidity but, like culture, only provides circumstantial evidence. Commercial ELISAs have become available to detect toxin in the stool.

9

Spiral bacteria

Introduction

All of the pathogenic spirochaetes including *Leptospira*, *Treponema* and *Borrelia* are members of the family Spirochaetaceae. Treponemal diseases are discussed in more detail in Chapter 19.

Leptospira

Classification

The genus *Leptospira* is divided into two species, *L. interrogans* and *L. biflexa*. The two species are morphologically indistinguishable but differ in that *L. biflexa* is able to grow at a lower temperature and is resistant to 8-azaguanine. *Leptospira biflexa* contains environmental saprophytes that are found in water. *Leptospira interrogans* contains the organisms which are parasitic for mammals.

Leptospira spp. are aerobic, tightly coiled bacteria, 6–20 μm long and 0.1 μm wide with hooked ends. They are motile by virtue of two periplasmic flagella which are attached to either end of the body. Most leptospires can be cultivated on artificial media containing serum or bovine serum albumin and essential lipids. The organisms are poorly stained by Giemsa or Gram's stain and are more readily visualized by dark ground or phase contrast microscopy.

Leptospira interrogans are further subdivided into more than two hundred serovars on the basis of agglutination reactions. For

Table 9.1 Examples of Leptospira serogroups and preferred hosts

Serogroup	Host
L. icterohaemorrhagiae	Rodents
L. canicola	Dogs
L. hardjo	Cattle
L. australis	Rodents

simplicity the names of serovars are shortened apparently giving the status of species, thus *L. interrogans* var. *icterohaemorrhagiae* is often known as *L. icterohaemorrhagiae*. Serovars are grouped together in serogroups of closely related organisms.

Clinical importance

Individual serovars usually have a preferred mammalian host but can infect a wider range of animal species including humans. The reservoir of *L. icterohaemorrhagiae* (the causative organism of Weil's disease) is the rat and for *L. canicola* the dog (Table 9.1). Leptospires colonize the renal tubules of their natural host and are excreted in the urine. Humans usually become infected through occupational exposure to the animal urine, or water or soil contaminated by urine. The disease was once common among sewer workers before these risks were appreciated. Many patients become infected by contact with water in the countryside in the pursuit of water sports such as canoeing or wind-surfing. Agricultural and abattoir workers are also at increased risk of

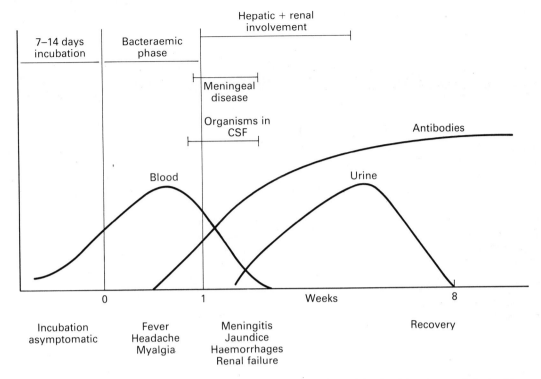

Figure 9.1 After the incubation period, leptospira are found in the blood associated with 'flu-like' symptoms. The meninges, liver and kidney may be involved in the next phase. (Adapted from *Gillies and Dodds Bacteriology Illustrated*)

infection depending on the animal and leptospires found in the environment.

Clinical leptospirosis affects three main organs – the central nervous system, the liver and the kidneys. The involvement of these organs and the severity of the disease differs with the infecting serovar. For example infection with *L. icterohaemorrhagiae* is usually more severe than with *L. hardjo*. The incubation period is usually 10 days but may be as much as a month. Clinical infection is divided into two phases – the bacteraemic phase where organisms can be found in the blood and the second phase where the leptospires disappear from the blood but may be found in the urine. The first phase is characterized by fever, headache, myalgia, conjunctivitis and abdominal pain. In many cases the second phase is asymptomatic even in Weil's disease. The clinical features of the second phase are variable depending on the infecting serovar. In some the picture is dominated by fever, uveitis and aseptic meningitis, but in others jaundice, haemorrhage, renal failure and myocarditis

can develop. This latter syndrome is more common in *L. icterohaemorrhagiae* infection where there may be a mortality of up to 10%. Death, when it occurs, is usually due to renal complications.

Laboratory diagnosis

If antimicrobial therapy is to have an influence on the outcome of this infection it must be instituted as early as possible.

Direct examination

Leptospires can be visualized in the blood of patients during the primary phase of the illness if the red cells are lysed and the organisms concentrated by differential centrifugation. These preparations are difficult to interpret and false-positive results are common. Freshly voided urine can be examined by dark ground microscopy for the presence of leptospires after the second week of illness. It is essential that this investigation is performed on fresh urine as the organisms are very sensitive to the effects of acid.

Culture

Leptospires can be cultured from the blood during the first week of illness. In the later stages of the infection urine can be cultured but the diagnostic yield is low as shedding may be intermittent. For the reasons stated above fresh urine should be cultured in medium to which an antibiotic supplement has been added, e.g. 5-fluorouracil and neomycin. Urine must be alkalinized and inoculated in serial dilutions.

Several liquid and solid media are available. Korthoff's medium consists of buffered salts, haemoglobin solutions, peptone and 10% rabbit serum. In Ellinghausen and McCullough medium the serum is replaced by bovine serum albumin, Tween 80 and a mineral and vitamin solution. Solid media can be made by the addition of agar to one of the broths.

Specimens should be incubated at 30°C for up to six weeks. Isolated leptospires should be identified by bacterial agglutination in a reference laboratory.

Serology

Antibodies begin to appear after the first week of illness, rise to a peak at one month and then begin to decline. A serological diagnosis can be made by measuring agglutinating antibodies in acute and convalescent sera (Fig. 9.1). In this technique a panel of leptospires of different serogroups are agglutinated with dilutions of the patient serum. More recently an enzyme-linked immunosorbent assay (ELISA) technique which detects IgG and IgM has become available which enables a diagnosis to be made either on a rise in IgG titre or with a single serum positive for IgM.

Antibiotic susceptibility

Leptospires are susceptible to penicillin, tetracyclines and aminoglycosides. Tetracycline has been shown to be superior in a controlled clinical trial and is also effective as a prophylactic agent.

Borrelia

Classification

Borrelia spp. are loosely coiled spiral bacteria 5–20 µm long and up to 0.5 µm wide. The cell wall consists of a plasma membrane, a peptidoglycan layer and an outer membrane. They have periplasmic flagella through which the organism gains its motility.

All *Borrelia* spp. are arthropod borne being transmitted by either lice, *Pediculus humanus*, or ticks of the genus *Ixodes* or *Ornithodorus*. Humans are the only reservoir of louse-borne relapsing fever (*B. recurrentis*), but the other organisms are transmitted when the natural cycle between tick and reservoir host (usually rodents) is interrupted by man. Borrelia infections arise sporadically throughout the world with individual species having a narrow geographical territory and host specificity. Epidemics of louse-borne relapsing fever can arise as a result of the disruption caused by war or mass migration. Tick-borne relapsing fever can be a threat to expeditions or military operations when the Borrelia-tick-rodent habitat is invaded.

Pathogenesis

In relapsing fever the borrelia invade the blood and produce an intense febrile response. The host produces antibodies which bring about fever lysis. The organism remains in the tissues and reinvades the blood again when antigenic variation of its outer membrane enables it to escape the activity of host antibody. This phenomenon is responsible for the relapsing course of infection. Relapsing fever is finally controlled when the organism exhausts its repertoire of antigenic variation (Fig. 9.2).

Lyme disease is caused by *B. burgdorferi* and transmitted to man by the bite of an Ixotid tick. After injection into the skin there is a local infection which migrates through the skin. The organisms are also disseminated throughout the body. Infection is characterized

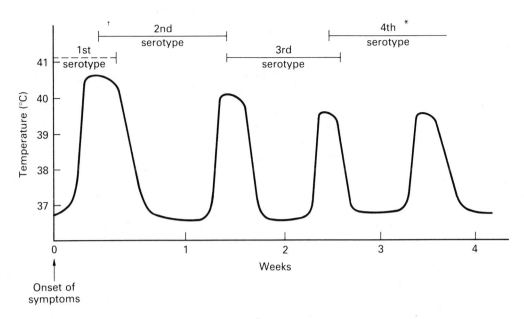

Figure 9.2 The natural history of relapsing fever showing fever pattern caused by succeeding waves of Borrelia of different serotypes

* The number of relapses varies (1–5) in *B. recurrentis* louse-borne infection and 0–13 in *B. duttoni, B. turicatae, B.hermsii* and *B. parkeri* tick-borne infection.

† Serotype 7 is the most common organism found on first relapse.

by an initial erythema chronicum migrans which may be followed by involvement of the central nervous system as meningitis, radiculoneuritis, or encephalitis. Attacks of arthritis, myocarditis and chronic atrophic dermatitis can develop months or years later.

The early symptoms of Lyme disease can be attributed to the acute infective process. The organism is able to persist in the tissues for many years and antibiotic therapy of late disease may bring about cure. The host immune response is important to the outcome of infection as patients with arthritis are more likely to express the HLA type DR4 (and also DR3).

Vincent's angina, an acute ulcerative condition of the mouth, is a synergistic infection of *B. vincentii* with oral fusobacteria (see p. 103).

Clinical significance

Relapsing fever

Louse-borne relapsing fever has a high mortality (up to 40%) compared to tick-borne disease in which it rarely exceeds 5%. Infection is characterized by high fever and rigors which last for three to six days and relapse about a week later. During the febrile period patients experience headaches, myalgia, tachycardia and hepatosplenomegaly. In a small proportion of patients a petechial rash may be present. Arrhythmias arising from myocarditis, cerebral haemorrhage or hepatic failure are the usual causes of death in fatal cases.

Lyme disease

Erythema chronicum migrans begins at the site of the bite in Lyme disease. It begins as a red macule or papule with a slowly expanding area of redness. The outer borders of this rash are a deeper red with a lighter centre. Secondary skin lesions can arise and conjunctivitis may also develop. During the acute phase of the illness the patient may experience headache, fever, and regional lymphadenopathy. The later stages of Lyme disease are characterized by attacks of arthritis usually in the large joints. Symptoms of meningitis, cranial nerve palsy and radiculitis may develop. Myocarditis which arises in the early phase of the disease may result in tachyarrhythmias or heart block. Acrodermatitis chronica atrophicans is a red skin lesion which can be sclerotic or atrophic arising from erythema chronica migrans or *de novo*.

Laboratory diagnosis

Microscopy

Relapsing fever can be diagnosed by demonstrating *Borrelia* in the peripheral blood during a febrile episode. Dark-ground microscopy can be used but the staining of thick or thin blood films with a Giemsa or Leishman's stain is simple to perform and easy to read.

Isolation

Borrelia spp., including *B. burgdorferi*, can be isolated in artificial culture using Barbour Stoener Kelly (BSK) medium. Isolation has no place in diagnosis, however, because of its low diagnostic yield. BSK medium is based on a tissue culture medium supplemented with bovine serum albumin, peptone and yeast extract, HEPES buffer, citrate, pyruvate, glucose, *N*-acetylglucosamine, and rabbit serum.

Serology

The variable antigenic nature of relapsing fever borrelias make serological diagnosis difficult. Lyme disease can be diagnosed by ELISA techniques. Concentrations of IgG rise slowly during the acute phase and IgM can be detected. In the later stages of infection much higher levels of IgG and IgM can be found. After successful treatment IgM becomes negative and IgG concentrations fall. Some patients have been diagnosed by culture of *Borellia* without an antibody response. Specific IgM can be detected in the CSF of patients with neurological complications.

False-negative results can be obtained early in the course of infection and cross-reacting antigens in other spirochaetes may result in false positives in patients with other infections.

Antibiotic susceptibility

Borrelias are susceptible to penicillins, cephalosporins, erythromycin, and tetracyclines. All of these agents are used for treatment of Lyme disease and a consensus therapeutic regimen is yet to emerge. Tetracycline is probably the drug of choice for the treatment of relapsing fever but penicillin and erythromycin are useful alternatives.

Spirillum minor

This is a Gram-negative spiral bacterium, 2–5 µm in length, 0.2–0.5 µm wide. It is motile by virtue of its two polar flagella. It is a commensal of rats, living in the nasopharynx. Infection is transmitted to man by the bite of a rat, hence the popular name of the infection 'rat-bite fever'.

After a two-week incubation period an inflammatory reaction is found at the site of the bite with accompanying regional lymphadenopathy and lymphangitis. There is a generalized maculopapular rash together with fever, headache and malaise. Endocarditis is the most serious complication which is responsible for the mortality associated with this condition. Recovery can occur without antibiotic therapy within two months. Rat-bite fever is diagnosed by demonstrating the organism in a preparation of blood or lymph node stained with Giemsa. This organism has not yet been cultivated *in vitro*. Treatment is usually with penicillin.

10

Medical mycology

Introduction

The isolation and identification of fungi is an important but often neglected part of medical microbiology. Fungi cause a wide range of different diseases, from superficial cutaneous infections with dermatophytes in the community to invasive *Candida* and *Aspergillus* in severely immunocompromised patients in the hospital environment.

Mycological investigation is often considered difficult and the natural province of a reference laboratory. This misconception arises because of the differences in the diagnostic approach required for mycology. The growth of fungal species is often slow, which brings it out of phase with the culture and antimicrobial susceptibility testing of routine bacteriology. Identification may require the use of stains and morphological criteria which are less definable than a positive result in a sugar fermentation or serological test. Attempts to make the diagnosis of fungal disease by serological means have proven elusive.

Many of the most important fungal pathogens, notably *Candida* spp. and *Aspergillus* spp., in the immunocompromised can also form part of the normal flora, which may lead to difficulty in interpretation of culture results. In addition, the classification of fungi is complex and not immediately clinically relevant, based as it is on the biology of reproductive mechanisms and hyphal morphology.

Definitions

Fungi can be divided into three main groups: the moulds, the yeasts, and dimorphic fungi. Yeasts are unicellular organisms that reproduce by budding. They have broadly similar microscopical appearances and are usually identified by biochemical techniques. They grow in solid media, with moist, creamy opaque colonies (Fig. 10.1).

The moulds grow as long tubular structures, known as hyphae, which grow together to form a network which is known as a mycelium. When moulds are isolated on solid media frothy, cotton wool-like colonies develop, some of which are pigmented. There is a diversity of colonial appearances which can be

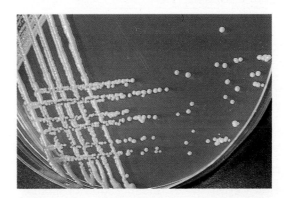

Figure 10.1 Butyrous white colonies typical of *Candida albicans*

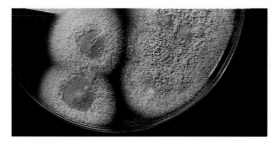

Figure 10.2   Colonies of *Aspergillus flavus*

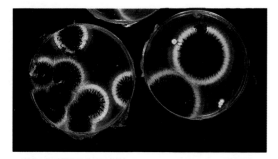

Figure 10.3   Colonies of *Aspergillus niger*

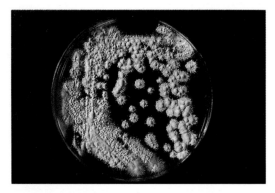

Figure 10.4   Culture of *Microsporum gypsum* on Dermatophyte Test Medium. Growth on this medium changes the indicator to red

helpful in identification (Figs 10.2 and 10.3). The hyphae grow into the medium (the vegetative mycelium) and above the medium (the aerial mycelium). The aerial mycelium gives rise to the fruiting bodies, which consist of asexual spores. Identification of moulds is often based on the morphology of the hyphae and the fruiting bodies (Fig. 10.4).

Some fungi are dimorphic, having both a yeast and hyphal stage in their life cycle. These are exhibited during growth under different conditions: mould-like growth occurs at 20°C and yeast-like growth at 37°C.

Moulds may propagate by the formation of spores and conidia. Spores reproduce either sexually by a process of meiosis and cell fusion or asexually by mitosis. Spores are of two types, sporangiospores and conidia. Sporangiospores develop asexually inside a special structure, the sporangium. Conidia are formed by differentiation of hyphal cells (arthrospores and chlamydospores) or from the hyphal tip. Conidia may be unicellular (microconidia) or multicellular (macroconidia) (Figs 10.5 and 10.6).

Fungi are eukaryotes containing a nucleus surrounded by a nuclear membrane, but many fungal cells are multinucleate. The cell wall is principally composed of chitin, which is a polymer of glucose and mannose and/or cellulose. The cell membrane contains sterols and fungi and are consequently resistant to many antibacterial antibiotics. They are susceptible, however, to antibiotics which interfere with sterol metabolism, such as the polyene group and imidazoles, or with DNA metabolism.

Classification

We have already divided fungi by one means of classification, that of moulds and yeasts. More formally, they are divided into four main groups: the Zygomycota, Ascomycota, Basidiomycota and Deuteromycota. The Zygomycota include organisms which have aseptate hyphae and reproduce asexually by spores inside a sporangium, and sexually by the production of zygospores. The Ascomycota have septate hyphae, produce conidia, or reproduce by means of ascospores produced within an ascus. The Basidiomycota have septate hyphae and reproduce asexually by conidia or sexually by means of basidiospores. The Deuteromycota, which include many of the medically important fungi, have septate hyphae and reproduce asexually with a production of conidia; they are not known to reproduce sexually. The clinically important fungi in these groups are shown in Table 10.1.

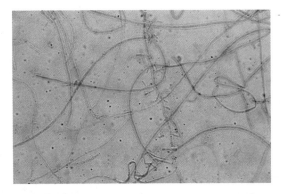

Figure 10.5 Monocellular microconidia of *Taenia rubrum*

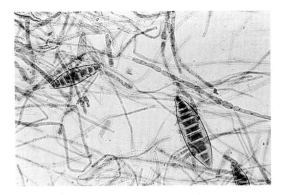

Figure 10.6 Macroconidia of *Microsporum canis*

Table 10.1 Examples of clinically important fungi

Immunocompromised patients	Dermatophytes	Systemic infections	Superficial and subcutaneous infections
Cryptococcus neoformans	Trichophyton mentagrophytes	Histoplasma capsulatum	Melassezia furfur
Candida spp.	Trichophyton tonserans	Histoplasma duboisii	Exophiala werneckii
Aspergillus spp.	Microsporum audouinii	Blastomyces dermatitidis	Madurella spp.
	Epidermophyton flocculosum	Coccidioides immitis	Sporotrichium schenckii

Clinical classification

A clinical classification is more valuable in the diagnostic microbiology laboratory as it separates the fungi into groups according to clinical relevance. Fortunately, this separation brings together organisms to which similar techniques for isolation and identification can be applied. Fungi can therefore be divided into three main groups: the cutaneous and subcutaneous group, which includes the species causing dermatophytosis, sporotrichosis and mycetoma. The opportunistic fungi are those species which cause disease in patients who are compromised as a result of coexistent medical conditions or medical therapy. These include aspergillosis, candidosis, cryptococcosis, etc. The final group are the systemic fungi which are primary pathogens. These include the causative agents of histoplasmosis, coccid-

ioidomycosis, paracoccidioidomycosis, blasto-mycosis, cryptococcosis and candidosis (see Table 10.1).

Opportunistic fungal infections

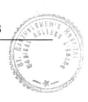

Candida

Classification

Candida spp. are members of the family Cryptococcaceae and are Deuteromycota ('fungi imperfecta' species without a recognized sexual form). Candidas are pathogens and saprophytes of animals and man. They are found as part of the normal flora of the mouth, gastrointestinal tract and genitourinary tracts and skin. They are also widely distributed in the environment and can be found on many plants. Most human infections are caused by *Candida albicans*, but other species, including *C. tropicalis*, *C. parapsilosis*, *C. glabrata*, *C. krusei* and *C. pseudotropicalis* can arise in clinical specimens and may cause disease (see below). The growth in pseudohyphae by *Candida* spp. is the only feature which separates this genus from *Torulopsis glabrata*. Sexual reproduction does occur in some *Candida* spp. notably *C. krusei* which is classified by its sexual stage *Issatchenkia orientalis*.

•Clinical importance

Candida spp. are frequent causes of invasive fungal infections in immunocompromised hosts. Most infections are caused by *C. albicans*, but other species, including *C. tropicalis*, *C. parapsilosis*, *C. glabrata*, and *C. pseudotropicalis* can occur. Some are important because of innate resistance to antifungal agents used in therapy or prophylaxis. *Candida krusei* is often resistant to fluconazole increasingly used in antifungal prophylaxis for severely immunocompromised patients and *C. lusitaniae* is resistant to amphotericin B.

These species are normal inhabitants of the human gut and are found on the skin and mucous membranes. They can be selected by the use of a broad spectrum of antibiotics. Patients with AIDS, neutropenia or those with severe combined immunodeficiency syndrome are highly susceptible to infection.

Candidas can infect the skin and nails and produce paronychia which is usually mild. Oral or vaginal thrush may follow a course of broad spectrum antibiotics or local steroid therapy. Patients complain of pharyngitis or a pruritic vaginal discharge and symptoms often resolve once the predisposing factor has been withdrawn or after a short course of antifungal chemotherapy.

In severely immunocompromised patients infection can take the form of severe oral thrush or oesophagitis which can result in pharyngitis, chest pain and severe weight loss due to dysphagia. This is one of the conditions which can be used to define AIDS in HIV-positive patients. Systemic invasion is common in neutropenic patients and those with normal immune function in intensive therapy units who have been treated with multiple courses of broad spectrum antibiotics and have indwelling intravascular lines.

Laboratory diagnosis

Microscopy

Microscopy of a wet preparation or Gram-stained smear can confirm the diagnosis of oral or vaginal thrush (Fig. 10.7).

Isolation

Candida spp. grow readily on simple laboratory media forming 1–2 mm white, butyrous colonies after 24–48 hours' incubation (Fig. 10.1). Like many other fungi growth can be obtained when the concentration of glucose is

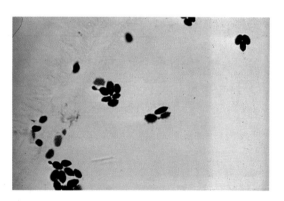

Figure 10.7 Gram stain of *Candida* spp. with budding daughter cells

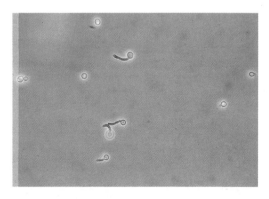

Figure 10.8 Germ tube formation in *Candida albicans*

increased to 5% at which level bacterial multiplication is inhibited. This is the basis for Sabouraud's dextrose agar. As this organism may form part of the normal flora and readily colonizes patients on broad spectrum antibiotics the significance of individual isolates can be determined only in relation to the whole clinical picture.

Identification

The simplest identification test for *C. albicans* is the demonstration of germ tube formation. Bovine serum is inoculated with part of a colony and incubated for two to four hours. A sample is examined under the microscope for the presence of small projection (the hyphal initial) which is known as the germ tube (Fig. 10.8).

Isolates can be subcultured on corn meal agar and the morphology studied after incubation at room temperature for up to 48 hours. The structures sought are blastoconidia, arthroconidia, pseudohyphae, true hyphae or chlamydospores.

Species identification can be made by biochemical techniques. Commercial biochemical identification techniques have recently been made available. Carbohydrate assimilation (auxanogram) tests can also be used. In an auxanogram growth in basal medium occurs only if the isolate is able to assimilate the test carbohydrate. Conventional tubes are incubated for up to three weeks at room temperature but commercial products are available which are incubated at 30°C and typically provide an identification after 48 hours.

Antibiotic susceptibility

Candida spp., with the exception of *C. lusitaniae*, are susceptible to amphotericin B. They are usually susceptible to the imidazoles such as ketoconazole, clotrimazole and fluconazole, and to 5-flucytosine.

Cryptococcus neoformans

Classification

The genus *Cryptococcus* is a member of the family Cryptococcaceae. *Cryptococcus neoformans* is the only species which regularly causes

infection in man. All cryptococci are obligate non-fermentative aerobes which grow well at 37°C. The sexual form has now been found and shown to be a basidiomycete with two species *Filobasidiella neoformans* and *F. bacillosporus*. Both cause a similar disease in the yeast form.

Cryptococcus neoformans is widely distributed in nature as a saprophyte and animal commensal. It is found in high concentration in pigeon faeces whose composition favours its growth.

Clinical importance

Before the development of the HIV epidemic cryptococcal infection was a rare cause of chronic lymphocytic meningitis. Patients were typically immunocompromised with lymphoma, steroids or cytotoxic therapy. It did infect immunocompetent patients with intense exposure, i.e. those in contact with bird droppings and pigeons. *Cryptococcus* is recognized as an important pathogen in AIDS patients, with up to 15% being infected.

The principal manifestation of cryptococcal infection is a subacute meningitis. Cryptococcal pneumonia and a fungaemic form causing shock is recognized.

Laboratory diagnosis

Microscopy

Cryptococci are readily visualized in a Gram-stained film of the CSF. If the CSF is mixed with India ink the organisms can be seen surrounded by a halo which consists of the polysaccharide capsule (Fig. 10.9). Not all isolates express a capsule and this technique is not sufficiently sensitive to be the sole rapid diagnostic method and should be used in conjunction with a latex test to detect capsular polysaccharide antigen.

Isolation

Cryptoccocus spp. are readily isolated on blood agar and unselective Sabouraud's agar without cyclohexamide. Large, white, butyrous colonies are seen after 24–48 hours' incubation at 37°C but may be delayed for up to five days.

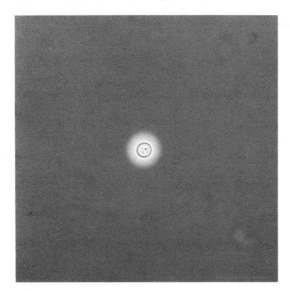

Figure 10.9   Cells of *Cryptococcus neoformans* surrounded by a halo of capsule in an India ink preparation

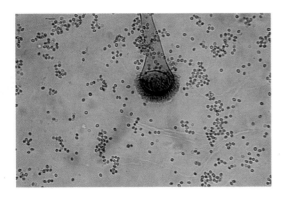

Figure 10.10   *Aspergillus* spp. conidospore with terminal phalliades

Identification

The identity of an isolate will be indicated by the characteristic variability of cell size and the capsule demonstrated with India ink. A presumptive identification can be made on the basis of a rapid urease positivity (by Christensen's method), phenol oxidase production and negative nitrate test. A definitive identification can be made with the methods described above for *Candida*.

Antibiotic susceptibility

Cryptococcus spp. are susceptible to amphotericin B, fluconazole and 5-flucytosine. Treatment with a 5-flucytosine allows the dose of amphotericin to be reduced.

Aspergillus spp.

Classification

There are several hundred *Aspergillus* spp. but only four are regularly associated with human infection: *A fumigatus*, *A niger*, *A. flavus*, and *A. terreus*. They grow with septate branching hyphae. Some of these may give rise to a long stalk-like, non-septate hypha arising from the specialized 'foot cell', which is topped by the conidiospore, the asexual reproductive structure. The conidiospore is bulbous and rows of cells called phialides form chains radiating from it. This feature can be used for distinguishing the species (Fig. 10.10).

Aspergillus spp. are free-living saprophytic organisms which are ubiquitous in the environment. Spores can be found in room air, unless air supply is ducted through HEPA filters.

Clinical importance

Aspergillus spp. may cause disease in non-immunocompromised patients without infection. In this circumstance inhalation of aspergillus spores give rise to a type 3 hypersensitivity reaction, with the clinical syndrome of 'Farmer's lung': fever dyspnoea and progressive lung fibrosis. In some patients, contact with *Aspergillus* spp. gives rise to a type 1 hypersensitivity reaction, leading to the syndrome of intermittent airways obstruction known as bronchopulmonary allergic aspergillosis. These patients are also colonized and positive sputum cultures can be obtained.

Patients with pre-existing anatomical abnormalities of the respiratory tract such as healed cavities or old tuberculosis can become colonized with aspergilli, giving rise to an aspergilloma, or 'fungus ball'. In neutropenic patients, aspergillus infection typically begins in the lungs, and fatal disseminated disease can develop. Other sites, including the paranasal sinuses, skin, central nervous system and eye may be infected.

Table 10.2   Systemic mycoses

Species	Geographic distribution	Clinical syndromes
Histoplasma capsulatum	C, SE and SW USA	Pulmonary, cutaneous disseminated infection
H. capsulatum var *duboisii*	Africa	Cutaneous lesions, multiple disseminated lesions, pulmonary involvement
Blastomyces dermatitidis	S USA	Acute or chronic pulmonary infection, cutaneous lesions and osteomyelitis
Coccidioides immitis	SW USA, Mexico, Central and South America	Pulmonary infection, acute and chronic progressive skin and soft tissue
Paracoccidioides brasiliensis	Central and South America	Acute or chronic pulmonary, or disseminated infection

Laboratory diagnosis

Sputum culture is of limited value as up to 20% of normal subjects will have a positive culture and is often negative in patients with infection. A positive culture in the presence of clinical evidence of disease in a predisposed patient would support the diagnosis. A representative alveolar specimen can be obtained by bronchoalveolar lavage where a positive isolate is diagnostic (98% specificity) but it lacks sensitivity.

Bronchopulmonary aspergillosis and Farmer's lung can be diagnosed by detection of precipitating antibody by countercurrent immunoelectrophoresis (CIE). Serological diagnosis is not helpful in immunocompromised patients who are unable to respond to infection with an antibody response. Attempts to detect aspergillus antigens have focused on galactomannan, although some initially encouraging results have been reported, successful diagnosis requires weekly serum specimens.

Many other fungi can affect the severely immunocompromised, including the zycomyocetes. Infections with these organisms are found in the elderly patients and those with poorly controlled diabetes mellitus, chronic alcoholism, or severe immunocompromise due to organ transplantation. Infection may take the form of invasion of the nose and paranasal sinuses, which may disseminate into the eyes and brain. Pulmonary disease may occur and the organism can be disseminated and infect other tissues.

The main species implicated are *Mucor*, *Rhizopus* and *Absidia* spp. They grow readily at 30°C on enriched media but many species are inhibited by cyclohexamide. Identification of the isolate is by morphological criteria.

Systemic fungal infections

Classification

The aetiological agents of systemic mycosis are dimorphic fungi. Like other dimorphic fungi, when grown at 25–30°C they take the form of a mould, but at 37°C, they grow in a yeast-like form. There are five main species: *Histoplasma capsulatum*, *H. capsulatum* var. *duboisii*, *Blastomyces dermatitidis*, *Coccidioides immitis*, and *Paracoccidioides brasiliensis*. They have a defined geographical distribution, being found in southwest USA, South America and Africa (Table 10.2).

Clinical importance

The organisms are found in soil, particularly in subtropical, semi-arid environments. Infection is common in endemic areas and is acquired by the respiratory route. Fortunately, the majority of infections are asymptomatic and self-limiting. Clinically severe disease may occur in the immunocompromised, which has made histoplasmosis a more important pathogen as the prevalence of HIV infection has risen in endemic areas. Histoplasmosis takes many forms and can be classified according to site and duration of infection or whether it is a primary infection or a reactivation. In this respect and in many others, histoplasmosis resembles tuberculosis, with which it is often confused. Primary infection is usually pulmonary, but primary cutaneous infection also occurs. Dissemination may develop in very young infants and those suffering from cellular immunodeficiency.

In African histoplasmosis (caused by *H. capsulatum* var. *duboisii*) pulmonary symptoms are less common and bone and skin lesions predominate. Blastomycosis also causes localized or self-limiting pulmonary disease. Chronic progressive forms also may develop affecting the lung, skin, bone, prostate, epidymidis and meninges. Osteomyelitis develops in up to one-third of patients. Coccidiodomycosis causes either self-limiting pulmonary lesions, progressive pulmonary disease, or disseminated infection in the skin or bones.

Paracoccidioidomycosis predominantly infects males because oestrogens inhibit the transformation from the mould to the yeast form. Clinical disease takes the form of acute or chronic pneumonia, or disseminated infection.

Laboratory diagnosis

All of these organisms are ACDP category 3 pathogens and all specimens in which they may be present should be handled in a containment level 3 facility. Wet preparations of sputum, CSF, urine, pus or skin scrapings can be examined microscopically. Sputum can be stained with Giemsa to show yeast-like cells inside macrophages. The pathogens are readily visualized in a Papanicolou-stained smear of sputum which can be useful for rapid diagnosis. Buffy coat macrophages or bone marrow aspirate can be stained with Wright's or Giemsa stain and may show intracellular *Histoplasma* (Fig. 10.11).

Isolation and identification

The dimorphic fungi can be cultivated in media such as Sabouraud's which does not contain cyclohexamide (some species are sensitive). Plates or culture bottles should be incubated at 30°C and retained for up to six weeks. The fungi may also be isolated from blood and grow well on media normally used

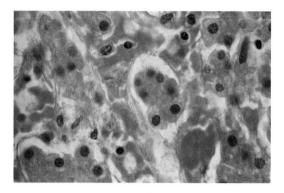

Figure 10.11   *Histoplasma capsulatum* like other systemic fungi is capable of causing disseminated disease. *Histoplasma capsulatum* can be seen here in the liver

in manual and automated systems. A superior recovery has been reported for the lysis centrifugation method (see Chapter 14).

Species identification is based on the morphology of conidia and chlamydospores found in the mycelial form. To differentiate *H. capsulatum* from saprophytic moulds conversion to the yeast form is necessary. Conversion is induced by subculturing the mycelial form in a rich medium such as brain heart infusion with cysteine at 37°C.

Serological diagnosis

The diagnosis of systemic mycosis can be made by detecting specific antibodies by CIE. This is an especially valuable investigation in patients who do not normally live in endemic areas.

Superficial mycoses

Introduction

Superficial mycoses are those caused by fungi that infect keratin which is found in the skin, hair, and nails. They rarely cause serious disease but are of medical importance because of chronic pruritus and pigmentary changes which occur. Infections can be caused by both yeasts and moulds.

Table 10.3   Examples of dermatophytes infecting man

Anthrophilic	Zoophilic	Geophilic
Epidemophyton floccosum	M. canis	M. fulvium
Microsporum audouinii	T. mentagrophytes	M. racemosum
Trichophyton mentagrophytes (var. interdigitale)	T. verrusocum	
T. rubrum		
T. tonsurans		

Dermatophytes

Classification

Three species of filamentous fungi are implicated in dermatophytosis: *Epidermophyton*, *Microsporum* and *Trichophyton*. Previously all were fungi imperfecti but the sexual stages of *Trichophyton* and *Microsporum* have been discovered and they are now classified as Ascomycetes.

The dermatophytes can be conveniently classified into three groups on the basis of their reservoir and host preference. Anthropophilic species are those which have man as their major host. The zoophilic pathogens infect animals and geophilic organisms are found in the soil but may infect animals or man.

Dermatophytes are transmitted by close contact and the organisms may spread rapidly within families or enclosed communities. Transmission of geophilic species is rare, but outbreaks of human infection have been reported. Transmission of zoophilic species also requires close contact, so infections are found in pet owners, farmers and vets. Examples of the three groups of organisms are found in Table 10.3.

Clinical importance

The dermatophytes are the cause of ringworm, so called because it takes the form of red, scaly, patch-like lesions which spread outwards leaving a pale healed centre. The lesions are rarely painful but can be very itchy. The cosmetic appearances are also important to the patient. Some species, notably those of animal origin, produce a more intense inflammatory reaction with pustular lesions or a larger inflammatory mass known as a kerion.

Infection of the nails is chronic and produces discoloration and thickening. Scalp infection leads to scaling and inflammation with hair loss which may sometimes be associated with scarring. Lesions of the skin and hair should be examined under u.v. light as a characteristic fluorescence may be found with some species.

Dermatophyte infection can be clinically classified by anatomical location, e.g. tinea capitis, tinea barbae. These different clinical entities tend to be caused by different species but the division is not absolute so the value of this classification is limited.

Laboratory diagnosis

Specimens

Scrapings of infected skin, hair and clippings from nails should be sent dry to the laboratory. They should be sent in an envelope rather than a tube in which moisture will collect and allow the multiplication of bacterial contaminants.

Microscopy

Skin, hair and nails are clarified for microscopy by gently heating in a solution of potassium hydroxide. Nails require a higher concentration for this effect. Preparations are then examined for the presence of the typical branching hyphal elements (Fig. 10.12).

Isolation

Dermatophytes grow readily on Sabouraud's dextrose agar. As all are resistant to the action

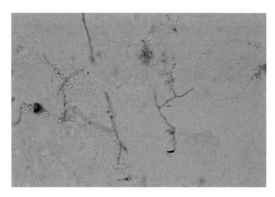

Figure 10.12 Hyphae can be seen in preparations of skin under microscopy

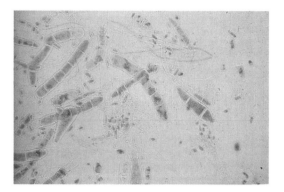

Figure 10.13 Macroconidia of *Trichophyton*

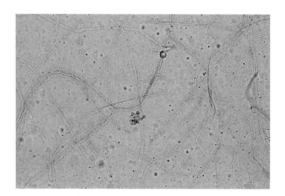

Figure 10.14 Microconidia of *Trichophyton mentagrophytes*

of cyclohexamide this is incorporated as a selective agent. Chloramphenicol and gentamicin can also be used for selection when bacterial contamination is likely. Dermatophyte test medium incorporates all three of these agents together with an indicator which detects the rise in pH consequent on the growth of dermatophytes. Cultures are incubated at 30°C for up to four weeks.

Identification

Full identification is made on the basis of colonial morphology, microscopic appearance, physiological and biochemical testing. The colonial morphology of these pathogens is variable and some examples are shown in Figures 10.5 and 10.6 and Table 10.4.

Mycelial preparations can be stained by lactophenol cotton blue and examined microscopically for the morphology of the conidia and chlamydospores (Figs 10.13 and 10.14).

Other tests which may be valuable include the hair perforation test where an uninfected hair is placed on a colony and incubated for up to two weeks. The hair is examined, as above, to detect penetration of the hyphae into the hair. Urea hydrolysis can be used to distinguish *T. rubrum* (negative) from *T. mentagrophytes* (positive). *Microsporum audouinii* grows poorly on a medium of polished rice grains in comparison to the other dermatophytes, including the morphologically similar *M. canis*.

Antibiotic susceptibility

The dermatophytes are typically sensitive to the imidazoles and griseofulvin. The latter drug must be given over extended periods as it affects fungi only in the keratinized layers as it is incorporated.

Other superficial fungal infections

Pityriasis versicolor is an infection of the stratum corneum caused by the yeast *Malassezia furfur*. Infection is characterized by brown, scaly macules on the trunk or upper arms. In areas exposed to the sun, hypopigmented lesions are seen as the infected skin fails to tan. In patients with AIDS, severe dermatitis may develop. Diagnosis is usually made clinically.

Tinea nigra, caused by *Exophiala werneckii*, is characterized by black, non-scaly macules on

Table 10.4 Characteristics of dermatophytes useful in identification

Species	Colonial morphology	Conidia
Epidermophyton floccosum	Powdery, green/khaki colonies; white tufts	Pear-shaped macroconidia
Trichophyton interdigitalis	White, powdery colonies, later cream centre	Abundant microconidia on hyphae; cylindrical macroconidia
T. rubrum	White, fluffy colonies; red/brown on reverse	Microconidia on sides of hyphae; macroconidia rare except granular colonies; long and cylindrical
Microsporum audouinii	Sparse, white, fluffy colony with salmon/brown on reverse	Microconidia long and on hyphae; macroconidia rare
T. mentagrophytes	White, powdery colony; dark brown/red on reverse	Spiral hyphae seen; multiple microconidia found in clusters on hyphae; macroconidia cylindrical and thin-walled
M. canis	White, buff with aerial mycelium; yellow/orange on reverse	Macroconidia large and fusiform with thick walls

the hands. It is most commonly found in central South America and the Caribbean. Black peidra caused by *Peidraia hortae* is a superficial infection characterized by hard, dark-brown nodules attached to the hairshafts. Black peidra is typically found in warm, moist tropics. White peidra, caused by *Trichosporon beigelii*, is characterized by soft white or greenish nodules on hair shafts. Infection is found in South America and the Far East and it only rarely occurs in northern America or Europe. Disseminated infection has been reported in patients with severe immunosuppression.

Mycetoma

The mycetomas are chronic, granulomatous lesions usually found in the foot or the hand. Infection arises as the result of inoculation of the causative organism into the subcutaneous tissues. It is therefore a more common disease among those who walk barefoot. The lesions are chronic and indurated, characterized by swelling and discharging sinuses. Deeper invasion and destruction of muscle and bone develops with chronicity. The pus present in these patients is often granular, with white or black grains. The colour of the grains depends on the species of fungus present. Mycetoma may also be caused by Actinomycetes (see Chapter 8).

The fungi most commonly associated with mycetoma are *Madurella mycetomatis*, *M. grisea*, *Pseudallescheria boydii*, and *Leptosphaeria senegalensis*.

The diagnosis is made by microscopic examination of pus or biopsy specimens together with culture on bacteriological media and Sabouraud's agar with chloramphenicol and cyclohexamide. Organisms isolated in culture can be identified on morphological criteria and the results of carbohydrate and nitrate utilization tests.

Sporotrichosis

Sporotrichosis is a chronic subcutaneous granulomatous infection caused by *Sporotrichium schenckii*. This dimorphic fungus grows in a yeast form in the host and at 37°C on blood cysteine glucose agar. *Sporotrichium schenckii* is an environmental saprophyte found in soil and plants. Cutaneous sporotrichosis is usually found in the young and extracutaneous infection in older patients. There is usually a history of exposure to the soil, e.g. farming or gardening.

The cutaneous lesions begin as a small red papule which darkens and intermittently discharges a serosanguinous exudate. Ulcers may develop and new lesions arise along the path of the lymphatics. Infection in the skin may spread to distant sites. Extracutaneous disease, when it occurs, is usually located in the main weight bearing bones and joints. The natural history is indolent but destruction of joints with loss of function will occur if the correct diagnosis is not made. Pulmonary infection is less common and meningitis a very rare complication.

Cutaneous infection is treated with local application of potassium iodide, but itraconazole may prove beneficial. Extracutaneous disease is usually treated with amphotericin B.

Parasitology

Introduction

Parasitology was once the province of special-ist laboratories in schools of tropical medicine. Freely available foreign travel means that millions of people travel to tropical countries where 'exotic diseases' may be contracted. The result of this social change is that acute malaria is now a more common diagnosis than infec-tive endocarditis in the UK. Each laboratory and microbiologist must be familiar with the diagnosis of malaria and other common tropi-cal parasites. In addition there is increasing recognition of the importance of parasites found in temperate countries. The increased population of patients who are severely immunocompromised as a result of cytotoxic drugs, steroids, organ transplantation and AIDS has resulted in a higher prevalence of toxoplasma, pneumocystis, and cryptosporid-ium infections. This chapter will focus on the major parasitic infections which are commonly diagnosed in a developed world laboratory.

Parasitic infections which present with fever

Malaria

Classification

There are four species which infect man. They are protozoa of the Plasmodidiae family, and members of the genus *Plasmodium*. The four species have different characteristics both in the type of red cells they may invade and the clinical symptoms they elicit.

Life cycle

Malaria is transmitted through the bite of the female anopheline mosquito. The mosquito injects sporozoites which are transported in the venous blood to the liver where they multiply for a varying period of time depending on species. This period, exo-erythrocytic schizo-gony, corresponds clinically to the incubation period. The hepatocytes rupture releasing merozoites into the peripheral blood and these go on to invade erythrocytes. The parasite grows (trophozoite stage) inside the red cell and undergoes erythrocytic schizogony forming a schizont. The process of division, or schizo-gony, usually occurs in the peripheral blood with the exception of *P. falciparum* where it takes place in the tissue capillaries. Merozoites are released and new red cells are invaded. After a time this parasitic cycle becomes synchronized and intermittent fevers occur. However, in non-immune patients infected with *P. falciparum*, high parasitaemia and severe complications are likely to occur before periodic fever becomes established. The trophozoite may also develop into gametocytes with the formation of female and male gameto-cytes. These stages, part of the sexual cycle, are taken up with the female anophelene mosquito in her blood meal. The parasites are set free in the mosquito stomach and the mature gameto-cyte undergoes further development. This divides into four or eight gametes, each of which forms a long thread-like structure,

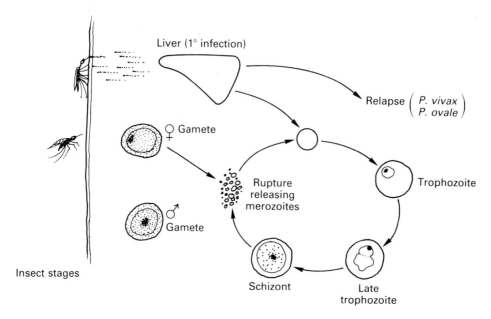

Figure 11.1   Life cycle of malaria

flagellum. The female gametocyte undergoes maturation and forms the macrogamete; the male gamete is called the microgamete. Fertilization takes place to form the zygote; this undergoes maturation through the ookinete stage which migrates through the stomach wall and develops into a cyst. The oocyst develops and spindle-shaped sporozoites develop. The cyst bursts liberating sporozoites into the body cavity from which they migrate to reach the salivary gland. The life cycle is completed when the next blood meal is taken (Fig. 11.1).

Of the four species, *P. falciparum* is the most important pathogen and is capable of causing death in a very short time in immunologically naive subjects (Table 11.1). The reasons for this difference are not fully understood but it is thought that the ability of this species to multiply rapidly in red cells of all ages may result in very high parasitaemia. In addition *P. falciparum* adheres to capillary endothelium, and this phenomenon also occurs in the brain with serious consequences. *Plasmodium falciparum* has the ability to stimulate macrophages to release cytokines such as tumour necrosis factor and these mediators can cause fever and shock.

Clinical importance

Falciparum malaria is one of the most important causes of morbidity and mortality for children under the age of five in endemic areas. Infection is characterized by fever, the course of which is divided into three stages: the cold, the hot, and the sweating stages. These stages are rarely seen in patients from non-endemic countries. In the early stage of illness fevers are high and irregular, but may begin to arise on alternate days in *P. falciparum*, *P. vivax* and *P. ovale* (tertian) or each three days *P. malariae* (quartan). In patients from non-endemic countries infected with *P. falciparum*, however, serious complications

Table 11.1   Complications of acute *P. falciparum* malaria

Cerebral malaria
Renal failure
Pulmonary oedema
Acute haemolysis
Hypotensive (algid) malaria
Chronic anaemia
Acute haemolysis

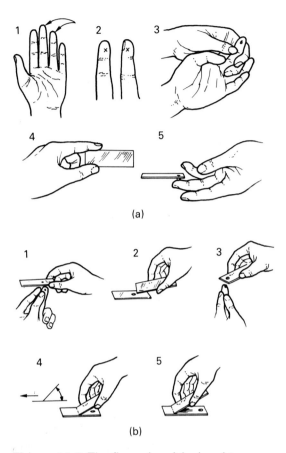

(a)

(b)

Figure 11.2 The finger is pricked and two drops of blood placed on the slide. One is spread over an area of 1 cm² (thick film) (b1 and 2) and the other spread with a second clean glass slide (b4 and 5) (thin film)

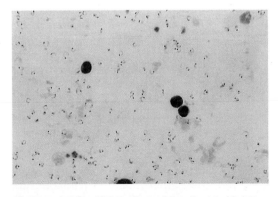

Figure 11.3 Thick film stained with Field's stain showing trophozoites of *P. falciparum*

are likely to have developed before this stage has been reached. Patients may also complain of cough, severe headache, vomiting and diarrhoea. There is often little to find on examination but splenomegaly is common in children and non-immune subjects. Patients may, in addition, be pale and slightly cyanosed.

Acute falciparum malaria is potentially fatal if not rapidly treated and is complicated by cerebral symptoms, anaemia, acute renal failure, or hypotension (see Table 11.1).

Diagnosis of malaria

Direct microscopy

Malaria may be readily diagnosed by the demonstration of parasites inside red blood cells. Specimens of capillary blood should be taken at the height of the fever and up to four hours afterwards. Only a small amount of blood is required and a complete examination can be performed on finger prick specimens by the technique illustrated (Fig. 11.2).

Thick and thin blood films should be examined in all patients where the diagnosis is suspected. These films serve different diagnostic purposes. The thick film acts to concentrate as many red cells as possible as the cells are lysed in the hypotonic stain used and the parasites and white cells are stained, showing up against the background of red cell debris (Fig. 11.3). The thin film enables a confident species diagnosis to be made and an accurate parasite count to be performed.

The severity of *P. falciparum* infections is judged in part on clinical assessment and the degree of parasitaemia. High parasite counts indicate that severe complications could develop and may indicate the need for intravenous quinine therapy. Exchange transfusion has recently been shown to be an important life-saving technique when the parasite count is very high and complications are present.

Speciation of malaria

There is much mystique attached to the speciation of malaria, but it is not difficult if some simple rules are followed. The microscopist should observe a number of features: size of the red cells, the presence and appearance of

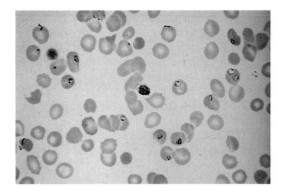

Figure 11.4 *Plasmodium falciparum*: a high parasitaemia with accole forms, double infections and a pre-schizont in the middle of the field. This is not usually found in the peripheral blood and indicates a very severe infection

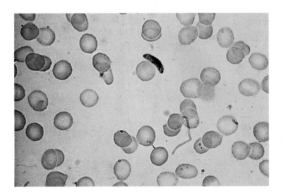

Figure 11.5 Gametocyte (sexual stage) of *P. falciparum*

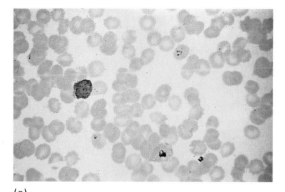

(a)

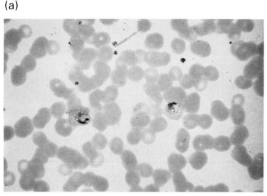

(b)

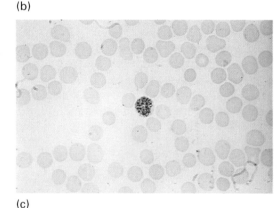

(c)

Figure 11.6 (*a*) Two trophozoites of *P. vivax* and Schuffner's dots can be seen in the lower red cell together with a gametocyte of *P. vivax*. (*b*) 'Amoeboid' trophozoites of *P. vivax*. (*c*) Schizont of *P. vivax*

dots in the red cell, the percentage parasite count, and the morphology of the trophozoites. The morphology of schizonts and gametocytes if present will assist identification. In *P. falciparum* infections parasitaemia may exceed 2.5%, and trophozoites usually appear as thin rings inside normal sized erythrocytes. Accole forms and multiple rings may be found (Fig. 11.4) but schizonts are not usually seen in the peripheral blood and if present indicate serious disease. In contrast, *P. vivax* has larger amoeboid trophozoites found in erythrocytes which are larger than normal and have fine dots evenly distributed in the cytoplasm (Schuffner's dots). Schizonts and gametocytes are often seen (Fig. 11.5). The features of these and the other malaria parasites are summarised in Table 11.2 and illustrated in Figures 11.4–11.7.

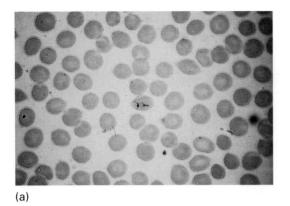

(a)

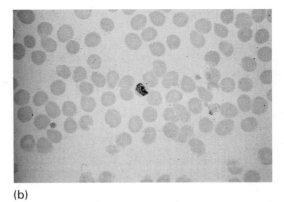

(b)

Figure 11.7 (*a*) Trophozoite of *Plasmodium ovale*: oval red cell with James' dots. (*b*) Band form trophozoite of *P. malariae*

Measuring parasitaemia

A high parasite count is associated with an increased morbidity and mortality, thus measurement of parasitaemia is a simple test for the severity of malaria. There are two main ways to measure the parasite count.

The percentage parasite count can be determined by the number of parasitized red cells out of 1000. The absolute parasite count is obtained by multiplying the percentage count by the red cell count.

An alternative method is to count the number of malaria parasites against the number of white cells in a thick blood film. The absolute parasite counts are made by multiplying the number of parasites per 100 white cells by the white blood cell count.

New diagnostic techniques

Several new techniques have been developed for the diagnosis of malaria. These include the use of monoclonal antibodies for antigen detection, enzyme-linked immunosorbent assays (ELISAs), and immunoradiometric assays (IRMAs). Gene probes to detect a repeating sequence in the malaria parasites has been described and polymerase chain reaction (PCRs) are being developed. None of these techniques yet exceed the sensitivity and specificity and low cost of thick and thin blood film examination by an experienced observer. They have much to offer, however, in epidemiologi-cal surveys and in diagnostic laboratories which have less experience of malaria diagnosis.

The 'QBC' diagnostic system uses fluorescein staining and a capillary tube examined microscopically for rapid field diagnosis. This method uses a simplified u.v. source and malaria parasites take up the stain and fluoresce in the u.v. light. The technique reduces the time required to examine individual specimens and has proven easy to learn and applicable in laboratories in developed and developing countries.

A number of serological techniques have been applied to the diagnosis of malaria, including indirect fluorescent antibody method and radioimmunoassay techniques. The presence of antibodies for malaria is of value in diagnosis in very few cases. It may be useful to screen blood donors, although a simpler, more cost effective way is to exclude all of the donors who have recently travelled to the tropics. The presence of antibodies to malaria would indicate exposure to malaria.

Antimalarial sensitivity

The species diagnosis is also important in pointing to the correct chemotherapeutic agents. Many *P. falciparum* parasites are now resistant to chloroquine, whereas the other species remain sensitive. Infection of the other malaria parasites results in a benign course

Table 11.2 Characteristics of the life-cycle stages of malaria parasites infecting man

Species	Red cell size	Special features of red cells	Trophozoites	Schizonts	Gametocytes
P. falciparum	Normal; high parasite counts occur	Maurer's clefts	Early trophozoites are thin rings; accole forms double chromatin dots, multiple trophozoites/RBC Amoeboid forms	Rarely found in peripheral blood	Crescent-shaped; pigment present
P. vivax	Larger, irregular; <2% parasitaemia	Schufner's dots	Fine pigment in cytoplasm	Large, round and irregular; scanty pigment	Large, round and irregular; scanty pigment
P. ovale	Large/oval; <1% parasitaemia	James' dots	Small, compact	Small, compact; scanty pigment	Small, round; nucleus on one side
P. malaria	Smaller; <1% parasitaemia	–	Band and bird's eye forms	Small, compact; abundant yellow pigment	Small, round/oval compact

Table 11.3 Classification of filaria parasites

Species	Disease	Diagnostic specimen for microfilaria
Wuchereria bancrofti	Lymphatic filariasis	Peripheral blood
Brugia malayi		
Mansonella spp.	Often asymptomatic	Peripheral blood
Loa loa	'Calabar swellings'	Peripheral blood
Onchocerca volvulus	'River blindness', chronic pruritus	Skin snips

and a fatal infection is rare in immunocompetent patients. *Plasmodium falciparum* and *P. malariae* do not have a dormant liver stage (hypnozoite) and thus, once the acute infection is treated no further therapy is necessary. In contrast *P. vivax* and *P. ovale* survive in the liver after acute infection and may result in relapse if not treated with primaquine. (NB: Glucose-6-phosphate status must be determined.)

Many new antimalarial agents have been described in response to the difficulties posed by chloroquine resistance. These include halofantrine, mefloquine and artimisinine; each is active against chloroquine-resistant *P. falciparum* and are gaining their place in antimalarial chemotherapy.

Filaria

Classification and clinical importance

Filaria are not commonly encountered in UK microbiological practice. They may be classified as follows: lymphatic filaria; *Brugia malayi*, and *Wuchereria bancrofti*, skin filaria *Onchocerca volvulus*, and loiasis (*Loa loa*) (Table 11.3).

Lymphatic filariasis is characterized by acute attacks of fever and lymphoedema which may be complicated by secondary bacterial infection. With repeated attacks the lymphatic system is permanently damaged resulting in local lymphoedema in the leg (to give elephantiasis), scrotum, or abnormal connections with the ureter to give chyluria.

Onchocerciasis, which is also known as 'river blindness', results from the inflammatory response to the migration of microfilaria in the eye. Adult worms are located in nodules and microfilaria migrate in the skin resulting in pruritus and dry thickened skin. More seriously the microfilaria migrate in the eye and the resulting inflammation causes blindness. Loiasis is less damaging and is often diagnosed on the basis of fleeting subcutaneous swellings known as Calabar swellings. Infection may be associated with fever and abnormalities of renal function.

Laboratory diagnosis

Specimens

The laboratory diagnosis of lymphatic filariasis is dependent on identifying microfilaria in the peripheral blood. Their presence in blood is synchronized with the feeding habits of the insect vector and thus they are found during the period which the vector is most likely to bite. Ten millilitres of blood must be taken at this time into citrate containers. If the result is initially negative the investigation may be repeated after the patient is given 50 mg of diethylcarbamazine to increase the number of microfilaria in the blood. The collected blood is concentrated by passing it through a polycarbonate membrane with a 5 μm pore size. The microfilaria are retained by the filter which can be transferred to a glass slide, stained and viewed under the light microscope (Fig. 11.8).

In onchocerciasis 'skin snips' or 'pinch biopsies' should be taken from any affected area together with two samples from over the shoulder blade, two from the buttocks and two from the thigh. It is important that the specimen is bloodless or parasites may be difficult or impossible to visualize. Individual pieces of skin are placed in saline in wells of a microtitre plate and incubated at room temperature. The wells are observed from time to time (and

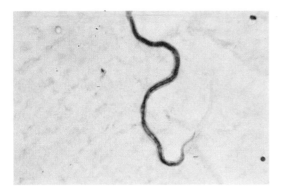

Figure 11.8   Filaria with a sheath and nuclei which do not go to the end of the tail

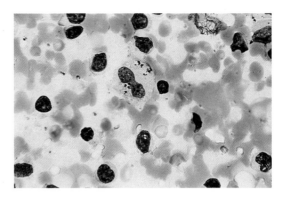

Figure 11.9   Amastigotes of *Leishmania donovani* inside macrophage cells

overnight) for the presence of microfilaria which migrate from the skin sample into the surrounding liquid. The microfilaria which have emerged from the skin sample can be fixed and stained for identification. When skin snips are negative the patient can be given a dose of 50 mg of diethylcarbamazine. This is known as the Mazotti test. A positive Mazotti test can have a clinical and parasitological result. Patients with onchocerciasis will note an increase in itch in the infected areas of skin which may also become reddened and oedematous. Skin snips taken during a test are more likely to be positive.

Identification of filaria

Microfilaria are identified on the basis of their size, the presence or absence of a sheath when stained by haematoxylin and eosin, and the pattern of nuclei in the tail of the microfilaria (see Fig. 11.9).

Serological diagnosis

Serological techniques for antibody detection have been described. One ELISA method uses the microfilaria of *Brugia pahangi* in the solid phase. This is a sensitive means of detecting antibodies to filaria species but it is impossible to distinguish between the species due to the presence of cross-reacting antigens.

Recent work indicates that many patients with filariasis have circulating phosphoryl-choline-containing antigen and diagnosis based on this principle is undergoing clinical evaluation.

Leishmania

Classification and clinical importance

Leishmania are intracellular protozoan parasites which are transmitted to man by the bite of a sandfly of the *Plebotomus* genus if in the Old World or *Lutzomya* if in the New World. They are part of the Kinetoplastida family which also include the trypanosomes. Leishmania are injected in the human host in the flagellate promastigote form where they are taken up by macrophages and other phagocytic cells of the reticuloendothelial system. They transform into the intracellular form, the amastigote (Fig. 11.9). There are more than seven species and there is a simple, clinical classification based on the three forms of clinical leishmaniasis.

Visceral leishmaniasis is caused by *L. donovani* and *L. infantum*, and is endemic in the Mediterranean, the Indian subcontinent, Africa, and Central and South America. Infection is characterized by fever, weight loss, anorexia, anaemia and hepatosplenomegaly. The parasite immunosuppresses the patient and there is production of large quantities of inappropriate low affinity antibody with the effect that they are susceptible to bacterial infections from which the patient eventually succumbs, about eighteen months after infection. Fever and weight loss are due to the action of macrophage-derived cytokines.

Cutaneous leishmaniasis is caused by *L. tropica*, *L. major*, *L. aethiopica*, *L. mexicana*, and *L. braziliensis*. Infection produces chronic discrete granulomatous skin lesions at the site

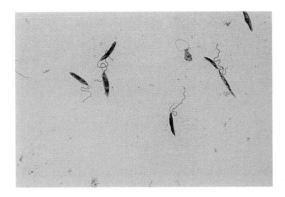

Figure 11.10   Promastigotes of *L. donovani*

of infection. Healing with scarring occurs and the patient is subsequently immune. Mucocutaneous leishmaniasis is more serious causing destructive lesions in the mouth and nose. This form may be caused by *L. aethiopica* and *L. braziliensis* and can arise after a long latent period.

In patients who have reduced cell-mediated immunity cutaneous lesions may become disseminated and visceral leishmaniasis becomes very difficult to treat. This is an increasing problem where HIV-infected individuals live in leishmania endemic areas.

Laboratory diagnosis

The diagnosis of all forms of leishmaniasis depends on demonstration of parasites in infected tissues. Bone marrow or splenic aspirate (if the clinicians are familiar with the technique) or lymph node aspirate should be obtained and stained with Giemsa. In cutaneous disease a slit skin smear may be diagnostic, otherwise a skin biopsy should be obtained and a morphological diagnosis made on impression smear or histological section. Leishmania found inside macrophages may be recognized by the presence of the nucleus and a small kinetoplast (Fig. 11.9). Leishmania may be cultured on various media including Schneider's and N-N-N medium where the promastigote form is seen (Fig. 11.10). Serological evidence of infection can be obtained by indirect fluorescent antibody test (IFAT), ELISA or direct agglutination, although these investigations are usually only performed in reference laboratories.

Trypanosomes

Classification and clinical importance

Trypanosomes are kinetoplastida and there are two species (one with two biovars) which are pathogenic for man.

Trypanosoma cruzi is found in South and Central America and transmitted to man by the triatomid or 'kissing' bug. Infection is followed by acute febrile illness, a latent period and later visceral complications: achalasia, cardiac arrhythmias, megacolon, and peripheral neurological signs.

Trypanosoma brucei has two biovars pathogenic for man, *T. brucei* var. *gambiense* responsible for West African sleeping sickness, and *T. brucei* var. *rhodesiense* which causes the more acute East African sleeping sickness. Infection is transmitted to man by the bite of a fly of the *Glossina* species (tsetse fly). There is an initial inflammatory response with regional lymphadenopathy at the site of the bite (the trypanosomal chancre) and a latent period followed by attacks of fever which may be associated with a rash. Finally invasion of the CNS takes place and mental function deteriorates where the patient initiates little voluntary movement. Death may occur as a result of encephalitis or bacterial infections due in part to the inanition of the patient and the immunosuppression caused by the parasite.

Laboratory diagnosis

South American trypanosomiasis is diagnosed by visualization of parasites in blood during the acute phase (Fig. 11.11) or by serology in the latent or chronic phase. The sensitivity of microscopy can be enhanced by culture of the parasites on N-N-N medium. Xenodiagnosis is a variation on culture. Uninfected bugs are allowed to feed on the arm of a patient and are then sacrificed after two weeks. The contents of the bugs' intestines are examined microscopically for the presence of parasites.

African trypanosomiasis is diagnosed by demonstrating the parasite in the peripheral blood or in lymph node aspirates (Fig. 11.12). It is important to determine whether infection has reached the CNS as the usual anti-trypanosome drugs, suramin and pentamidine, do not cross the blood–brain barrier. If

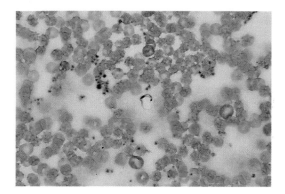

Figure 11.11 South American trypanosomes

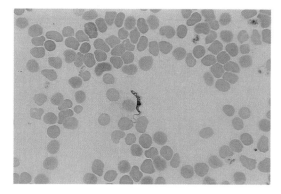

(*a*)

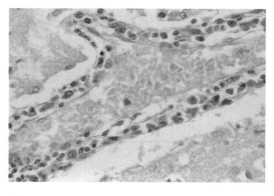

(*b*)

Figure 11.12 (*a*) African trypanosomes. (*b*) Brain infected with African trypanosomes

infection is diagnosed the systemic disease should be treated before lumbar puncture is performed to reduce the risk of introducing viable trypanosomes into the CSF. Serological methods are available but are of limited value in acute diagnosis.

Toxoplasmosis

Classification and clinical importance

Toxoplasma gondii is an obligate intracellular parasite with a wide host range. The sexual stages of the life cycle only occur in the definitive host which are members of the cat family. Man becomes infected by eating undercooked meat, or food which has become contaminated by cat faeces. Infection is common in the UK, but even more common in cultures where undercooked meat is often eaten. *Toxoplasma gondii* is well adapted to the human host and infection rarely results in clinical illness. In some patients an infectious mononucleosis syndrome may develop with fever and lymphadenopathy. This may be complicated by myocarditis.

Toxoplasmosis is of more significance to the unborn child where transplacental infection may result in mental retardation and ocular lesions. Prenatal infection only occurs during acute primary infection in the mother. Toxoplasmosis has also proven a significant pathogen in patients who are severely immunosuppressed as a result of transplantation (usually heart or bone marrow). In AIDS patients reactivation of latent foci in the brain results in a space-occupying lesion and resultant neurological deficits (Fig. 11.13).

Laboratory diagnosis

Toxoplasma may be cultured from infected tissue in a cell culture system or in mice. This is slow and insensitive, however, and poses a significant infection hazard and is rarely practicable in a routine laboratory. Diagnosis of toxoplasmosis, therefore, depends on serology.

Serum can be screened by an agglutination test, either latex agglutination or indirect haemagglutination which detects both IgG and IgM. Positive sera can then be selected for IgM detection by either an antibody capture ELISA or immunosorbent agglutination assay (ISAGA). The definitive test is the Sabin-Feldman dye test which utilizes live *Toxoplasma* tachyzoites, and because of this the test is limited to reference centres.

In the immunocompromised host most clinical toxoplasmosis arises as a result of reactivation of latent infection. Serology is of little value

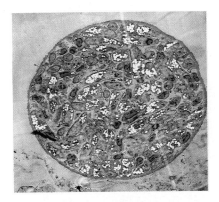

Figure 11.13 Cyst of *Toxoplasma gondii* in the brain (of a mouse)

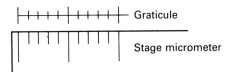

Figure 11.14

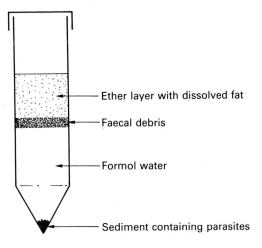

Figure 11.15

as raised titres of IgG antibody are always present and an IgM response does not develop. Toxoplasmosis poses a risk to the fetus during acute infection. Transplacental infection can only be proved if fetal IgM is obtained.

Antibiotic susceptibility

Toxoplasma gondii is inhibited by folate antagonists such as sulphadiazine, pyramethamine, by dapsone, clindamycin, spiramicin and the newer macrolides.

Intestinal parasites

Diagnosis of intestinal parasites

Macroscopic appearance

A report of the macroscopic appearance of the specimen should be made noting the colour, consistency and presence of blood, pus or mucus. Taeniasis, ascariasis and threadworm infection may also be diagnosed on macroscopic appearance of worms or segments in the stool.

Microscopy

The simplest method of detecting faecal parasites is to examine a saline-wet preparation where approximately 1 mg faeces is thoroughly mixed with normal saline. In order to obtain the best diagnostic yield from the examination of the faeces it is essential to scan the whole of a cover-slip systematically with both the ×10 and ×40 objectives. The ×10 objective is used to identify possible parasites, and the ×40 to demonstrate the detail necessary to identify the species. A drop of Lugol's iodine can be added to stain cytoplasmic glycogen. The identification of a parasite is made on the basis of characteristic morphology and size. Size may be determined by measuring the parasite with a calibrated graticule placed in the eye-piece (Fig. 11.14).

Formol-ether concentration

Concentration methods may be required to detect the presence of faecal parasites. This is essential when parasite numbers are likely to be low, e.g. in travellers with helminthic infections where worm burdens are often low, in infection where egg numbers are often low (e.g. taeniasis and schistosomiasis), to test cure, and to count parasite numbers in epidemiological surveys.

The formol-ether concentration technique can be used to concentrate parasitic cysts and ova in faeces. Other concentration methods, such as the zinc sulphate, saturated NaCl or sugar flotation techniques may be used but these do not concentrate all parasitic species with equal efficiency. In the formol-ether technique faeces are strained to remove large faecal debris. The formalin fixes the parasites and kills contaminating bacteria. Faecal debris is separated in a layer below the ether component which also serves to dissolve faecal fat (Fig. 11.15). The result is that parasitic cysts and ova are concentrated in the pellet in a preparation which is easier to examine because of the removal of faecal fat and debris.

Calibration of an eye-piece graticule

Accurately measuring the size of cysts and ova found in faecal preparation is the most important method of establishing the parasite's identity. To ensure accurate measurement the eye-piece graticule should be calibrated with the aid of a stage micrometer. The micrometer is placed on the microscope stage and the microscope focused on the micrometer scale with the ×10 objective (see Fig. 11.14). The stage is moved so that a large division of the graticule scale is aligned with the 0 line of the micrometer. The point at which the divisions of the graticule and micrometer are next aligned is noted and the number of micrometer divisions divided by the number of graticule divisions. The size of parasitic cysts can be calculated by multiplying the number of graticule divisions measured by the parasite by the number obtained in the calibration.

Normal faecal debris

Faeces contain many objects which may be mistaken for parasites, such as pollen grains, hair, muscle fibres, starch grains and even air bubbles!

Intestinal protozoa

Amoebae

Entamoeba histolytica is the major pathogenic amoeba of the gastrointestinal tract. Ingested cysts develop into vegetative amoebae in the colon. During their passage through the colon the trophozoites encyst into a form adapted for survival in the environment. *Entamoeba histolytica* infection may result in acute amoebic dysentery which is characterized by gradual onset with low or no fever and copious bulky offensive smelling stools with blood and mucus (see bacterial dysentery). Many patients have only mild symptoms or may be asymptomatic. In some cases intestinal infection can be overwhelming with severe colitis. In untreated or inadequately treated infection recurrent attacks of dysenteric symptoms may occur.

Entamoeba histolytica may invade beyond the intestine resulting in liver abscess and abdominal amoebomas. Rarely abscesses can be found in other organs including the lung and the brain.

There are three main clinical syndromes where a laboratory diagnosis is sought: acute amoebic dysentery; recurrent (chronic) infection or invasive disease (amoebic liver abscess, etc.).

Acute amoebic dysentery

The diagnosis of acute amoebic dysentery can be established by finding trophozoites of *E. histolytica* in fluid stool or in scrapings from rectal ulcers taken at sigmoidoscopic examination.

Specimens should be examined immediately, preferably on a heated stage, as the characteristic amoeboid movement of the trophozoite is lost as the specimen cools. Trophozoites should be sought with the ×10 objective and identified by their characteristic movement with pseudopodia. *Entamoeba histolytica* trophozoites may be distinguished from commensal amoebae such as *E. coli* by the presence of ingested red cells in the cytoplasm: trophozoites of non-pathogenic amoebae are found in faeces but do not ingest red cells.

Serology is of limited value in the diagnosis of acute amoebic dysentery as less than 50% of patients will have raised antibody titres. In addition, the presence of raised titres in a patient from an endemic country may relate to a previous infection.

Chronic amoebiasis

Faeces should be processed by the formol-ether concentration technique. 'Hot stools'

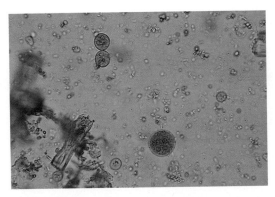

Figure 11.16 Cysts of *Entamoeba coli* and *E. histolytica* in stools

(i.e. freshly excreted) are unnecessary as trophozoites are unlikely to be found. As in the case of acute infection serological testing is not diagnostic. Cysts of *E. histolytica* must be differentiated from non-pathogens by determining the size and morphology. The distinguishing morphological features are the number of nuclei and size and shape of the chromatid body (see Table 11.4). The nuclei are more easily visualized using an iodine stain and the chromatid body can be demonstrated by staining (Burrow's or Sarguant's stain).

Entamoeba histolytica has no more than four nuclei, although young cysts may contain only one or two. In contrast between four and eight nuclei can be visualized in *E. coli*. The chromatoid bar of *E. histolytica* is short and broad with rounded ends compared with a needle-like structure in *E. coli* (Fig. 11.16: it may be difficult to see).

Invasive amoebiasis

Amoebic abscesses are often found in the absence of intestinal parasites, nonetheless faeces should be examined. The diagnosis is supported by finding a peripheral neutrophil leucocytosis and, in the case of amoebic liver abscess (ALA), a raised concentration of alkaline phosphatase in serum. Imaging of the liver and other organs by ultrasound and CT scanning can suggest the diagnosis.

In almost all patients anti-amoeba antibodies can be detected. The cellulose acetate precipitation (CAP) technique is a rapid method for use in ALA. Antibodies determined by this method are present during the acute phase of the infection but decline and disappear about three months after successful treatment. Antibodies can also be detected using an IFAT method. After invasive amoebic infection antibody concentrations are slower to rise than those detected by cellulose acetate precipitation CAP but remain positive for a prolonged period.

Giardia lamblia

Life cycle and habitat

Infection with *Giardia lamblia* occurs world-wide especially where poor sanitation allows water supplies and food to be contaminated with *Giardia* cysts. The life cycle is simple and man is the only host. Ingested infective cysts excyst to form flagellate trophozoites in the jejunum and multiply there by binary fission. They attach themselves strongly to the intestinal wall by a sucking disc and absorb nutrition. As the parasite passes down the intestine the trophozoite develops into the cyst form and is excreted in the faeces.

Clinical importance

Infection with *G. lamblia* is characterized by anorexia, crampy abdominal pain, borborygmi and flatus accompanied by bulky, offensive and fatty stools. Patients may lose weight and there may be an associated lactose intolerance or fat malabsorption. Relapse will occur if the patient is inadequately treated.

Laboratory diagnosis

The diagnosis of giardiasis can be established by finding cysts of *G. lamblia* in stools. A minimum of three stools should be examined as the shedding of giardia cysts is intermittent (diagnostic yield from one stool approx. 60%, three stools approx. 90%).

In cases with severe diarrhoea giardia trophozoites can sometimes be seen. To detect these a drop of a mucoid specimen should be placed on a glass slide and covered with a cover slip to make a thin preparation. The trophozoites have a characteristic concave shape (9–20 µm) with rotating motility ('the floating leaf'). Preparations may be stained by Fields, Wright's or Giemsa stain.

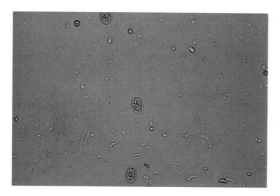

Figure 11.17   Cysts of *Giardia lamblia* in stools

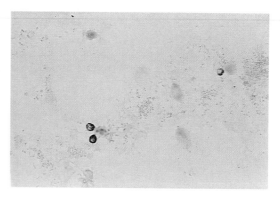

Figure 11.18   Ziehl-Neelsen preparation of stool showing *Cryptosporium parvum*

Faeces should be concentrated by the formol-ether technique and *Giardia* cysts are identified by size and shape: the cysts are oval measuring 10–12 µm $\times$ 6 µm, an axoneme can be seen in the cytoplasm (Fig. 11.17). An increased diagnostic yield may be obtained by using a direct immunofluorescent technique which utilizes monoclonal antibodies to *Giardia*. Several commercial test kits are available.

Jejunal contents can be obtained by aspiration, or 'Enterotest' string test. A preparation should be examined immediately for the presence of motile *Giardia* trophozoites, and stained with Giemsa. An ELISA technique detecting *Giardia* antigen in stool has been described but has not gained acceptance as a routine technique in diagnostic laboratories.

Cryptosporidium parvum

This coccidian parasite has recently been recognized as an important cause of human infection causing acute profuse watery diarrhoea in children. The symptoms last for between five and 10 days and resolve spontaneously. In patients who are severely immunocompromised such as those with AIDS an effective immune response does not develop and severe diarrhoea continues without resolution. Generalized acute infections may also occur in this patient group. There is currently no effective therapy, although some patients may benefit from treatment with spiramycin or azithromycin.

Cryptosporidiosis should be sought routinely in children with diarrhoea, and in all HIV-positive patients with diarrhoea. Infected patients usually produce high numbers of cysts and thus a concentration technique is not required. A direct smear should be made and stained with the cold Ziehl-Neelsen stain or an auramine phenol technique (Fig. 11.18). *Cryptosporidium parvum* can be transmitted to humans via water.

Cryptosporidia are 5 µm oval-round cysts which are acid fast. Direct immunofluorescence methods for faecal examination are available commercially.

Isospora belli

Isospora belli is another coccidian parasite which causes a self-limiting diarrhoeal disease. It is an uncommon pathogen in temperature zones, but may be acquired in tropical countries. In AIDS patients the parasite behaves in a similar manner to cryptosporidium and may not be eliminated. Cysts may be found in faeces but are less numerous than in *Cryptosporidium* infections. The formol-ether concentration technique should therefore be used. The oocysts can be detected with the $\times$10 objective and identified with the $\times$40 objective. *Isospora belli* oocysts are oval 32 $\times$ 16 µm. Immature cysts, which predominate in faeces, have a single zygote (Fig. 11.19). Two zygotes may be seen in mature oocysts.

Non-pathogenic protozoa in faeces

Many non-pathogenic protozoa may be found in human faeces. It is essential that these are

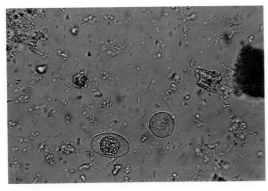

Figure 11.19 Unstained preparation of stool with cysts of *Isospora belli*

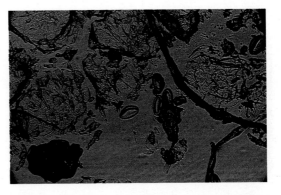

Figure 11.20 Sellotape preparation from a child with pinworm: *Enterobius vermicularis*

correctly identified and their non-pathogenic nature reported to clinicians (Table 11.4). Studies of isoenzyme patterns (zymodemes), have indicated that only some *E. histolytica* are associated with disease, these non-pathogenic zymodemes predominate in *E. histolytica* originating in the UK. '*E. histolytica*' with non-pathogenic zymodemes have been renamed *E. dispar*. Methods to determine zymodeme type require culture of amoebic trophozoites and starch gel electrophoresis together with detection systems for several enzymes. This is only available as a research technique.

Intestinal helminths

Introduction

Intestinal helminths are of considerable importance world-wide as a cause of chronic morbid-

ity. Fortunately heavy helminth infections are uncommon in developed countries. A more usual clinical situation is to discover helminth eggs incidentally, or as part of a screening procedure for travellers returning from endemic countries.

Threadworms

Enterobius vermicularis is a common parasite world-wide. It may be difficult to treat, and patients may suffer recurrent infections. *E. vermicularis* eggs are found in greatest numbers on the perianal skin shortly after going to bed or early in the morning before bathing. A Sellotape swab may be used to collect eggs from the perianal area. This consists of a microscope slide with a piece of adhesive tape fixed to one end. The tape is then folded over a tongue depressor exposing the sticky side, and forming a swab. This is pressed against several areas of

Table 11.4 Differentiation of intestinal parasitic cysts

Species	Size (μm)	Nuclei	Other features
Entamoeba histolytica	10–15	1–4	Blunt-ended chromatid bar in immature cyst
E. hartmanni	7–9	1–4	Blunt-ended chromatid bar in immature cyst
E. coli	16–30	1–8	Needle-like chromatid bar may be seen
Iod amoeba butschlii	9–15	1	Large glycogen vacuole in iodine preparation
Endolimax nana	6–9	4 (star-like)	–
Giardia lamblia	Oval (10 × 6)	4 (not seen)	Central axoneme
Chilomastix mesnili	Lemon-shaped 5–7	1	Cystosome

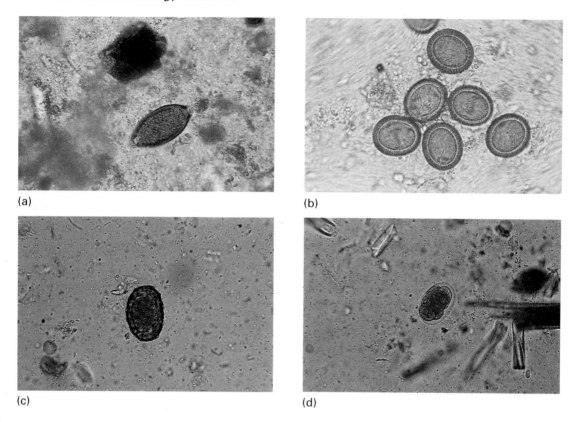

Figure 11.21   (*a*) Eggs of *Trichuris trichuria*. (*b*) Taenia eggs showing hooklets within. (*c*) Eggs of *Ascaris* spp. (*d*) Hookworm eggs

perianal skin in order to collect *E. vermicularis* eggs. The swab is then unfolded and stuck down to the microscope slide and smoothed with cotton. The slide is then examined microscopically (Fig. 11.20).

Hookworms

There are two main species of hookworm infecting man: *Ancylostoma duodenale* and *Necator americanus*. They cause disease by competing for nutrients, and by taking blood from the host which results in iron deficiency. Serious malnutrition can develop in heavy infections. Diagnosis is by demonstration of the characteristic eggs in the faeces (Fig. 11.21). The species can be distinguished only if ·the stools are cultures as for strongyloides and the hatching filariform larvae examined for their different morphology.

Trichuris and ascaris

Both of these species have a world-wide distribution and are very common. They cause disease by competing for nutrients with the host and in heavy infections signs of intestinal obstruction or rectal prolapse may be seen. Large numbers of eggs are produced and are therefore readily seen on examination of faecal specimens (see Fig. 11.21).

Strongyloides stercoralis

Strongyloides stercoralis differs from most other helminths in that it is able to multiply inside the human host. Strongyloides infection is usually lifelong with recurrent episodes of cutaneous larva migrans: larvae track under the skin leaving an inflammatory trail which is first oedematous and then red and itchy, fading over 48 hours. Soldiers who became infected while prisoners of war in the Far East are still being diagnosed as having active infection more than 40 years later.

In circumstances where the cell-mediated immunity is compromised uncontrolled multiplication takes place and severe generalized strongyloides (hyperinfection syndrome) infection (often accompanied with Gram-negative septicaemia) can occur. This syndrome can arise after commencement of steroid therapy, organ transplantation or in patients with HTLV 1 infection.

Laboratory diagnosis

Specimens

The laboratory diagnosis of strongyloidiasis can be made by examination of faeces for the presence of larvae, examination of intestinal string, and by serology. Rhabditiform larvae are rarely seen in saline-wet preparations, but may be found in specimens of mucus. Strongyloides are concentrated effectively by the formol-ether method but are killed by the formalin making the non-motile larvae difficult to see. Larvae are large and unsheathed 200–300 μm long and 15 μm across. There is a bulged oesophagus with a short buccal cavity. These features are used to distinguish *Strongyloides* from hookworm species.

In cases where strongyloidiasis is suspected a sample of faeces should be cultured with activated charcoal at room temperature for one week. The rhabtidiform larvae multiply and develop into filariform larvae which will migrate into fluid surrounding the culture. Fluid should be aspirated by pasteur pipette and examined microscopically. (*Caution*: filariform larvae are able to infect through normal skin.)

String test

The duodenal string test consists of a nylon thread with a weight which is contained within a gelatin capsule. One end is taped to the patient's cheek and the capsule swallowed. After two to three hours the string is recovered. If it is bile-stained, implying passage into the duodenum and jejunum, examination is worthwhile. The string is placed in a conical-bottomed tube or bottle, vortex mixed with physiological saline and centrifuged. The deposit is then examined for the presence of motile rhabitiform larvae.

Serological techniques

Several ELISA techniques have been described to detect antibodies to strongyloides and are usually more sensitive than culture or microscopy. *Strongyloides ratti* antigen has been used as the solid phase antigen. Although a sensitive method there is substantial cross-reaction between antibodies to *Strongyloides* and *Filaria*.

Taenia saginata and *Taenia solium*

These cestodes (platyhelminths) are the beef and pork tapeworms respectively: the intermediate host are cattle and pigs respectively. Man becomes infected by eating 'measly meat' which contains the intermediate cystic stage. Infection may be acquired world-wide in countries with inadequate meat inspection facilities. The pork tapeworm is rarely found in exclusively Islamic countries. After ingestion the cysts develop in the human host to a tapeworm which usually causes little symptoms in most patients. The pork tapeworm differs from the beef worm in that man can also act as the intermediate host and it is this phenomenon which is of most medical significance. The cystic stages are distributed throughout the tissues giving rise to cutaneous, subcutaneous and muscle lumps, but more seriously space-occupying lesions in the brain or spinal cord where they may cause seizures or transverse myelitis. This syndrome is known as cysticercosis.

Laboratory diagnosis

The diagnosis of an intestinal tapeworm is made by finding the characteristic eggs in the faeces. Occasionally whole or part of a tapeworm may be passed. The species may be identified by counting the number of lateral branches to the central uterine stem (15–20 in *T. saginata* and 7–13 in *T. solium*). When cysticercosis is suspected the diagnosis is often made on the basis of X-ray and CT-scan appearances. ELISA assays for measurement of anti-cysticercus antibody have proven to be a valuable adjunct to diagnosis.

Other cestode infections

There are two species mainly responsible for human hydatid disease *Echinococcus granulosis* and *E. multilocularis*. The diminutive tapeworms are found in the intestine of domestic and wild canids and the eggs passed in the faeces. The intermediate host of *E. granulosis* is the sheep who ingest the eggs and multiple cysts develop in the liver and lungs where the sexual stages take place. The cycle is complete when canids eat the tissues of infected sheep. Human hydatid disease occurs when man replaces sheep in the life cycle. *Echinococcus multilocularis* is found in foxes, wolves and dogs and small rodents as the intermediate hosts.

The symptoms and signs of hydatid disease are due to the effects of space-occupying lesions in the liver, lungs, abdominal cavity or CNS. *Echinococcus multilocularis* cysts lack a clear cyst wall in the human host and the 'cyst' may ramify widely in the tissue making operative intervention difficult.

The diagnosis is made on the basis of ultrasound and CT-scanning evidence of cysts supported by serological investigations for both specific antibody and in some centres hydatid antigen. Hydatid cysts may be removed operatively after a course of anthelminthic treatment has been given. The viability of the protoscolices can be determined by mixing the fluid with eosin: viable protoscolices will exclude the eosin (Fig. 11.22).

Schistosomiasis

There are three main species affecting humans, *Schistosoma mansoni*, *S. haematobium* and *S. japonicum*. *Schistosoma mansoni* is found in Africa and South America, and *S. haematobium* only in Africa; *S. japonicum* is least common and is confined to the Far East.

Humans become infected when schistosome cercaria penetrate the skin. Once inside the body they develop into male and female adult worms and after migration may be found in the veins of the superior or inferior mesenteric

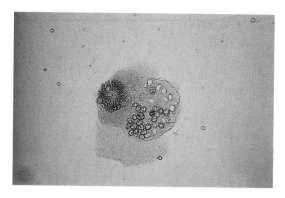

Figure 11.22   Protoscolices of echinococcus

plexus or the vesical plexus depending on the species.

The initial illness is characterized by fever, mild hepatosplenomegaly, skin rash and arthralgia – known as Katayama fever. When egg laying begins there may be an episode of bloody diarrhoea or haematuria. Later, in heavy infection, the fibrotic reaction to schistosome eggs deposited in the liver results in hepatic fibrosis and portal hypertension. Eggs in other sites may cause fibrotic changes in the lungs, the bladder (in the case of *S. haematobium*) and space-occupying lesions in the brain and spinal cord.

Laboratory diagnosis

In developed countries most of the patients are returning travellers in whom heavy worm burdens and severe pathology are rarely found. The diagnosis of schistosomiasis can be established by demonstrating the presence of schistosome eggs in stool, urine, rectal snips or other tissue biopsy or by finding serological evidence of infection together with eosinophilia and appropriate clinical signs.

When faecal samples are consistently negative and schistosomiasis is suspected rectal biopsy may provide a positive diagnosis.

Schistosoma haematobium adults are found in the veins of the vesical plexus and eggs are expelled into the urine. Urine should be collected at mid-day and 10 ml passed through a polycarbonate filter (12–14 µm). It is then examined under a light microscope for the presence of trapped schistosome eggs (Fig. 11.23).

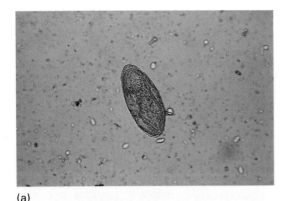

(a)

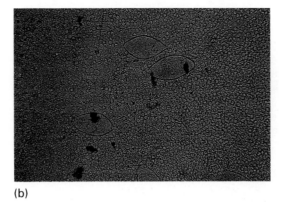

(b)

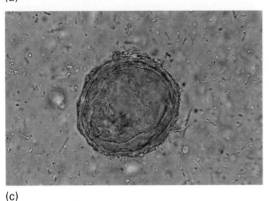

(c)

Figure 11.23 (*a*) Eggs of *Schistosoma mansoni* with lateral spine. (*b*) *S. haematobium* eggs with terminal spine. (*c*) *S. japonicum* egg

Several ELISA techniques have been described for the detection of antibodies to schistosoma. Soluble egg antigens (usually of *S. mansoni*) are used for the solid phase, and a number of other highly purified antigens are being evaluated. Serology is of most value in patients with suspected schistosomiasis who have had a defined exposure, e.g. returned travellers.

Toxocariasis

Toxocara canis is a canine ascarid parasite which causes visceral larva migrans or ocular granulomas when humans become infected. Eggs excreted in the faeces of dogs require two weeks' incubation in the soil before they are infective. Infection is common in children who have poor hand hygiene and in those who are occupationally exposed to dogs at the time of whelping.

The parasite is unable to develop through its full life cycle in the human host and develop-ment is halted at the second L$_2$ stage. Larvae migrate through the tissues and the inflamma-tory response to their presence is responsible for the symptoms and signs of the disease. Visceral larva migrans is characterized by fever, cough, bronchospasm, abdominal pain, lymphadenopathy, and hepatosplenomegaly. When a larva lodges in the retina a granuloma develops and if this is centrally placed complete loss of vision will follow.

As toxocara is unable to complete its life cycle in humans eggs cannot be found in the faeces but a serological diagnosis is easily made using an ELISA which uses excreted antigen in the solid phase.

Trichinosis

Trichinella spiralis is a parasite of carnivores with a wide host range. Humans become infected when they eat undercooked meat, often pork or bear. Adult worms live in the intestine for up to two months and the female produces larvae which migrate to skeletal muscle where they invade, develop and encyst.

Early infection may be marked by mild diarrhoea and fever myositis, periorbital oedema and eosinophilia. A definitive diagnosis is made by demonstrating the parasite in a muscle biopsy. Antibodies begin to rise four weeks after infection and can be detected by direct immunofluorescence.

Liver flukes

The two main liver flukes infecting man are *Fasciola hepatica* which has a world-wide distribution and *Clonorchis sinensis* which is found in South-East Asia. Fasciola infection is acquired by ingestion of aquatic vegetation which has been contaminated by an intermediate stage (encysted metacercaria). The metacercaria migrate to the liver and adults develop. Disease results from liver damage and the effects of ectopic worms. *Clonorchis* is acquired by eating undercooked fish which have metacercaria encysted under their scales.

Diagnosis of both infections is by demonstrating the characteristic eggs in the faeces. Pseudofascioliasis can be diagnosed if a patient has recently consumed infected cattle or sheep as the eggs contained in the meal will pass through the intestine.

Pneumocystis carinii

Taxonomy

The taxonomic position of *Pneumocystis* is not clear. Its life cycle of trophozoite and cyst stages resembles that of a protozoan, it responds to 'anti-protozoal' but not antifungal agents and microtubular structure and membrane fusion function similar to protozoa. The pneumocystis 16_s and 18_s rRNA sequence is more similar to fungal than some protozoa species. Like fungi *Pneumocystis* is sensitive to candin antibiotics and has a separate dihydrofolate reductase and dihydropteroate synthetase.

Clinical importance

Pneumocystis carinii infection was once a very rare cause of pneumonia in the immuno-compromised and severely malnourished. The AIDS epidemic was detected in part because of an increase in requests for pentamidine to treat young men with this condition. It was thought that pneumocystis infection was acquired at an early age and that subsequent immunocompromise allowed latent infection to re-emerge. There is, however, evidence that infection can be transmitted from person to person.

The conditions associated with developing *P. carinii* are cyclosporin and steroid therapy, T-cell lymphomas and HTLV-1-associated leukaemia. HIV infected patients are not likely to develop infection until the CD4 count falls below $0.2 \times 10^9/l$.

Patients present with a dry cough and increasing dyspnoea over days or weeks. They may experience difficulty in taking a deep breath but rarely have pleuritic pain. Patients are usually febrile at presentation but sweats are rare. There are few clinical signs on examination of the chest but other stigmata of AIDS may be present.

Pneumocystis carinii is an important presenting and AIDS-defining condition. It is an important cause of mortality and morbidity. Although much work has been performed in describing major antigens of *P. carinii* the pathogenesis of the disease remains obscure.

Laboratory diagnosis

The clinical diagnosis of pneumocystis infection is supported by X-ray appearance of the chest which can be highly variable, arterial blood gases and exercise oximetry.

Specimens

Sputum is rarely produced and has a low diagnostic yield when available. Specimens can be obtained by bronchoalveolar lavage. Sputum may be induced when the patient inhales a nebulized solution of hypertonic saline. The mucoid material which is coughed up can be used for microscopical diagnosis. Sensitivity of this technique in comparison to bronchoalveolar lavage is up to 55% when performed by experienced ward and laboratory staff.

Direct microscopy

The cysts of *Pneumocystis* are stained by

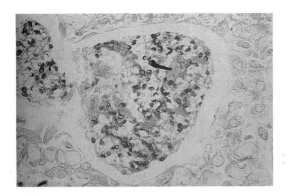

Figure 11.24 Lung stained with Grocott stain. *Pneumocystis carinii* shown as black cyst-like structures

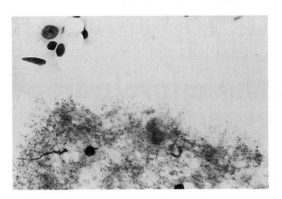

Figure 11.25 Trophozoites of *Pneumocystis carinii* from a bronchoalveolar lavage of an AIDS patient. (Stained with Giemsa)

Table 11.5 Examples of helminth eggs found in human specimens

Species	Size (microns)	Special features
Hookworm	50–60 × 40–45	Thin shelled
Ascaris lumbricoides	50–70 × 40–50	Thin
Taenia spp.	30–40 × 20–30	Thick, round shell
Trichuris trichuria	50–55 × 22–24	Double speculum
Enterobius vermicularis	45–50 × 25–30	D-shaped
Schistosoma mansoni	115–175 × 45–70	Lateral spine
S. japonicum	70–100 × 55–65	Spine scarcely visible
Fasciola hepatica	130–150 × 60–90	Operculum
Clonorchis sinensis (Opisthorchis)	27–35 × 12–20	Operculum and small, terminal spine
S. haematobium	110–170 × 40–70	Terminal spine

Papanicolou, methenamine-silver (Fig. 11.24), and toluidine blue. The trophozoites may be stained by Giemsa or Dif-Quik (Fig. 11.25). Monoclonal antibodies which bind to the surface of *Pneumocystis* have been successfully used in a direct fluorescence test. It is a more expensive and time consuming test to perform and cross-reactions with *Aspergillus* and *Candida* have been described.

Serology

Antibody detection is of little diagnostic value as many patients have antibodies to *Pneumocystis* and patients sufficiently immunocompromised to be at risk of this infection are usually unable to mount a significant antibody response.

Antigen detection methods have been described but have suffered from significant problems with false-positive results. Methods based on the polymerase chain reaction have been described and promise much for the future.

Antibiotic susceptibility

Pneumocystis carinii is susceptible to folate antagonists such as sulphamethoxazole, trimethoprim, pyramethamine, dapsone. It is also sensitive to pentamidine which may be given parenterally or by aerosol for prophylaxis. Promising results have also been obtained with a combination of primaquine and clindamycin.

12

The microbiology laboratory: organization and quality assurance

Microbiology staff

Clinical microbiologist

The clinical microbiologist has a central role in the investigation of patients with infection. This includes advising on appropriate specimens, their collection and transportation to the laboratory and supervision of laboratory examination. Once the results have been obtained, the clinical microbiologist must interpret the results to clinical colleagues and advise on appropriate therapeutic measures to be taken or further investigations to be performed.

In the UK, the role of the clinical microbiologist is unique. Their function, in the hospital setting, is similar in nature to that of infectious diseases physicians in the USA consulting on the investigation and treatment of patients with infections. In addition to these responsibilities, clinical microbiologists manage the laboratory in collaboration with scientific staff, using their knowledge of the clinical problems posed to plan laboratory investigations so that the most rapid and effective laboratory reports are provided.

Medical laboratory scientific officers (MLSOs)

The main role of the MLSO is to examine clinical specimens according to agreed laboratory protocols. It is, thus, that the burden to provide rapid accurate reproducible results falls mainly on the MLSOs and this usually includes the provision of an 'out of hours' service.

In addition, senior MLSOs manage laboratory house-keeping: ordering equipment, reagents, maintenance, supervising collection of specimens and safe disposal of waste. They also have a major role in ensuring adequate quality control of laboratory media and reagents used in the examination of specimens. In some hospitals they also play a role in the control of hospital infection, investigating ward outbreaks and offering advice on methods of preventing spread of micro-organisms.

Scientific officers

In some laboratories a third group of microbiology staff is employed: scientific officers. Their role is often to develop new laboratory techniques, plan and execute the introduction of techniques and evaluate the quality of work. Senior scientific officers may act as laboratory managers and in the absence of a clinically qualified microbiologist provide advice to clinicians.

In addition to these three main groups, all laboratories need the support of clerical and administrative staff who receive, register specimens and dispatch completed reports to wards and general practitioners. Porters, cleaners, and maintenance engineers all play a part in the smooth running of the laboratory.

Control of infection officer

The control of infection officer for a hospital is usually one of the consultant microbiologists or a consultant in communicable diseases control. The post holder is normally the chairman of the control of infection committee which meets regularly to discuss matters relating to controlling the transmission of infection in the hospital environment. It is not possible to state what is in the remit of the group as it must be free to tackle all subjects which may be relevant. The likely spectrum of topics is diverse ranging from nurses' uniforms, through provision of side room accommodation and boarding of patients to engineering matters such as the plumbing system or cooling towers which might act as a reservoir for legionellas, and the control of clinical waste.

The control of infection officer is responsible for the production of guidelines for the prevention of nosocomial infection. When outbreaks of infection occur it is the responsibility of the control of infection officer to coordinate the investigation and control measures required. To execute these duties fully and to provide advice to hospital management on projects which will have a bearing on infection in the hospital it is inevitable that attendance at many meetings will be necessary when, for example, new service developments, buildings or extensions are being planned.

Control of infection nurse

The control of infection nurse is administratively responsible to nursing management but operationally responsible to the control of infection officer. The control of infection nurse is responsible for supervising the implementation of the control of infection guidelines, and plays a key part in investigating potential outbreaks and liaising with the nursing staff on the wards so that infected patients are placed in the correct isolation facilities. In addition, he or she collects data on transmission of infection, and provides advice to the junior medical and nursing staff on clinical procedures such as urinary catheterization or care of intravenous lines. As a result the control of infection nurse will have a major role in the education of members of staff in control of infection practice.

Accreditation

Individual users of the microbiology laboratory are usually not in a position to judge the quality of the results provided. To ensure that pathology services are of a high quality many countries have set up national accreditation schemes. In the USA this role is discharged by the Federal Drugs Administration, and in the UK by Clinical Pathology Accreditation (CPA), a company jointly owned by pathology professional bodies, several Royal Colleges, and Health Services Associations.

Accreditation seeks to audit externally departmental organization and quality assurance programmes. Pathology laboratories apply for accreditation by confirming fulfilment of standards laid down by the accrediting body. All disciplines of the pathology apply as a whole or in isolation. Accreditation is awarded provisionally and confirmed after a later site visit when compliance with the standards is validated by inspection. This accreditation visit is performed by inspectors who will usually work in pairs, a consultant or similar grade scientist, and a senior medical laboratory scientific officer. In a pathology department with the four main specialties, four teams will visit on a single day with one of the team acting as chairman. As well as inspecting for compliance with the accreditation standards confidential opinions will be sought from users and hospital managers. After a satisfactory site visit accreditation is granted but if problems are detected full accreditation is withheld until these are resolved. An appeal can be made to the CPA board if there is a disagreement with the decisions of the inspectors.

Accreditation standards

A total of 44 standards has been set divided into six headings. These relate to the organization and administration, staffing and direction, facilities and equipment, policies and protocols, staff development and education, and quality evaluation.

Medical audit

Over recent years there has been an attempt to develop systems to evaluate the quality of medical services provided. In the setting of pathology the areas of concern are with access of users to the service, and the availability of results in a time frame which facilitates clinical decisions. It is also concerned with the use of resources and the process of work. In addition audit seeks to uncover the impact of the laboratory service has on patient care and its influence on patient well-being.

Microbiologists may also participate in the audit of other clinical specialties where topics related to infection are discussed. In some institutions it may be possible to establish a multidisciplinary infection audit team which includes microbiologists, infection diseases specialists, other clinicians and the control of infection staff.

Laboratory controls

The diagnostic process is complicated and many controls are necessary to ensure the best results. These controls are of different types: i.e. there are process and batch controls and audit procedures. The nomenclature of the controls applied in laboratories can be confusing but some of these are set out below.

Quality assessment

This term is often confused with quality control as quality is usually assessed by the processing of externally supplied specimens which have become colloquially known as 'quality control specimens'. All quality assessment schemes are broadly based on WHO criteria for such services.

The UK has a national system of quality assessment, the National External Quality Assessment Scheme (NEQAS), which is employed by microbiology laboratories and other pathology disciplines. Specimens are sent to participating laboratories which contain any pathogen except those in Hazard Group 4. These specimens must be examined by normal laboratory protocols. Organisms included are those which most laboratories should be able to identify but the frequency of distribution will not reflect their prevalence in UK practice as more emphasis must be given to pathogens of public health importance which only occur rarely such as *C. diphtheriae* or *V. cholerae*. Schemes for syphilis serology, antimicrobial assay, parasitology, mycology and tuberculosis microscopy are also available.

Individual specimens are subject to internal quality control at NEQAS as specimens are sent to geographically diverse locations, processed to demonstrate whether the expected results are obtained and posted back to the base laboratory. In addition duplicate samples are available to laboratories which have failed to correctly identify the organism. A detailed breakdown of the results obtained together with teaching material is sent to each participating laboratory.

The essential components of the scheme are that it is national in that specimens are sent to most laboratories within the country and thus results can be compared with peer laboratories. This also allows the scheme to investigate the effects of individual technologies on results when in addition to the result the means whereby they are obtained are also reported. It is confidential: this enables laboratories to participate without fear of censure so that when deficiencies are found they may be speedily rectified.

External quality assessment is not without difficulties. It is more difficult to disguise external preserved specimens so there is a danger that laboratory staff may deal with these specimens in a different manner than from routine specimens. Any special treatment afforded to these specimens does, in part, reduce their value in determining the quality of service for 'normal specimens'. Special processing is also likely to develop as a form of competition between laboratories or as a means of ensuring that the laboratory gets the result right. In this context the right result may be the wrong one if it points to areas where basic laboratory practice could be improved.

Good laboratory practice

Good laboratory practice refers to the organizational aspects of laboratory management which are needed to ensure good quality results are consistently produced. It includes the provision of laboratory manuals, a documented programme of calibration and maintenance for laboratory equipment and a staff training and development programme.

To ensure good laboratory practice a series of detailed protocols must be written. These include standard operating procedures (SOPs) for the use and maintenance of equipment which detail the way in which equipment is to be used, calibration and records, and the maintenance cycle. Standard operating procedures should also include the work of non-technical staff including clerical, portering and cleaning staff. A laboratory methods manual should be available at the point of use detailing all the methods used at that work station.

A safety manual must be written in a way that is comprehensible to all grades of staff and explains the action necessary to ensure a safe working environment. A copy must be given to all members of staff and it is advisable that they certify its receipt and that they understand the information it contains. Senior technical staff should be available to explain the manual and the instructions it contains.

Laboratory manual

The laboratory manual should be drawn up by the senior MLSOs and should provide a detailed method for performing each laboratory test. The manual should be signed and dated by the senior staff and regularly reviewed so that individual tests do not become outdated or subject to 'protocol drift'. (Protocol drift is where small changes are made in a procedure on an *ad hoc* basis without alteration in the laboratory manual.) The inevitable result of protocol drift is inconsistent results and confusion for new and trainee staff. The manual should provide a standard of practice which can be monitored by senior MLSOs.

Each method should include details of the materials required for the technique and this should include details of the shelf-life, stock control and quality control of each component. The equipment required must also be clearly stated and reference should be made to the standard operating procedure to be employed in using this equipment. The specimen

required for the test should be defined together with methods for assessing suitability for processing where relevant (e.g. sputum, see p. 181).

The methods must be simply written so that it could be performed by new staff. By writing the method for beginners no prior knowledge is assumed and the final result is likely to be clearer. The results which can be obtained and how these results are to be interpreted must be clearly described. A clear reporting strategy must be recorded, i.e. what isolates are reported and what sensitivities performed.

Quality control

Quality control refers to the control of materials, media and tests performed in a microbiology laboratory. Each laboratory must have a comprehensive system of quality control for each of its diagnostic activities. This includes the production of media, identification tests, antibiotic susceptibility tests, antibiotic assays and serological techniques. Considerations of quality control in these areas will be discussed in more detail in the relevant chapters. We will focus here mainly on the steps required for quality control of microbiological media.

Quality control of media

The quality of microbiological media is central to the value of a laboratory. An enrichment medium which is insufficiently nutritious to support the target pathogen will result in many false-negative cultures. A similar situation will arise if a selective medium is too inhibitory suppressing the pathogen as well as the normal flora. If, however, the medium is not sufficiently inhibitory commensal organisms will overgrow the plate obscuring the pathogen sought.

The quality of media can be controlled in two ways: process control and batch control. It is the latter which is often referred to as quality control. Process control depends on having a set of standard operating procedures for operation of equipment used in media production, sterilization, methods and recipes describing the production of medium whether this be from a commercial manufacturer or

Table 12.1 Examples of control organisms for quality control of laboratory medium

Culture medium	Control organism(s)	Expected reaction
Brain heart infusion	*Staph. aureus* NCTC 6571	Growth in 24 hours
Blood agar	*Strep. pyogenes* ATCC 19615	Small clear grey beta-haemolytic colonies
Crystal violet blood agar	*S. pyogenes* (selected) *S. aureus* (inhibited)	Beta-haemolysis No growth
MacConkey agar	*Escherichia coli* NCTC 10418 *Proteus* spp. NCTC 10823 *Streptococcus*	Pink colonies Pale colonies Growth inhibited
Xylose lysine desoxycholate	*E. coli* *S. typhimurium* NCTC 12023 *Sh. sonnei* ATCC 25931 *Streptococcus* spp.	Yellow colonies Pale colonies Red colonies Inhibited
Selenite F broth	*S. typhimurium* *E. coli*	Growth No growth
Urea broth	*Proteus vulgaris* *E. coli*	Pink colour 4–6 hours No change
New York City medium	*N. gonorrhoeae* NCTC 8375 *Proteus vulgaris* NCTC 4175	Luxuriant growth Inhibited

made up in-house. The quality of reagents which goes into the medium including water pH and ion content must also be clearly set out and methods for measurement and if necessary rejection of batches laid down.

In batch control two areas must be considered: the physical characteristics of the medium and its microbiological performance.

Physical characteristics must include the appearance of the medium: a blood agar plate in which the red cells have settled is not satisfactory for testing haemolysis. The physical appearance and the limits of variation should be described in the method. The medium should have an adequate gel, growth will be poor and the colonies small if the gel is too hard; conversely soft medium is difficult to work with as it has a tendency to tear.

Medium should be controlled in its pH as deviations in this important criterion will result in poor growth in pH-sensitive organisms. This can be tested with a simple pH meter. Isolation and identification media must be reliably sterile, thus samples from each batch poured should be tested for sterility at 37°C and at room temperature before the batch is released.

The shelf-life of media should be established and a stock control system instituted to ensure only in-date stock is used.

The microbiological performance of media should be controlled with a panel of standard organisms. These may be established locally but it is better to use those recommended in standard textbooks, by the PHLS or by the American NCCLS. Stocks of control organisms can be obtained from the National Collection of Type Cultures and American Type Culture Collection.

Standard cultures are used to ensure that medium is sufficiently nutritious to support the growth of fastidious pathogens. This may be achieved by performing a viable count of an overnight growth of a control organism or by the Miles and Misra technique or counting the colonies after a standardized plating method. In addition to demonstrating adequate nutritional support characteristic appearances or reactions should be present, e.g. beta-haemolysis or coloured colonies due to indicator changes. For selective media the ability to suppress unwanted organisms should be demonstrated in parallel to support for the target organisms. Some examples of control organisms are found in Table 12.1.

13

Safety in the laboratory

Introduction

A microbiology laboratory deals with large numbers of clinical specimens, many of which contain human pathogens. Indeed, it is the job of a microbiology laboratory to isolate pathogens, often in large numbers. So, far from avoiding infectious agents, the microbiologist is bent on seeking them. There is a danger, however, that pathogens may be approached with insufficient respect, as if with familiarity there is also immunity.

In the past safety has often held a low priority in hospitals and laboratories. This contrasts with some industries, notably the airlines where the emphasis on safety has led to the development of a 'safety culture'. The Control of Substances Hazardous to Health Act has brought in regulations which have forced safety to the top of the agenda in laboratories.

Many countries have national codes to reduce the risk of laboratory acquired infection. In the UK the report of the committee chaired by Sir James Howie formed the basis of laboratory safety guidelines. This has now been revised in the light of the changes which have taken place in diagnostic laboratories and the equipment that they use (*Safe working and the prevention of infection in clinical laboratories*, see Further reading).

It is also important that microbiology laboratories widen their perspective. Although there is an inevitable focus on biological hazard many toxic chemicals are used, and other physical hazards such as radiation and fire must be considered.

Control of substances hazardous to health (COSHH)

The COSHH regulations were introduced to limit the exposure of workers to hazardous substances. A substance hazardous to health is defined as 'any natural or artificial substance: solid, liquid or vapour or hazardous microorganism'.

The essence of the regulations is to evaluate the hazard of each procedure, to plan methods to eliminate or reduce that hazard and monitor any exposure to hazardous substances. If a hazard is unavoidable a health surveillance programme must be built into the protocol.

The assessment of risk (the COSHH assessment) must be made by a competent person, e.g. a senior MLSO or scientist. It must be written, available to the workers and subject to regular review. The preparation of these assessments is an opportunity for discussion in the workplace which will orientate the whole staff to the priority of safety.

The act requires that employers ensure that the control measures are properly used and that safety equipment, personal protective equipment and controls are properly maintained. It is required that 'all necessary information, instruction and training' are provided to employees.

These regulations require a significant amount of paperwork and organization. A number of manuals published by major chemical companies have simplified the completion of COSHH assessments.

Table 13.1 Examples of bacteria, viruses, protozoan and fungi defined by hazard group (according to Advisory Committee for Dangerous Pathogens)

Hazard group	Bacteria	Viruses	Fungi	Parasites
4	–	Lassa fever virus Ebola virus	–	–
3	*Mycobacterium* *tuberculosis* *Coxiella burnetti* *S. typhi*	Japanese B encephalitis virus Rabies virus	*Histoplasma capsulatum* *Coccidioides immitis* *Paracoccidioides brasiliensis*	Leishmania* *Trypanosoma cruzi* *Naegleria* spp.
2	*Bacteroides* spp. *Staph. aureus* *E. coli*	Adenovirus Measles virus Mumps virus	*Candida albicans* *Aspergillus flavus* *Aspergillus fumigatus*	*Plasmodium* spp. *Pneumocystis carinii* *E. histolytica*

* Safety cabinet is not essential.

Developing a safety policy

In developing a satisfactory safety system, the main areas for consideration are:

1 Assessment of the risks of transmission of infection
2 The design of the laboratory and equipment which will facilitate safe handling of pathogens
3 Development of laboratory protocols which have safety procedures built in
4 Effective decontamination of pathogenic material
5 Monitoring of safety
6 Education of staff and occupational health

Assessment of risks

Each procedure within the laboratory can be examined to assess the risk of transmitting infection and to plan methods which minimize those risks. When the pathogens found in clinical specimens are known it is wise to remember that more than one pathogen may be present. Knowledge of likely pathogens together with their route of transmission enables appropriate techniques to be considered.

Classification of pathogens

It is fundamental to safe working practices that pathogens are correctly categorized. The Advisory Committee for Dangerous Pathogens (ACDP) is charged with advising laboratory workers of the hazards of micro-organisms in the UK, and other countries have similar systems. The ACDP has adopted four hazard groups and these are described briefly below (Table 13.1).

Category 1: An organism that is most unlikely to cause human disease.

Category 2: An organism that may cause human disease and that might be a hazard to laboratory workers but is unlikely to spread in the community. Laboratory exposure rarely produces infection and effective prophylaxis or treatment is usually available.

Category 3: An organism that may cause severe human disease and presents a serious hazard to laboratory workers. It may present a risk of spread to the community, but there is usually effective prophylaxis or effective treatment is available.

Category 4: An organism that causes severe human disease and is a serious hazard to laboratory workers. It may present a high risk of spread to the community and there is usually no effective prophylaxis or treatment (see Table 13.1).

Routes of transmission

There are four main routes of transmission which occur within a laboratory.

Oral transmission

The acquisition of an infective agent in the laboratory via the oral route may occur, especially when intestinal pathogens are isolated in pure culture. For some organisms such as *Shigella* spp. the infective dose is very low.

Aerosols

Organisms which are capable of invading the body via the respiratory tract may cause infection in laboratory areas if aerosols containing such organisms are produced in the course of laboratory work. Laboratory practice should be reviewed to minimize the risk of aerosol production (see below).

Laboratories should have negative pressure (airflows from the corridor into the laboratory). Organisms which are readily transmitted by the aerosol route, e.g. *M. tuberculosis*, should be manipulated in a safety cabinet located in a special laboratory or a suite of laboratories should be set aside for this purpose. This is discussed in more detail below.

Parenteral

Some organisms only pose a risk within the laboratory if inoculated through the skin. This can occur when specimens or cultures are accidentally injected with a needle or when accidents occur with sharp materials such as broken glass. A few organisms such as *Leptospira*, *Treponema* and the rhabditiform larvae of *Strongyloides* are capable of invading through intact skin.

Mucosal

Organisms may be transmitted through mucosal surfaces by splashing into the eye; these are generally the same sort of organisms which are transmitted by the parenteral route. Mucosal splashing can occur at any time when fluids are being manipulated, especially when pipetting, while washing enzyme-linked immunosorbent assay (ELISA) plates, or dropping materials into liquid.

Reducing the risk of oral transmission

Oral transmission is minimized by ensuring separation between work and recreation areas. For this reason, laboratory areas must be separated from rest rooms where food may be eaten. Food must not be brought into, or consumed in, laboratory areas. There must be no smoking, chewing, or drinking, and cosmetics should not be applied while in laboratory areas. Mouth pipetting should not take place. Where appropriate, latex gloves should be worn. Laboratory coats of the Howie type (coats which are closed to the neck with press studs and have elasticated cuffs) should be worn within the laboratory and should be removed before leaving. Laboratory workers should wash their hands whenever they are known to have been contaminated and before leaving the laboratory.

Reducing the risk of aerosol transmission

There are a number of basic microbiological techniques and procedures in which aerosols may be readily generated. These include homogenization of tissues with mechanical or manual grinders or similar techniques. Aerosols may also be generated by careless use of bacteriological loops, especially if they are large and poorly made. Aerosols may be created when loops are made to vibrate during use. To minimize these risks, the loop should be 2–3 mm in diameter and completely closed. Nichrome wire is usual but another alternative is platinum wire which vibrates much less during use. Flaming of loops may result in spattering small droplets of bacteriological cultures. There is little evidence that significant aerosols are created in this way but to reduce these potential risks, a number of different micro-incinerators have been designed, both gas and electric (Fig. 13.1).

Aerosols are generated when hot loops are plunged into liquid cultures. This may be simply prevented by using a loop which has been allowed to cool fully. Aerosols may also be generated during slide agglutination, especially if the organism, saline and antiserum are mixed too vigorously. When agglutinations are performed on hazardous

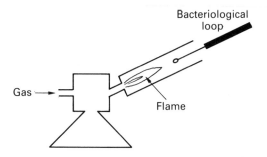

Figure 13.1 Micro-incinerators reduce the risk of viable organism 'spilling' when the loop is flamed

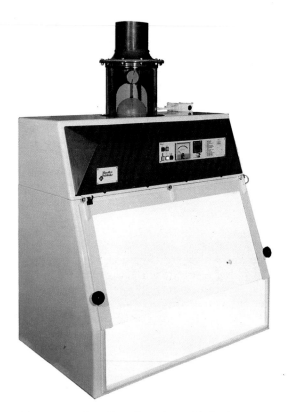

Figure 13.2 Class I cabinet. Air is drawn into the cabinet and exhausted through a HEPA filter

micro-organisms (category 3) they should be performed in a safety cabinet. Formol saline (10%) can also be used to reduce these risks.

When a catalase test is performed by adding a drop of hydrogen peroxide on a glass slide, the bubbling of positive organisms may result in dispersal of organisms into the air. A simple method of preventing this is to touch the tip of a capillary tube containing hydrogen peroxide onto the suspect colony. If catalase is present in the organism, bubbles rise inside the tube and remain there (see Fig. 2.3).

When specimens or cultures contain hazardous organisms which may be transmitted via the respiratory route (category 3) are being examined in the laboratory, manipulations should take place within a Class I safety cabinet conforming to BS 5726 in a separate laboratory room (containment level 3 laboratory) (Fig. 13.2 and Table 13.2).

The high energy involved in centrifugation may result in generation of aerosols if the specimen containers break during a run. Centrifugation of patient materials containing pathogens transmitted via the respiratory route should be performed in sealed centrifuge buckets, which will contain any aerosol generated. The sealed buckets should be opened inside a Class I safety cabinet.

Reducing the risk of parenteral transmission

Many organisms such as hepatitis B virus, HIV, and trypanosomes are transmitted via the parenteral route. The risk of transmission can be reduced by ensuring that latex gloves are worn at all times when specimens or cultures of organisms known to be transmitted by this route are handled. This prevents the

Table 13.2 Summary of characteristics of microbiological safety cabinets

	Pathogens	Inflow	Outflow	Protection of work	Protection of worker
Class I	2, 3	Room air	HEPA filtered	+/−	++
Class II	2, 3	Room air HEPA filtered	HEPA filtered	++	+
Class III	2, 3, 4	HEPA filtered air	HEPA filtered	++	+++

accidental inoculation through small cuts and abrasions which may unknowingly be present. Laboratory procedures should be carefully reviewed to minimize the use of needles, scalpels and other sharp instruments. Where possible plastics should replace glass and specimens should be decontaminated whenever this can be done without compromising the results of any investigation (e.g. formalinizing CSF for cell counts).

The use of sharps and the accidental breakage of glass equipment is inevitable. It is important that adequate sharps containers are available. There are many commercial sharps containers which are made of robust plastic or cardboard and can retain liquids.

Reducing the risk of mucosal transmission

Organisms may be transmitted after splashing specimens or cultures into the eye. Techniques should be examined to prevent splashing and eye protection should be worn where possible.

Structural aspects of safety

Laboratory safety is facilitated by a well-designed laboratory suite. Attention must be paid to the materials employed in floors, walls and benching, in the provision of services including water supply and ventilation.

High containment facilities (level 3) must be provided for any laboratory likely to isolate organisms in Hazard Group 3 or which examines specimens which might contain such organisms (e.g. sputum). A laboratory suite may contain many laboratories and facilities, such as media preparation rooms, autoclave facilities, an incubator room, and a cold room. Each of the individual laboratories within the clinical microbiology suite should conform to containment level 2 or containment level 3 (ACDP regulations).

Several features are common to both levels of containment. Laboratories should be of an adequate size, with 24 m³ for each laboratory worker. Where walls may be splashed with biological materials, they should be impervious to chemicals used in the laboratory. The laboratory should be easy to clean and bench surfaces should be impervious to water and resistant to acids, alkalis, solvents and commonly used disinfectants. Suitable materi-

als for benches include laminates. Traditional teak benching is no longer recommended but where it is already in place it must be fully sealed and adequately repaired where cracking has occurred. Laminates have the advantage that they may be moulded at front and rear to prevent liquid spillage.

Care must be taken to ensure that benches are at a comfortable working height. Fatigue and backache caused by uncomfortable working positions will predispose to accidents.

Laboratory floors should be seamless, impermeable to liquids and resistant to acids, alkalis, and solvents used within the laboratory areas.

A wash hand basin and coat-hooks should be located near the laboratory exit. Taps should be of the type which may be operated without the use of the hands. Access to the laboratory should be limited to designated members of staff.

Special requirements of containment level 3

A containment level 3 laboratory should be sited away from the main work of the department and access limited to authorized personnel who are trained in the use of the room and in the manipulation of Hazard Group 3 organisms. The doors should be locked when not in use. A continuous airflow into the laboratory must be maintained when work is in progress. A system must operate to prevent positive pressurization of the room if the extraction fans fail. Reversed airflows into the ventilation system must also be prevented.

The laboratory should be equipped with glass panels so that those working within can be seen in case there is an accident. A biohazard sign designating the laboratory as containment level 3 must be displayed along with a list of those authorized to use the laboratory.

The laboratory should contain sufficient equipment for all of the techniques to be carried out including a centrifuge with sealed buckets, incubators, refrigerator, and deep freeze. Adequate storage within the laboratory should also be available so that workers are not required to leave the laboratory frequently to replenish supplies. A microbiological safety of class 1 or class 3 conforming to BS 5726 must be available and all procedures where cultures or specimens are manipulated must be performed in this cabinet. It should be exhausted through a HEPA filter to the outside air. The laboratory should be sealable so that it can be fumigated.

The ventilation system of a containment level 3 room must be carefully designed so that it will not compete with the airflows across the face of the safety cabinets in use in the room.

Safety cabinets

There are three main types of safety cabinets: Class I, II, and III, not to be confused with the four hazard groups, e.g. Class I cabinets are used for category 3 pathogens (see Table 13.2).

Class I cabinets

Class I cabinets or exhaust protective cabinets (BS 5726) are simple in design, with air being drawn through the face of the cabinet and out through the HEPA filter to the outside air (see Fig. 13.2). The extraction fan is located at the end of the trunking as this will ensure that it is always under a negative pressure in the event of a leak. Excessive length and 90° turns should be avoided as these interfere with the airflow.

The cabinets should be carefully located within the room to prevent disturbances in the airflow caused by passing workers or competition with other cabinets or the ventilation system. The airflow across the face of the cabinet should be 0.7–1 m/second and this can be confirmed with an anemometer. The containment afforded by the cabinet should be checked regularly. This can be done by a biological method where *Bacillus globigii* is released inside the safety cabinet and culture media exposed outside the cabinet to detect escape. This organism has yellow colonies which are easily detected. The ratio of spores generated to the number which escapes is used to calculate the British Standard Protection Factor. The spore test is rarely used in routine laboratories.

A more practical method and thus more frequently used is the potassium iodide method. In the latter method, the challenge aerosol is potassium iodide and the detection system is a pair of centrifugal air samplers on which membrane filters are placed. After the nebulizer is run the filters are placed in a

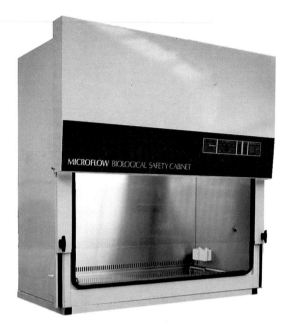

Figure 13.3 Class II cabinet air flows into the cabinet and filter air flows down over the work protecting the operator and the work

solution of potassium chloride and hydrochloric acid, which makes the drops of potassium iodide visible. The protection factor can be calculated in the same way as in the spore method.

Safety cabinets may be decontaminated by fumigation with formaldehyde or adding water to a mixture of formaldehyde and potassium permanganate. Some cabinets, especially Class II cabinets, may recirculate to room air. Decontamination of such cabinets is difficult as special arrangements must be made to disperse the formaldehyde gas after decontamination is complete.

Class II cabinets

Air is drawn into the cabinet and through a HEPA filter and downwards onto the work surface. A portion of the filtered air is extracted (Fig. 13.3). Class II microbiological safety cabinets provide protection to the operator and also to the work. They are, therefore, suitable for tissue culture, where contamination of cell-line is minimized.

through glove ports (Fig. 13.4). This type of cabinet provides maximum protection to the worker from aerosol hazard. Some argue that the need to manipulate all materials and equipment with gloved hands increases the risk of accidental self-inoculation when needles and other sharp implements must be used.

Containment level 4

Containment level 4 laboratories are rare and usually localized at national reference or research laboratories. They are operated on the basis of complete security of the material used in the laboratory. Laboratory workers change fully before entering the laboratory in an air-lock while work is contained in Class III cabinets and there is a negative pressure between the laboratory, the air-lock and the outside. Air enters through HEPA filters and is extracted through a pair of HEPA filters. A double-sided inter-locked autoclave ensures that all material leaving the laboratory is rendered safe. The worker should be visible within the laboratory through glass panels and an intercom or telephone system provided with an additional competent person available to assist in emergencies. Respirators must be available for this contingency.

Decontamination

Autoclaves

One of the major problems in microbiology laboratories is the large quantity of infected waste which is produced. All material must be rendered safe before leaving the laboratory. For solid waste, this is most easily achieved by autoclaving. Adequate records of autoclaving temperatures and cycle durations must be kept, together with spore tests on the autoclave, to ensure that all materials being sent from the laboratory have been adequately decontaminated.

Once sterile the waste is then transported for incineration. It is esential that transport of all infected waste is supervised by a member of staff who is trained to handle microbiological material.

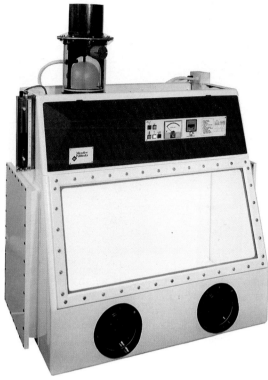

(a)

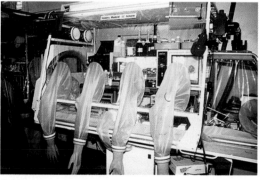

(b)

Figure 13.4 (*a*) Class III cabinet. (*b*) Self-contained laboratory within a Class III cabinet for processing specimens from patients with haemorrhagic fevers

Class III cabinets

These are similar in clinical design to Class I cabinets. However, air is drawn into the cabinet and exhausted through a HEPA filter. It is fully enclosed and the operator works

Table 13.3 Chemical disinfectants in common use in the laboratory

| | | Activity against organisms | | |
Class of agent	Bacteria	Fungi	Viruses	Mycobacteria
Phenolics (e.g. Hycolin)	+++	+++	+/−	+++
Hypochlorites (e.g. Chloros)	++	++	+++	−
Aldehydes (e.g. formaldehyde)	+++	+++	+++	+++*
Glutaraldehyde	+++	+++	+++	+++**

* Fumigation safety cabinets
** Disinfect equipment

Chemical disinfection

Discard jars should contain the appropriate disinfectant at the correct 'in use' dilution. A system should be enforced which ensures that the discard jars are changed daily. The most commonly used disinfectants are phenolic-based compounds (e.g. Hycolin), hypochlorites (e.g. Chloros), and glutaraldehyde. Their spectrum of activity is set out in Table 13.3.

It is essential that the appropriate disinfectants are immediately available to deal with spills within the laboratory area and for disinfecting bench surfaces when the working day is finished.

Safety monitoring

Under the Health and Safety at Work Act, responsibility for safety is vested in the head of department and the employer.

Training and monitoring

The Health and Safety at Work Act places an obligation on the employer to provide a safe working environment. This includes a provision of a general statement of safety policy, a written organization, and arrangements implementing safety policies. To achieve this, each laboratory should generate its own local rules which will be drawn up in consultation with the local safety committee and union safety representatives. These rules should include the following:

Safety officer

The head of department is legally responsible for safety within the workplace but may appoint someone to assist in this task. The duties of the safety officer include advising the head of the department on the safety matters, facilitating translation of the main aims of the safety protocol into day-to-day working practice, identifying potential hazards, monitoring safety standards, and educating members of laboratory staff.

Local rules (safety manual)

These must include clear instruction for the disposal of potentially infected material. It should also include details of disinfection of laboratory equipment, identifying the most appropriate means whereby this may be achieved. The correct disinfectants for each disinfection procedure must be identified together with the appropriate dilution.

Simple safety guidelines for ancillary staff, contractors, and visiting workers should be written. The vaccination requirements and any screening procedures to identify the immune status of individuals must be stated, together with the arrangements for medical surveillance through occupational health schemes. A card should also be provided to workers, identifying them and their duties in the microbiology department so that their usual medical attendant can be made aware of particular hazards which may have been acquired during the course of their work.

Training

A training officer should be identified within the laboratory. This person should have skills in communication so that the requirements of laboratory safety can be explained to staff and that they can be motivated to follow the protocols. Each worker within the laboratory area should be trained in the procedures they are expected to perform in their work and be advised of the biological hazards and the way in which these can be minimized. All new entrants to the laboratory area should receive safety training and should not be permitted to work with biological materials until the safety officer is satisfied with their ability to do so. New procedures and modification to protocols introduced to the laboratory should be accompanied by a training period before they are introduced to routine use. Regular refresher courses are required to update staff on routine technical procedures, such as disinfection of safety cabinets, role of disinfectants, management of spills, etc. Many laboratories have regular teaching seminars. It is good policy that a safety seminar is included in such a series on a regular basis.

Safety audits

Every written laboratory method is subject to 'protocol drift'. However, the passage of time, shortcuts, and misinterpretations result in a change in basic procedures. If such protocol drift is not to result in biological hazard, a system of safety audits must be undertaken on a regular basis. These provide the opportunity to monitor the safety system of the laboratory, to inspect laboratory maintenance records, e.g. confirm that the microbiological safety cabinets provide a sufficient degree of protection. It also provides an opportunity to ensure that lists of pathogens and inventories of freezers, chemical cupboards, and all COSHH assessments are in date. As well as this, the safety audit raises the profile of safety and gives an opportunity to remind all workers of the implications of safety in their day-to-day work.

The safety audit should be performed without prior consultation and at a time when the laboratory is operating fully. This will enable the dispassionate eye to identify previously unseen hazards and ensure that the 'worst case' rather than the 'best face' is seen.

The safety audit should wherever possible be performed by the department head or another senior member of staff to emphasize the priority placed on safe working practices.

Universal precautions

The term universal precautions refers to a system of infection control measures which are applied to the hospital environment to prevent the transmission of parenteral infectious agents. The impetus for their development was the expanding HIV epidemic.

The basic premise on which these precautions are based is that parenterally transmissible viruses are common in the community and that patients cannot be identified in advance. This contrasts with the approach which categorizes patients and gives special treatment to them. There are many objections to the latter policy. There is an objection to stigmatizing patients, and also the special treatment they are afforded often means second class treatment for themselves and their specimens.

The major effect on laboratories is the disappearance of biohazard labels. Universal precautions should have little impact on a microbiology laboratory as the need to prevent transmission of parenteral infection is well known and the necessary procedures should already be in place. However, the decision of a hospital to institute a system of universal precautions should prompt the laboratory to reassess all safety precautions.

14

Collection of blood for culture

Introduction

In most clinical situations where bacteraemia is suspected the organisms are intermittently present in the blood, e.g. in cholangitis. The bacteraemia of infective endocarditis and intravenous line sepsis is by contrast more continuous.

Fever is the pathophysiological response to the presence of bacteria or their breakdown products. Bacterial components such as lipopolysaccharide stimulate the production of cytokines such as interleukin 1 and tumor necrosis factor (TNF) by macrophages. Cytokines mediate the metabolic changes and febrile response associated with infection. Fever is at the end of the response to bacteraemia so samples from patients with intermittent fevers should be taken while the temperature is rising or as soon after the spike of fever as possible. The timing of blood sampling in suspected endocarditis and i.v. line sepsis is not so critical (Fig. 14.1).

Principles of blood culture

The major purpose of blood culture is to detect organisms circulating in the peripheral blood of patients with undiagnosed infection. To achieve this blood culture media should be sufficiently rich to allow the growth of the most fastidious pathogens which may be found in the peripheral blood.

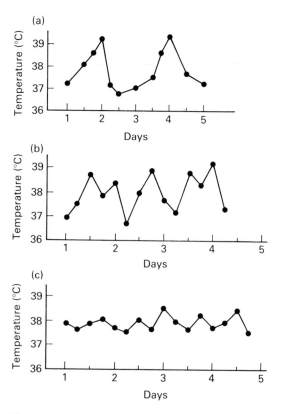

Figure 14.1 The pattern of fever is a valuable indicator to the diagnosis. (*a*) The typical 'tertian' fever of *P. vivax* malaria with peaks on alternate days. (*b*) Swinging fever often found in occult abscess or TB. (*c*) The low grade continuous pyrexia of endocarditis or line-related sepsis

Blood culture is more than simply the collection of specimens, the inoculation of blood culture medium, and subculture. Septicaemia is one of the most important life-threatening conditions and therefore the rapid detection of positive culture and identification of the likely pathogens as early as possible is an important aim. Consequently blood culture must be seen as encompassing a whole system which includes the consideration of a number of different points.

1 Provision of a culture medium or media which is sufficiently rich to encourage the growth of the most fastidious organisms present in peripheral blood.
2 Education of the medical staff on proper means of collecting blood cultures and minimizing skin contamination.
3 Rapid transmission of specimens to laboratory and culture under proper conditions of temperature and atmosphere.
4 Absence of substances which interfere with bacterial growth, e.g. antibiotics.
5 Early detection of positive cultures and provisional identification of likely pathogens and rapid communication of these results to clinician.
6 Minimization of laboratory-induced contamination.
7 Final bacterial identification and sensitivity testing.
8 Audit of the blood culture system to review sensitivity and specificity of the investigation.

Number

The yield of positive cultures is best when two samples are taken not less than one hour apart. Above this number the diagnostic yield does not improve and the risk of confusion due to false-positive results from skin or laboratory containments increases. As well as this examining a large number of negative cultures is wasteful of time and material resources. The value of blood culture as the principal means of detecting serious sepsis is reduced if it becomes a 'routine' investigation taken without adequate laboratory-ward liaison.

Volume

There are often as few as one colony forming units (cfu) bacteria per ml of blood and in cases of continuous bacteraemia the number may be lower still. The volume of blood cultured is therefore of critical importance in ensuring reliable and sensitive results. Not less than 10 ml of blood should be collected and there is an increased diagnostic yield with each millilitre of blood up to approximately 30 ml collected. In continuous bacteraemia it is especially important to collect a large volume of blood.

In neonatal infection where there is a higher density of bacteria a smaller volume of blood may yield positive results.

It is important that the volume of blood is not too high as this will remove the dilution effect of the blood culture medium which reduces the antibacterial effects of the collected blood. A 1 : 10 dilution is probably optimal for both Gram-positive and Gram-negative pathogens.

Site and skin preparation

Blood samples for culture should always be collected from a peripheral vein. Samples may be collected from indwelling intravenous devices but should always be accompanied by a peripheral sample to allow a proper interpretation of isolates such as *S. epidermidis* which may colonize these devices.

To reduce the risk of introducing contaminating skin commensals the venepuncture site should be selected to provide easy venous access, and be thoroughly disinfected.

The operator should wear a pair of disposable sterile gloves, and use a 'no touch' technique throughout. Some authors argue that the wearing of gloves may increase the risk of contamination by reducing manual dexterity. If ungloved hands are used they must be thoroughly clean and the 'no touch' technique must be rigorous. The increasing prevalence of HIV infection means that blood sampling should be performed by gloved hands.

Media for blood culture

Aerobic media

Simple media: nutrient or glucose broths can be used for blood culture as the addition of blood makes the final medium rich. The bottles should be vented to encourage the growth of strictly aerobic species such as *P. aeruginosa*. Glucose (0.1–0.5%) may be added to enhance the growth of streptococci, but the value of this practice has been questioned. Higher concentrations of glucose (>1.0%) can lead to death of the culture due to excessive acid production.

Liquoid (polyathenol sulphonate) acts to inhibit the bactericidal effect of blood. It does inhibit the growth of a number of organisms, however, including *N. meningitidis*, *N. gonorrhoeae*, *Streptobacillus moniliformis* and several anaerobic species including *Peptostreptococcus*. This adverse effect can be reversed for *Neisseria* spp. by the incorporation of 1% gelatin in the medium.

Biphasic medium (Casteñeda method) is valuable in the isolation of *Brucella* spp. This employs a solid agar slope together with a liquid phase (see Fig. 6.5) of the same medium (such as tryptose soy, serum-dextrose, and liver infusion broth). The bottle is inspected daily and if no colonies are seen is tipped over so that the solid phase is inoculated (see p. 76). This technique reduces the risk of contamination during the extended incubation which is often necessary to culture brucella. Another advantage is that the sealed bottle provides a degree of containment for this category 3 organism which readily causes laboratory acquired infection.

Anaerobic media

In laboratories where two or three different bottles are used for blood culture, one of these should be of a composition which will encourage the growth of anaerobic organisms. Media which are used for this purpose include Brewer's thioglycolate, fastidious anaerobe broth, Robertson's cooked meat with brain heart infusion broth and thiol broth. Thiol broth and fastidious anaerobe broth give excellent results.

Liquoid is not usually added to anaerobic broths because of its inhibitory effects on some species of anaerobic cocci. Reducing substances, usually thioglycolate salts, are added to maintain a low redox potential. Not all of these additions are beneficial, some thioglycolate has been shown first to enhance and then kill a growing *Bacteroides* culture.

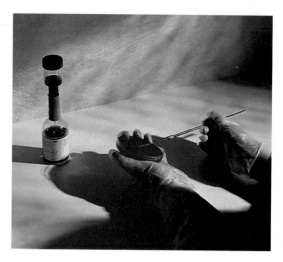

Figure 14.2 'Signal' blood culture bottle being subcultured

To ensure a high yield of anaerobic organisms specimens should be sent to the laboratory with the minimum of delay. The culture bottles should be incubated in an anaerobic atmosphere with the caps loosened. An anaerobic cabinet is especially valuable for this purpose.

Blood culture sets

Whatever media are chosen there is an inevitable compromise of the yield of fastidious organisms obtainable. To overcome this blood is inoculated into several bottles each of which are capable of giving a high diagnostic yield for a particular group of bacteria, for example anaerobes. It is now unusual for a single blood culture bottle to be used, however a commercial blood culture system (Signal, Oxoid, England) does do this (see below and Fig. 14.2).

Some laboratory protocols include a medium which is incubated in 10% CO_2 atmosphere with the top loosened to enhance the possibility of isolating capnophiles such as some *Haemophilus* spp. and *Brucella* spp. Venting in CO_2 will also enhance the yield of a wide range of organisms including *Neisseria, Escherichia, Pseudomonas, Staphylococcus,* and *Klebsiella*.

The simplest set would, therefore, consist of a vented aerobic bottle incubated in a 10%

CO_2 atmosphere together with a specific anaerobic broth.

Other sets might include an additional unvented aerobic bottle, which might be a diphasic medium (see Fig. 6.2).

It is important, whatever the composition of the conventional blood culture set, that medium made available to the wards is as fresh as possible. It is important that stock is carefully controlled so that blood from septicaemic patients is inoculated into fresh medium supplies of blood culture sets being supplied through a central distribution point. They should be clearly date stamped and not dispensed or used if this date is passed.

Laboratory examination of blood culture

Duration of incubation

The duration of incubation for a blood culture should be determined by the clinical information provided. In most cases where septicaemia is suspected almost all significant pathogens are detected before seven days' incubation. In contrast positive culture can be delayed for up to three weeks in the case of brucellosis. Extended periods of incubation are also required in cases of pyrexia of uncertain origin or endocarditis when more unusual slow growing bacteria, e.g. *H. aphrophilus* and *C. hominis* are a possibility. A positive culture can also be delayed in cases of typhoid fever. Thus, the clinical microbiologist should carefully select the blood culture specimens which will be incubated for a prolonged period.

It is equally important to provide significant and negative results as early as possible. Examination and subculture of a large number of negative cultures necessarily reduces the time that can be spent on each individual specimen and therefore reduce the overall quality of the blood culture system.

Detection of a positive culture

From the clinician's point of view the most valuable report is that which provides a significant positive result at the earliest possible time. There are many different ways to detect positive blood cultures and it is in this area that major advances have been made in automating this time-consuming process by detecting early signs of bacterial multiplications.

There are two major manual systems and an increasing number of automated systems:

Manual systems

1   The daily inspection of blood culture bottles in which the blood has clearly sedimented and is undisturbed. Growth may be detected by noting the presence of turbidity, production of gas and, rarely, development of microcolonies on top of the blood layer. A sample of the culture is taken, a Gram stain performed and it is plated on a range of media and incubated in aerobic and anaerobic conditions. This approach will detect positive cultures which have more than 10^6 colony forming units/ml. However, some bacteria such as *N. meningitidis*, *H. influenzae* and anaerobic streptococci may fail to cause turbidity until higher concentrations are reached. Any system which includes macroscopic examination should also include blind subculture of all bottles as part of the protocol otherwise a number of infections caused by these organisms will be missed.

In addition to this, individual specimens thought likely to be positive because of the clinical circumstances may be examined microscopically. If Gram stain is used the result may provide help in guiding antimicrobial chemotherapy. The sensitivity of Gram stain is between 10^5 and 10^6 colony forming units/ml. The sensitivity may be enhanced by staining with acridine orange which detects approximately 10^4 colony forming units/ml.

2   Blind subculture. Routine subculture to aerobic media, six to 12 hours after receipt, may yield 36% of all positive isolates subsequently identified. A second subculture between 12 and 17 hours increases this yield to 63% of all isolates. A laboratory which adopts the blind subculture strategy would routinely subculture blood cultures twice per day in the first 24 hours to give the earliest possible yield.

The role of routine blind anaerobic subculture is less clear. Some studies indicate that most clinically significant anaerobic aspects are detected by visual inspection followed by subculture. However, some anaerobic streptococci may not produce turbidity in the blood culture bottle until they are present in very large numbers.

Many laboratories adopt a strategy of routinely subculturing blood culture samples at the end of incubation. The results of trials are contradictory, but one might conclude that since most positive isolates are detected early in the course of incubation that little additional information will be obtained by routine terminal subculture. More importantly it may increase the risk of laboratory-based contaminants and may serve to produce misleading reports.

Automated systems

These systems are beneficial by automating the laborious process of detecting bacterial growth in blood culture, and therefore has an important role in reducing tedious subculture, and controlling costs. In addition since only those bottles with a high likelihood of a positive result are subcultured, laboratory-introduced contaminants are reduced. The most widely applied method is one in which CO_2 produced by growing cultures is detected.

Two methods have been used:

1   Radiometric method: BACTEC 403 system. The media contain substances in which some of the carbon atoms (^{12}C) are replaced by ^{14}C. When bacterial multiplication takes place carbon dioxide is produced, some of which is radiolabelled. The BACTEC system detects this CO_2 by sampling the head space of the bottle and passing it through a detection system. The machine produces a result which indicates the bottles which require subculture.

The BACTEC 403 system has undergone extensive trials and is now widely accepted. It is at least equivalent to conventional blood culture systems in sensitivity and reduces the time it takes before a positive result is reported. Some studies suggest that the BACTEC system may be superior to conventional blood culture methods in its detection of fungaemia. In addition, the radiometric system can be modified to detect the growth of mycobacteria when ^{14}C palmitate is incorporated into a mycobacterial growth medium. This has proved particularly valuable in the diagnosis of disseminated mycobacteria in AIDS patients.

2   Carbon dioxide produced by the growing culture can also be detected using infrared detection. This updated version of the BACTEC system (BACTEC MR-660) has many advantages over the radiometric system, not at least by simplifying the disposal of spent blood culture bottles and obviating the need for radioactive precautions.

3   More recent developments use a CO_2 sensitive membrane incorporated into the bottle. The production of CO_2 is detected as a colour change which is detected automatically. The advantage of this system is that cultures are continuously monitored, reducing the time lag to positive diagnosis.

In addition, the new system has superior computerized data handling facilities and is able to process a larger number of specimens.

As well as being useful in detecting positive blood cultures radiometric CO_2 systems can be modified to perform rapid sensitivity tests for slow growing organisms such as mycobacteria.

Impedance

The products of metabolism of a growing bacterial culture will produce alterations in the flow of an alternating current culture applied to the medium. This phenomenon can be used to detect growing cultures and a commercial system using the method of this system has been produced. One advantage of using this system is the detection of growth by continuous on-line monitoring of electrical impedance and conductance in the culture fluid. Like the systems detecting CO_2 production impedance measurement can be used for rapid sensitivity testing.

Redox potential

In this method inoculated blood cultures are inserted into a silo where two electrodes (one gold and the other aluminium) within the bottom rubber bung pierce a membrane and enter the culture medium. This system operates like a small battery where a voltage is produced when Al^{3+} ions dissolve in the medium and electrons travel to the gold electrode. There they reduce substances in the medium. A metabolizing organism present in the culture will cause a change in the concentration of reducible substances in the medium causing a decline in the voltage which is detected by the computer.

Antigen detection

Some organisms are rapidly killed in blood culture due to products of their own metabolism. This may result in false-negative blood culture. *Streptococcus pneumoniae* is particularly sensitive to this effect. In patients in which pneumococcal infection is suspected the blood culture supernatant fluid can be used in a pneumococcal antigen detection test, e.g. countercurrent immunoelectrophoresis (CIE) or latex test enabling a positive diagnosis test to be made of the absence in viable organisms.

It is useful to detect antigens in patients with positive cultures when Gram staining demonstrates Gram-positive cocci. A centrifuged deposit can be examined for the presence of coagulase, and streptococcal latex agglutinations performed which can give an early indication of the species of Gram-positive coccus isolated.

Gas-liquid chromatography

The presence of anaerobes in a blood culture can be established by attempting to detect the products of anaerobic metabolism by gas-liquid chromatography. This technique is time consuming but may result in a positive diagnosis being made more rapidly. However, it detects only the presence of anaerobes but does not identify them and therefore is of limited clinical value.

Contamination of blood cultures

Contaminating organisms can be found in up to 12% of blood cultures. An isolate should be considered suspect if an organism of low virulence such as *S. epidermidis*, non-diphtheria corynebacterium or *Bacillus* spp. is isolated from one bottle of a set. However, in some cases, when only small numbers of organisms are present in the blood, chance may distribute them to one bottle. Similarly significant bacteraemia with two separate species such as *Bacteroides fragilis* and *Escherichia coli* does occur and is usually associated with a poor prognosis. Mixed growths, however, including *S. epidermidis* and/or diphtheroids are likely to indicate a skin origin for the bacteria.

The diagnosis of the contaminated blood culture can be made only after thorough clinical evaluation of the patient's condition. With modern medical practice many patients are immunocompromised or may have long-term indwelling prosthetic devices such as Hickman catheters, and these may be colonized with organisms from the skin – *S. epidermidis* or diphtheroids. Before organisms are discarded as contaminants the patient should be seen and a history taken; the presence of fever and relevant clinical signs should be sought. The site of the blood culture must be established (whether the blood culture was taken from a peripheral vein or through an intravenous canula) and whether the skin was adequately prepared. The microbiologist should take the investigation of potential contaminant organisms as an opportunity for educating clinicians in the proper method of disinfecting the skin. Further blood cultures should be requested to confirm the absence of bacteraemia. The laboratory should monitor the rate of those non-significant isolates so that any upward trend can be investigated. There may, for example, be a breakdown in laboratory protocols resulting in contamination at the bench or it may be that individual clinicians are neglecting the proper collection procedures.

Contamination of blood cultures may occur in the ward or in the laboratory. The major opportunity for contamination of blood culture occurs when blood is withdrawn for culture. The microbiology laboratory should produce a protocol for taking of a blood culture including a method for skin disinfection. To ensure that this information is communicated to clinicians, regular training sessions must be held to teach staff taking up an appointment for the first time. Contaminating organisms can also be introduced at a time when blood is injected into the blood culture bottle if the top of the blood culture bottle is not sterile. The venesector should always inoculate blood cultures before providing blood samples for haematology and clinical chemistry, otherwise it is possible for contaminating organisms such as *Acinetobacter* and *Flavobacteria* to be transferred.

The risk of contaminating blood cultures in the laboratory increases with the number of manipulations which are performed. Subculture should be performed in a large room with still air or in a Class I or Class II microbiological safety cabinet. Laminar flow cabinets where the airflow is directed into the face of the operator should not be used. (See Safety in Laboratories, Chapter 13.)

If a wire loop is used for subculture it should be of sufficient length so that the handle does not need to touch the rim of the bottle. When the rim of the bottle is flamed the bottle should be carried to the flame in an upright position, otherwise organisms suspended in the air will be drawn into the bottle. Techniques which increase the number of manipulations such as the lysis centrifugation technique and antimicrobial removal devices result in higher contamination rates. These techniques should be closely monitored to ensure that laboratory contaminants are kept to a minimum.

Removal of antibiotics in blood

Organisms are present at low concentration in the blood of patients with bacteraemia and some are fastidious. It is important therefore that the antibacterial effect of serum is neutralized. This is usually achieved by dilution in the medium (see above) or the addition of liquid. Some patients, however, may have received antibiotics before blood culture has been performed and an attempt can be made to inactivate the antimicrobial agents. Broad spectrum beta-lactamases may be added to the medium in the laboratory after inoculation. The addition of *p*-amino benzoic acid will oppose the action of sulphonamides and thymidine will neutralize the effects of trimethoprim. Antimicrobial removal devices have been devised. These consist of anion exchange resins added to the medium. They are relatively expensive and some authors

consider that their use reduces the numbers of significant positive isolates. They have not yet achieved a place in routine blood culture technique. All of these processes result in an increased manipulation of the specimen and may result in higher contamination rates.

Concentration techniques

Lysis centrifugation

This method uses anticoagulated venous blood to which a lysis agent is added. The bacteria are centrifuged and the deposit is then plated on solid media. This technique will result in more rapid detection in bacteraemia and fungaemia. This technique is commercially available (Isolator Dupont) and is relatively expensive. Care must be taken if higher contamination rates are not to be found due to the increased manipulation.

Lysis filtration

In this technique anticoagulated venous blood is passed through a filter. The filter is washed and divided and parts are placed on different media which may then be cultured under appropriate atmospheric conditions. This technique has the advantage of growing the organism as colonies on solid media from the outset and from removing bacteria from the presence of the potentially inhibiting substances within the blood. It is time consuming and expensive and may increase the contamination rate. It is not yet commercially available.

Investigation of pyrexia of uncertain origin

Introduction

Pyrexia of uncertain origin (PUO) is a term which may be defined in a number of ways. A useful definition is, 'Fever greater than 38°C for more than five days for which there is no obvious cause'. This definition excludes patients with transient fevers and trivial infections and focuses on those in which there is true diagnostic uncertainty.

Aetiology

There are three groups of causes of PUO:

- Infections
- Inflammatory conditions (e.g. collagen vascular diseases)
- Malignant disease

Infections make up approximately 30% of published series, malignant disease 15% and collagen vascular diseases 20%.

PUOs can be subdivided into 'acute' and 'chronic', although in practice these definitions are more relevant to published reviews than individual patients. In acute PUO infection is a more likely diagnosis with viral causes prominent. In chronic PUO inflammatory disorders such as systemic lupus erythematosus or rheumatoid arthritis, and malignant diseases such as lymphomas make up a larger proportion of cases. Of the infective causes in chronic PUO bacterial infections such as tuberculosis and endocarditis, and parasitic infections such as toxoplasmosis become more important.

Investigation of PUO

The investigation of PUO is dependent on an initial thorough clinical history and physical examination, a fever chart, and a systematic plan of laboratory and radiological examination. The history taking should be repeated as patients will bring to mind important information at subsequent interviews. In a case of PUO the patient's condition may change from day to day so thorough physical examination should be repeated.

The history

Duration of fever, diurnal variation or periodicity should be sought. In vivax malaria fever may occur on alternate days (tertian), and in TB or lymphoma drenching sweats at night may be reported. Associated symptoms should be sought – rash or joint pain. Thorough systematic enquiry may provide a pointer to a source of sepsis: recurrent cough, TB.

Present and past medications including blood transfusions should be recorded and an inquiry made into intravenous drug abuse. Evidence of treated or partially treated tuberculosis, or a cardiac valve lesion which may point to endocarditis should be sought. Autoimmune disease may have a familial component and contact with family members with infectious diseases may be revealed. Gynaecological and contraceptive history should be detailed, e.g. presence of an intrauterine contraceptive device.

The history should include personal details including racial origin as some conditions such as Familial Mediterranean fever are more common in some races, i.e. people of the Mediterranean basin or Ashkenazi Jews. A history of sexual orientation and exposure may indicate a risk of acute or chronic sexually transmitted disease including HIV infection. Occupation must be detailed as many infections may be occupationally acquired, e.g. leptospirosis in sewer workers and brucellosis in abattoir workers. Hobby activities should be explored as these may bring the patient into contact with specific infections, e.g. ramblers with Lyme disease or pigeon fanciers with ornithosis. Regular or intensive contact with animals should be recorded, dogs pointing to toxocarisasis, for example.

A detailed travel history is essential and should date back at least a year. Although there are cases of malaria occurring after 30 years most occur within one year of return from a country where malaria is endemic. Remember travel history does not just mean travel to exotic locations like Bali or Kenya. Some infections would be difficult to diagnose without a travel clue, e.g. leishmaniasis acquired in Portugal, Lyme disease in New England, brucellosis in the Middle East.

Physical examination

The physical examination should be complete but a number of areas should be studied carefully (see Table 14.1).

Trials of therapy

In some situations there may be a strong clinical suspicion of tuberculosis, without a clear

Table 14.1 Examples of clinical signs which should be sought in cases of pyrexia of uncertain origin

System	Sign
Sinuses/teeth	Occult abscesses
Skin	Rashes, nodules, petechiae, splinter haemorrhages
Lymph nodes	Generalized, localized, regional nodes denoting primary site of sepsis
Hepatosplenomegaly	Evidence of liver metastases Splenic enlargement 　mild 　moderate 　large
Joints	Symmetrical arthropathy: rheumatoid arthritis, etc. Lumbosacral tenderness: brucellosis, TB
Cardiovascular system	Murmurs of infective endocarditis, rheumatic fever, pericardial rub
Chest	Consolidation, pleural rub or effusion
Testes/scrotum	Chronic orchitis, testicular tumour
Eyes	Collagen vascular disease, conjunctivitis: Reiter's syndrome
Mouth	Candidiasis: buccal ulceration

diagnosis. In this instance a trial of therapy may be employed. Isoniazid and ethambutol should be administered for this purpose as they will have no effect on other bacterial infections. The response should be closely monitored by regular fever measurement and sequential ESR or C-reactive protein (CRP) estimations.

Investigations

The investigative effort has been made more easy by improvements in imaging techniques. Investigation should be divided into three main phases:

Phase 1. Initial screen: taken on all PUO patients
Phase 2. Directed examinations
Phase 3. Specialist investigations and imaging.

Phase 1

The initial screen should include haemoglobin, white cell count and differential, serum electrolytes, liver enzymes, chest X-ray sputum culture including culture for mycobacteria,

MSU for microscopy and culture, stool for culture and microscopy for parasitic ova and cysts. A specimen of serum should be saved on admission and when a second serum has been obtained tested for those infections suggested by the results of the initial screen to detect rising titres. Blood should be obtained for culture on at least three occasions. The serum should be tested for the presence of auto-antibodies, and the ESR or C-reactive protein concentration measured (Table 14.2).

Phase 2

The second group of investigations will be specific for each individual patient, being guided by the results of the history, clinical examination and initial investigations. An example of such a series of phase 2 investigations is illustrated in Table 14.3 which might be used in the case of a patient with a history of recent tropical travel, fever and eosinophilia.

Phase 3

The final group of investigations are the specialist imaging techniques such as

Table 14.2 Examples of investigations used in an initial screen

Haemoglobin, white cell count and differential blood count
Serum electrolytes
Liver enzymes
Chest X-ray
Sputum culture conventional and TB
MSU microscopy, biochemistry and culture
Acute serum saved
Blood culture ×3
Erythrocyte sedimentation rate, C-reactive protein
Auto-antibody screen
Blood coagulation

Table 14.3 Examples of critical pathways for some syndromes: tropical travel and eosinophila, modified by geographical exposure

Stool examination ×3
String test
Strongyloides culture
Serology
  schistosomiasis
  filariasis
  hydatid
  fasciola
  toxocara
  cysticercus
  strongyloides
Skin snips (onchocerciasis)
Whole blood for microfilaria
Mazzoti reaction

Table 14.4 Imaging and invasive investigations

Ultrasound abdomen, pelvis
CT scanning
MRI
Sinus/mandible X-ray
Liver biopsy
Bronchoalveolar lavage
Bone marrow
Liver or other organ specific biopsy
Mantoux and Mazzoti tests

computerized tomography (CT), magnetic resonance imaging (MRI) and ultrasound, and invasive investigations such as liver biopsy. The choice of these investigations will depend on the results of the first stages and re-examination of the clinical history and signs. The availability of ultrasound and CT scanning means that laparotomy is now rarely required for the diagnosis of PUO when in the past it was common (Table 14.4).

Elements of the initial screen should be repeated at intervals, and further blood cultures may be obtained.

Common diagnoses in PUO

Occult abscess is a common diagnosis in PUO and sites which should be excluded include: mandible, liver, sub-phrenic area, pelvic space. Osteomyelitis should be investigated with technetium, and labelled white cell scans.

Endocarditis is a diagnosis which may be found in patients without prior risk factors. Short courses of antimicrobials given in the community may cause initial false-negative blood culture. Repeated cardiac auscultation, and blood culture together with echocardiography may be necessary to make the diagnosis.

The biliary tract is a common source of occult sepsis. Endoscopic retrograde cannulation of the pancreatic duct (ERCP) may be both diagnostic and therapeutic allowing for the operative removal of biliary stones obstructing the biliary duct. Liver enzymes, ultrasound and CT scanning may be helpful. The urinary tract may be a source of sepsis without the classical symptoms of dysuria and frequency. The strict numerical classification of Kass may not strictly apply in all circumstances – an infection may be present with $<10^5$ cfu/ml.

Tuberculosis is of increasing importance with the HIV epidemic. The diversity of sites means that many specimens must be taken and cultured before TB can be confidently excluded. Mantoux testing, direct examination and culture of sputum, urine, gastric aspirate and bone marrow, liver biopsy may be required.

Mononucleosis: some patients have little lymphadenopathy with acute toxoplasmosis. Modern IgM ELISAs and immunohistochemistry make this more easy to diagnose.

Infection with human immunodeficiency virus should be excluded in all cases of PUO.

Other easy to forget conditions are *Borrelia* infections (including Lyme disease and relapsing fever), leptospirosis, sarcoidosis and other chronic granulomatous disease, parasitic diseases, malaria, Familial Mediterranean fever, lymphoma/leukaemia, factitious fever, renal cell carcinoma, Crohn's disease, hepatoma, ornithosis, Q fever, rheumatic fever, Still's disease, rheumatoid arthritis and systemic lupus erythematosus.

Examination of specimens from the central nervous system

Acute meningitis

Meningitis is an acute medical emergency in which laboratory examination of cerebral spinal fluid (CSF) plays a central role in establishing an aetiological diagnosis, and in guiding early antimicrobial chemotherapy.

Aetiology

Meningitis is an inflammation of the layers of tissue surrounding the brain. Infection can be carried to this site via the blood stream as part of a systemic infection, e.g. meningococcal meningitis or enterovirus infection. It can occur due to a tear in the outermost layer, the dura, which communicates with the outside, or through a fractured cribiform plate. Infection can also spread from sites of parameningeal suppuration such as acute or chronic otitis media or mastoiditis. Meningitis can also rarely arise following trauma or by rupture of a brain abscess into the ventricles (Table 15.1).

Meningitis is characterized by fever, headache and neck pain. This exhibits itself as an inability to flex the neck, 'neck stiffness', as this movement stretches the inflamed meninges and causes reflex muscle spasm. As the infection progresses the level of consciousness deteriorates.

Meningitis can be classified by its speed of development making the difference from the usual rapidly progressive pyogenic meningitides caused by the meningococcus or pneumococcus with infections with a more insidious onset such as tuberculous meningitis.

Table 15.1 Pathogens of the central nervous system

Helminths
Strongyloides stercoralis
Angiostrongylus cantonesis
Toxocara canis
Echinococcus spp.
Taenia solium

Protozoa
Toxoplasma gondii
Plasmodium falciparum
Trypanosoma brucei var. *gambiense* and var. *rhodesiense*

Fungi
Cryptococcus neoformans
Aspergillus spp.
Candida albicans

Bacteria
Escherichia coli
Streptococcus agalactiae
Haemophilus influenzae
Streptococcus pneumoniae
Listeria monocytogenes
Mycobacterium tuberculosis

Meningitis can be also classified according to causative pathogen or by the nature of the cellular response in the CSF into pyogenic or lymphocytic. Pyogenic meningitis is associated with an excess of polymorphs in the CSF and is most often caused by bacteria such as *N. meningitidis*, *S. pneumoniae* or *H. influenzae*. Lymphocytic meningitis is associated with viral infection, tuberculosis, syphilitic meningoencephalitis and leptospirosis. There are of course exceptions to these tidy rules. Early in the course of tuberculous meningitis the cellular response can be dominated by polymorphs. Similarly in pyogenic meningitis which is partially treated by antibiotics the major cell type can be lymphocytes.

Almost all bacteria have been found at some time as pathogens in the meninges but broad patterns of infection can be found, and are useful in planning empirical therapy when initial investigations do not identify a pathogen.

Neonatal meningitis

Neonates are very susceptible to pyogenic meningitis and are predisposed to infection when there is prolonged spontaneous rupture of the membranes, an operative delivery, prenatal infection of the mother (e.g. listeriosis), or where the infant is smaller than it should be for its gestational age (small for dates). The most frequent bacterial pathogens are *Streptococcus agalactiae* (group B streptococcus) and enterobacteria especially *Escherichia coli*. During this period the infant may also be infected with the meningococcus and the pneumococcus. The latter infection being more likely if there is a congenital immunodeficiency such as a complement deficiency or an abnormal communication between the skin and the meninges as in the case of a mid-line dermoid tumour.

Preschool age children

Over the age of six months antibodies to *H. influenzae* type b acquired from the mother transplacentally begin to wane, and this organism becomes the major pathogen, together with *N. meningitidis*.

Young adults

In young adult life *N. meningitidis* is the most common pathogen, but pneumococcal meningitis may occur in those predisposed by splenectomy, sickle cell disease (where there is a functional splenectomy), or where trauma has resulted in a tear in the dura. In the elderly, chronic bronchial sepsis, alcoholic liver disease and immunosuppression, either iatrogenic or as a result of coincidental disease, suggest that the pneumococcus is the most likely pathogen. *Listeria monocytogenes* can infect any age group but meningitis associated with a high mortality occurs in the elderly and immunosuppressed patients.

Other causes

Meningitis may be part of systemic infection with other bacterial pathogens, including *M. tuberculosis*. *Staphylococcus epidermidis* and other bacteria of relatively low pathogenicity can colonize indwelling ventricular shunts leading to a chronic infection.

Treponema pallidum gives rise to an acute meningo-encephalitis in the secondary phase of the disease but this diagnosis is now uncommon in developed countries. *Cryptococcus neoformans* was once a rare cause of meningitis, usually in patients with heavy exposure to birds and their droppings where *C. neoformans* is found in great quantity. It is now, however, much more common occurring in up to 15% of patients with AIDS.

Parasitic infections

Many parasites are capable of causing meningitis. A meningo-encephalitis meningitis is part of the pathogenic process preceding the late stages of African trypanosomiasis. In acute malaria caused by *P. falciparum* cerebral symptoms and signs may form a critical part of the disease. In patients with a lower state of consciousness who had recently travelled to areas where malaria is endemic *P. falciparum* malaria is an important differential diagnosis, although meningitis and signs of meningitis are not usually found.

Primary amoebic meningitis is caused by *Naegleria fowleri* and is acquired after bathing in stagnant water. This organism is a free-living amoeba whose normal habitat is fresh water and as such can be found in rivers, reservoirs and swimming pools. Infections are geographically restricted, the highest incidence occurring in Australia. Infection with *N. fowleri* is rapidly progressive and rarely responds to treatment.

Angiostrongylus cantonensis is a nematode which is a natural parasite of a Chinese species of snails. Infection can be transmitted to man causing an eosinophilic meningitis. Eosinophilic meningitis can also rarely occur due to the passage of migrating worms. *Toxocara canis* is the commonest cause of visceral larva migrans but this rarely gives rise to meningitis. Although rare gnathostomiasis and dirofilariasis can both give rise to meningitis in this way.

Strongyloides stercoralis larvae migrate in human tissues. If there is a fall in cell-mediated immunity strongyloides can multiply without control, giving rise to the hyperinfection syndrome. The passage of larvae from the gut bringing enteric Gram-negative organisms with them, can give rise to septicaemia and meningitis.

The prognosis of meningitis is very variable, at one extreme enterovirus meningitis rarely gives rise to serious complications, whereas the mortality from pneumococcal meningitis is rarely better than 20% in the best centres and can be as high as 60% in economically poor districts and in the developing world. Intermediate between these is *H. influenzae* and *N. meningitidis* where, with optimum therapy, mortality should be less than 5%.

Laboratory diagnosis

Collection of specimens

CSF should be collected in cases where the diagnosis of meningitis is suspected, provided the clinician is sure there is no raised intracranial pressure which is an absolute contraindication and the procedure will not result in delay in initiating therapy (in patients with a purpuric rash of meningococcal septicaemia). A description of the methods for performing a lumbar puncture are beyond the scope of this book. It is essential that the skin is adequately prepared to prevent contamination of the CSF specimen and the introduction of potential pathogens into the CSF.

Approximately 3–4 ml of CSF should be collected and this should be divided into three sterile containers. Clinicians should be aware of the urgency of a CSF examination and should ensure that specimens are transmitted to laboratory with minimal delay. It is preferable for them to bring it themselves so that they are able to act immediately on the result.

The microbiology laboratory should be alerted in advance to enable processing of the specimen to take place immediately on arrival.

Direct examination

The CSF should be examined macroscopically for xanthochromia and blood.

The specimen of the CSF should be centrifuged at 1800 g for approximately 10 minutes. The deposit is used to make three slides for microscopic examination, and the supernatant fluid can be sent for measurement of glucose and protein. The first slide should be stained by Gram's method and examined for pyogenic bacteria (Fig. 15.1) and the second with Giemsa stain so that the percentage of neutrophils and lymphocytes can be determined accurately. The third should be stained with Ziehl-Neelsen's stain, although this is frequently omitted if there is little in the clinical presentation to suggest tuberculous meningitis.

To prepare a slide for CSF specimen microscopic examination a circle should be drawn on the slide with a diamond marker and drops of the CSF deposit added. Each drop should be allowed to dry before the next drop is added. In this way the CSF is concentrated layer upon layer, maximizing the chances of obtaining a positive result. The sensitivity of direct examination may be increased by staining with acridine orange (see p. 163).

Cell count is an important diagnostic parameter (Table 15.2) assisting in the discrimination of viral and bacterial meningitis. The cell count

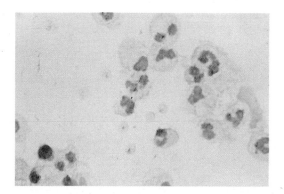

Figure 15.1 Cytospin preparation of CSF stained by Gram's stain showing a single Gram-positive coccus

Table 15.2

Type of meningitis	White cell count	CSF sugar/ blood sugar	Protein	Stain	Other techniques
Acute bacterial	High, often >0.5 × 19⁹/l; predominantly PMN	<40%*	Raised >0.4 g/l	Gram stain	Antigen detection; CSF lactate
Acute viral	Raised 0.005–0.5 × 10⁹/l; predominantly lymphocytes	Normal	Normal or slight	–	Request throat swab; faeces for viral culture
Tuberculosis	Raised 0.005–0.5 × 10⁹/l	<40%	Raised >0.4 g/l	Ziehl-Neelsen or auramine	Culture on Lowenstein-Jensen
Normal	<0.005 × 10⁹/l	≥40%	0.1–0.4 g/l	–	–
Cryptococcus neoformans	>0.005 × 10⁹/l - 0.5; predominantly lymphocytes	<40%	Raised >0.4	Gram stain, India ink or tolmudine blue	Cryptococcal capsular antigen
Syphilis	>0.005–0.5 × 10⁹/l	>40%	>0.4 g/l	–	VDRL positive; TPHA IgM positive
Subarachnoid	RBC/WBC in haemic proportions	>40%	>>0.4 g/l	–	Xanthochromis
Leptospirosis	0.005–0.5 × 10⁹/l	>40%	>0.4 g/l	Leptospira on dark ground	Leptospira serology

*Concurrent blood glucose should be taken

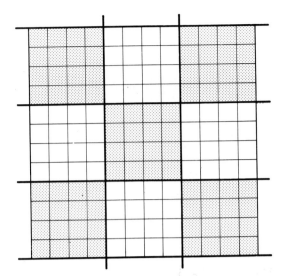

Figure 15.2 Fuchs–Rosenthal chamber. The coverslip is placed on firmly and the cells permitted to settle for 5 minutes. Five large squares (shaded) are counted. Number of cells counted = cells/mm^3

is performed with an unstained preparation of uncentrifuged CSF in a counting chamber of which there are several suitable for the purpose, e.g. those of Neubauer or Fuchs-Rosenthal (Fig. 15.2).

Additional staining methods

India ink

Cryptococcal meningitis is now a more common clinical entity due to the acquired immune deficiency syndrome. When cryptococcal meningitis is suspected an India ink preparation should be examined. A small drop of CSF deposit obtained after centrifugation should be placed on a microscope slide and mixed with a drop of India ink (neat commercial India ink from the artists' supply shop is quite satisfactory for the purpose). If India ink is unavailable, nigrosin at 200 g/l can be used. Cover with a coverslip and examine the preparation using the ×40 times objective. *Cryptococcus neoformans* will be seen as round or oval cells between 5 and 20 µm in diameter surrounded by a bright halo which represents the unstained capsule (see Fig.

10.9). The budding characteristic of yeast cells may also be seen. Remember that patients with cryptococcal meningitis rarely have large numbers of white cells in the CSF and it is possible for the inexperienced observer to mistake the yeast cells for lymphocytes.

Trypanosomiasis

Examination of the CSF is an important part of staging African trypanosomiasis. This disease has two phases: the first is the acute phase in which the parasite is localized in the blood stream and the patient suffers from fever, skin rashes and lymphadenopathy; the second cerebral phase is characterized by deteriorating mental function. Suramin, the main drug used for the treatment of trypanosomiasis, does not cross the blood–brain barrier and it is thus ineffective in the treatment of late disease. The CSF must, therefore, be examined to determine if it has become infected, in which case melarsaprol, which crosses the blood–brain barrier but has many serious adverse effects, must be used. CSF examination in these circumstances should not be performed until sufficient treatment has been given to ensure that trypanosomes have been cleared from the circulation to minimize the risk of them being inoculated into the peri-spinal space.

The CSF obtained must be examined within 15 minutes of its collection as trypanosomes rapidly lose their motility and disintegrate. The specimen should be examined with the ×40 objective, with the diaphragm sufficiently closed to give good contrast. Dark ground microscopy may be used if it is available.

If cerebral trypanosomiasis is suspected a Giemsa-stained preparation of the CSF deposit should be examined, this will facilitate the demonstration of trypanosomes and morula cells. These cells are slightly larger than erythrocytes, have many vacuoles and stain dark red.

Primary amoebic meningitis

Primary amoebic meningitis is a very rare condition associated with swimming in stagnant water. In this circumstance, direct examination of CSF demonstrates the absence

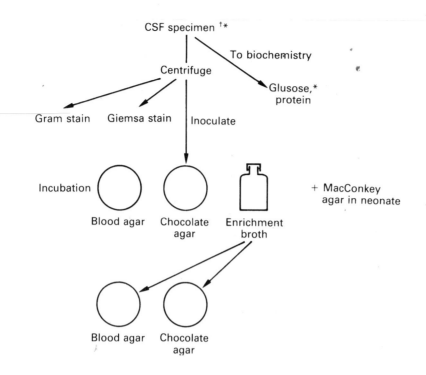

Figure 15.3
Processing of
specimens of
cerebrospinal fluid
(CSF)

* Concurrent blood glucose should be taken

† Concurrent blood cultures should be taken

of bacteria. *Naegleria* can be demonstrated using the ×10 objective in unstained preparations. The organisms are 22 by 7 µm and are rapidly motile. Unlike *Entomoeba histolytica*, they remain motile for several hours at room temperature and do not phagocytose red cells. They can be stained with Giemsa and haematoxylin but do not stain well by Gram's method.

Culture

The centrifuged deposit should be inoculated on chocolate agar and incubated in a humidified atmosphere and 10% CO_2, and on blood agar incubated aerobically. In addition, if the specimen has been obtained from a neonate (among whom *E. coli* meningitis is common) the specimen should be inoculated onto MacConkey's agar. An enrichment medium should also be inoculated and one such as

Robertson's cooked meat broth or Brewer's medium could be used. The enrichment medium should be subcultured after 24 hours on both blood and chocolate agar (Fig. 15.3).

Organisms may be cultivated only from the enrichment broth, and there is no problem of attaching significance to such an isolate if it is a primary pathogen such as *N. meningitidis*. If, however, the organism is a possible skin commensal the clinical condition should be reviewed to determine the significance of the isolate which may be of importance in a patient with an indwelling intraventricular shunt.

If tuberculous meningitis is suspected the CSF deposit should be inoculated on two slopes of Lowenstein-Jensen medium, one incorporating glycerol and another incorporating pyruvate, and into Kirchner's liquid medium for maximum diagnostic yield.

When cryptococcal meningitis is suspected Sabouraud's agar should also be added.

Antigen detection in the CSF

Detection of bacterial antigens in the CSF has been the subject of much research. This approach has the advantage that a rapid diagnosis is available usually within one hour of the specimen being submitted. In general, antigen detection, by whatever method employed is more sensitive than Gram staining, detecting approximately 10^3 organisms/ml compared with 10^5–10^6 organisms/ml. Antigen can be detected even after antimicrobial therapy has commenced and when direct microscopy is negative.

Most of the organisms that cause pyogenic meningitis have a polysaccharide capsule, for example *S. pneumoniae* and *N. meningitidis*. The polysaccharide which the organisms produce is not readily degraded in the body and thus it circulates in the serum for a number of days. It is excreted in the urine and bacterial antigens can be detected for up to two weeks. The appropriate specimens for bacterial antigen detection are, therefore, CSF, serum, and urine. The techniques utilized include countercurrent-immunoelectrophoresis, coagglutination, latex agglutination and enzyme-linked immunosorbent assay (ELISA). These methods are described in detail in Chapter 21.

The specificity of CSF antigen techniques is high but the sensitivity is variable. Sensitivity is higher in studies in developing countries than in developed countries; this is probably related to the severity of the meningitis (i.e. the number of organisms present in the CSF on presentation). Antigen concentration in the CSF can be directly related to the mortality for several pyogenic meningitides and has been used to plot the recovery of patients with pneumococcal meningitis.

Other investigations

Microbiological investigations are not the sole means of making a diagnosis of meningitis. CSF glucose and protein concentrations must also be measured. The concentration of glucose in the blood must also be measured to provide a ratio. In patients with bacterial meningitis the CSF glucose concentration is usually less than 40% of that found in the blood. Moreover, patients with a CSF glucose concentration of less than 1 mmol/l have a poorer prognosis than those with higher concentrations. Protein concentration is raised in bacterial meningitis; in tuberculous meningitis is can be very high. Other non-infective conditions can alter the results of both CSF glucose and protein. CSF glucose is lower in patients with lymphomas and leukaemia with cerebral invasion. Protein can be mildly elevated in multiple sclerosis and markedly raised if there is an obstruction in the free flow of CSF (Froin's syndrome).

Differentiation of bacterial and aseptic meningitis

The standard textbook definition of CSF findings in bacterial and viral meningitis is apparently straightforward, and is illustrated in Table 15.2. However, in partially treated pyogenic meningitis the predominant cell type may be the lymphocyte with minimal change in the CSF/blood glucose ratio. Similarly, the polymorph may be the predominant cell early in the course of viral or tuberculous meningitis.

Measurement of the concentration of CSF lactate can distinguish between viral and bacterial meningitis: patients with viral meningitis have normal concentrations of lactate while lactate concentrations in bacterial meningitis are elevated. Measurement of C-reactive protein (CRP) in the serum may help to distinguish bacterial from viral meningitis. CRP concentrations are elevated in bacterial meningitis but normal or only minimally raised in the case of viral disease. The measurement of CSF CRP is more specific but requires a very sensitive detection system as the concentrations found within CSF are much lower than those found in serum.

Brain abscess

A brain abscess is a pyogenic infection in the cerebral substance. Such infections arise from metastatic spread of sepsis from other sites. Chronic bronchial sepsis, as in the case of bronchiectasis, is an important predisposition. Primary haematogenous abscesses may arise and these are usually polymicrobial infections in which one of the organisms isolated is often 'S. milleri'. Infection may also spread from contiguous structures: frontal, mastoid or maxillary sinuses, or chronic otitis media. Brain abscess can also be the result of direct inoculation of organisms following a compound skull fracture or penetrating foreign body.

Brain abscesses present clinically with the signs of infection together with lowered consciousness level and signs of an intracerebral space-occupying lesion. Patients may complain of headache, and may vomit. Focal neurological signs may be present such as focal epileptic seizures or upper motor neurone lesions.

Bacterial flora

Brain abscesses are often polymicrobial especially when the organisms have their origin in the gastrointestinal tract or arise as a result of bronchiectasis. Anaerobic organisms are frequently involved including *Bacteroides* spp., *Porphyromonas* spp. and anaerobic cocci. *Streptococcus milleri* is often a component and other aerobic and facultative anaerobes found include *S. aureus* and *Proteus* spp.

Tuberculomas

Tuberculomas are small, caseous foci found in the brains of patients with miliary tuberculosis, which are often multiple. Individual tuberculomas may enlarge to produce mass effects. Fungal abscesses with *Aspergillus* usually occur only in severely immunocompromised patients such as those undergoing liver or bone marrow transplantation.

Parasites

Other infectious causes of mass lesions in the brain include cerebral toxoplasmosis which is an important cause of death in AIDS patients. *Entamoeba histolytica* infection can be complicated by metastatic abscesses of which the most common site is the liver, but amoebic brain abscesses do occur. Autochthonous infection with *T. solium* eggs gives rise to cysticercosis in which the intermediate stage of the parasite develops in the human host instead of the pig (the natural intermediate host). Cysticerci are found throughout the tissues but cerebral cysticerci are the main cause of morbidity and mortality. Cerebral hydatid disease may also mimic brain abscess, this is most likely to arise in *Echinococcus multilocularis* infection.

Diagnosis of brain abscess

The diagnosis of brain abscess is made on the basis of the clinical features of the condition and the use of imaging techniques such as CT scanning. Surgical evacuation of the abscess pus is a part of the therapeutic process and brain abscess pus should be processed to provide a bacteriological diagnosis which may point to the source of the sepsis, and to ensure that the empirical therapy started at the time of diagnosis is adequate. The specimen should be processed in the same way as a pus sample and these methods are discussed in more detail in Chapter 18. It must be emphasized that fastidious anaerobes which are poorly oxygen-tolerant play an important role in the aetiology of brain abscess and therefore if these organisms are to be cultured, gassed out medium and rapid transit to the laboratory, possibly using one of the anaerobic transport systems (see p. 94), is necessary.

Infections of the respiratory tract

Introduction

Acute lower respiratory tract infections are important causes of mortality world-wide. More than five million children under the age of five die of acute respiratory infections each year. Severe community-acquired lower respiratory tract infection is a common medical emergency and acute bacteraemic lobar pneumonia continues to have a high mortality even though active antibiotics are readily available. In milder cases infections of the respiratory tract are the cause of significant morbidity and consequent economic loss due to time off work. Postoperative chest infections have a significant mortality and prolong the patient's stay in hospital, which increases clinical costs.

Specimens from the respiratory tract are a numerically important part of the work processed by the UK laboratories. The difficulties of interpretation imposed by these specimens mean that the amount of clinical liaison is disproportionate to their number.

Specimens which are representative of infection in the alveoli cannot be easily obtained without contamination by nasopharyngeal secretions. The normal flora of the respiratory tract contains many organisms which can, under certain circumstances, act as pathogens (Table 16.1). Many of the respiratory tract pathogens are difficult to cultivate, requiring special media and extended periods of incubation (e.g. mycobacteria or aspergillus), or may not be cultivated with currently available techniques (e.g. *Pneumocystis carinii*).

Classification of lower respiratory tract infections

A large number of different microbial species are capable of invading the lungs and causing disease. Table 16.1 lists some of these but the list is not exclusive. In many instances the diagnosis and choice of therapy can be made only on an empirical basis. To simplify this process patients should be classified into clinical groups in which a particular range of pathogens are more likely.

Sputum

Direct microscopy

The inevitable delay imposed by the need to culture has prompted a search for reliable, rapid diagnostic techniques. The simplest is direct microscopic examination of clinical specimens, or centrifuged deposits of respiratory secretion stained by Gram's method.

The appearance of sheets of Gram-positive diplococci in lacunae of the capsule where the stain cannot penetrate may be diagnostic of pneumococcal infection (Fig. 16.1). A number of studies have reported the positive value of direct microscopic examination of expectorated sputum from patients with acute community-acquired pneumonia. Results obtained from this investigation correlate with more invasive techniques such as transtracheal aspiration. Other studies have found opposite

Table 16.1 Pathogens associated with acute lower respiratory tract infection

Patient type	Common pathogens	Routine diagnostic method	Specimen cross reference
Previously healthy adults	a *Streptococcus pneumoniae*	Culture	Sputum
	Staphylococcus aureus	Culture	Sputum
	b *Mycoplasma pneumoniae*	Serology	
	Chlamydia pneumoniae	Serology	Serum
	C. psittaci	Serology	
	Coxiella burnettii	Serology	
	Mycobacterium tuberculosis	Culture	Sputum
Older patients with chronic respiratory disease	c *Haemophilus influenzae*	Culture	Sputum
	S. pneumoniae	Culture	Sputum
	Legionella pneumophila	Culture/serology	Lavage/sputum
	M. kansasii	Culture	Sputum
Aspiration pneumonia, or pneumonia with bronchial obstruction	Groups a and c	Culture	Lavage
	Bacteroides spp. and *Porphyromonas* spp.		
Postoperative pneumonia and ITU patients	Groups a and c	Culture	Sputum (without dilution method)
	Enterobacteria and Pseudomonas		
Immunocompromised patients	*M. tuberculosis*	Culture	Sputum/lavage
	Pneumocystis carinii	Direct microscopy/DFA	Lavage/induced sputum
	Cytomegalovirus	Culture	Lavage
	Candida albicans	Culture	Lavage
	Aspergillus spp., etc.	Culture	Lavage

results and have questioned the value of the sputum microscopy.

A major advantage of a Gram stain of sputum is that it indicates the suitability of the specimen for culture. This is an essential part of any semi-quantitative method as salivary contamination with upper respiratory tract flora can confound the results of culture. The presence of polymorphonuclear leucocytes (PMNs) and alveolar macrophages suggests the presence of material of alveolar origin, and squamous epithelial cells indicate salivary contamination. Specimens with <10 squamous cells and >25 PMNs per ×10 field are likely to represent alveolar specimens and give results which correlate well with transtracheal aspiration.

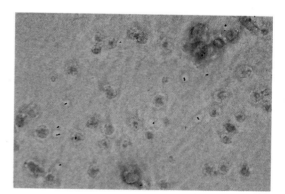

Figure 16.1 Gram-positive cocci typical of *S. pneumoniae* in sputum

Culture

Most patients with lower respiratory tract infection are treated in the community with empirical antibiotic therapy. Once these have been administered the possibility of obtaining a positive culture may fall by sixfold. Many patients are unable to produce a specimen of sputum; some find the process difficult to coordinate, or are too ill to generate the physical effort required. Even when a specimen of sputum can be obtained it is inevitably contaminated by oral flora. These other organisms may inhibit or obscure the growth of respiratory pathogens.

Invasive methods

The majority of patients with acute lower respiratory tract infections may be diagnosed and managed by clinical examination, chest X-ray and conventional sputum culture, but in those who are severely ill, or who are immuno-compromised and at risk of infection with a wide diversity of pathogens, more invasive techniques may be necessary.

Percutaneous transtracheal aspiration can be performed with local anaesthesia and a long intravenous cannula. It may be used on patients who are seriously ill or comatose, who have a pneumonia, and who are unable to produce sputum. Serious complications are rare except in the severely hypoxic and those with bleeding disorders. This technique, however, has, to a large extent, been replaced by broncho-alveolar lavage in which individual bronchopulmonary segments may be lavaged with sterile physiological solutions and the washings aspirated and submitted for micro-scopical examination and culture. This technique was originally used as a tool for obtaining secretions and cells from the lower respiratory tract in patients with lung carci-noma or occupational lung disease. It has proved to be of great value, however, in the diagnosis of patients with life-threatening pneumonia, especially in those who are immunocompromised. In addition, trans-bronchial biopsy can be performed and this may be beneficial in diagnosis of pulmonary infiltrates. Fifty to 100 ml of non-bacterio-static physiological saline is instilled sequen-tially three times and the fluid aspirated and pooled. The specimens are filtered through a sterile gauze pad and cultured semi-quantita-tively.

The specimen should be inoculated on blood and chocolate agar. Less than 10^5 colony-forming units of respiratory organisms are considered not to be significant but possibly due to oro-pharyngeal contamination. The specimen is centrifuged and the deposit diluted and used to inoculate buffered charcoal yeast extract (see below). Sabouraud's agar is also inoculated for the isolation and identification of fungal species including *Aspergillus* and *Candida*. A portion of the specimen should be prepared in a cytospin centrifuge and the deposit used for the detection of *Pneumocystis carinii* (see Chapter 11).

Semi-quantitative culture

A simpler more widely applicable technique is semi-quantitative culture which can be adopted where sputum samples are homoge-nized, diluted and viable counts performed. The value of these techniques is controversial and they suffer from practical disadvantages. Many of the substances used to homogenize sputum, such as *N*-acetyl cysteine and dithio-threitol, reduce the number of viable organ-isms making it imperative that laboratory protocols are adhered to strictly. Semi-quanti-tative methods simplify selection of colonies for identification and susceptibility testing and may assist in the interpretation of culture results.

This approach has proved valuable in a number of studies and correlates well with the results of transtracheal aspirates or broncho-alveolar lavage but is less useful in the diagno-sis of nosocomial Gram-negative pneumonia.

Media

Digested sputum is inoculated undiluted and diluted on chocolate agar, which favours the isolation of *H. influenzae*, and a plate made selective for *S. pneumoniae* such as oxolinic acid, blood agar, crystal violet blood agar, or gentamicin nalidixic acid blood agar. In patients where enterobacteria and *Pseudomonas* are important pathogens MacConkey agar should also be included in the set (Fig. 16.2).

To facilitate the selection of suspect *H. influenzae* and *S. pneumoniae* colonies discs of bacitracin and optichin can be placed on the chocolate and selective plate respectively (Fig. 16.3).

Nasopharyngeal aspiration

In children who do not usually produce sputum, aspirated samples of nasopharyngeal secretions have been used to obtain specimens for culture.

A soft, plastic tube attached to a sputum trap is passed into the nasopharynx via the nose. Gentle suction is applied so that nasopharyngeal secretions are aspirated into the sputum trap.

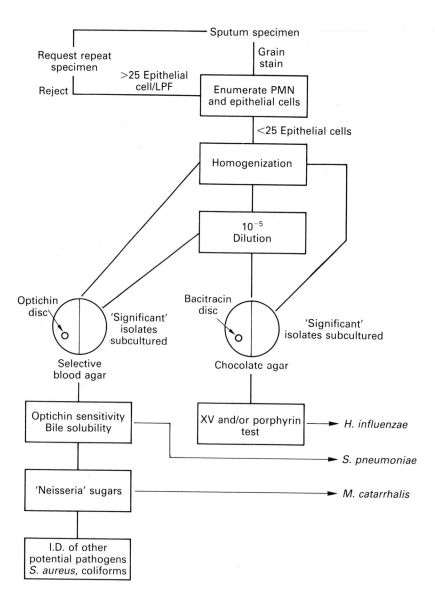

Figure 16.2
Diagram for processing of sputum specimens.

These may be cultured but the interpretation of the results is subject to the same difficulties as sputum samples already referred to above. Semi-quantitative culture of nasopharyngeal secretions can be correlated with the clinical signs of pneumonia in children. Bacterial counts greater than 10^4 cfu/ml of respiratory pathogens were found in 59% of clinically diagnosed bacterial infections compared with 18% of clinically non-bacterial infections.

Lung puncture

A pure culture of respiratory pathogens can be obtained from specimens obtained by lung puncture in patients with radiological consolidation. This technique is not widely applied because of fears of causing a pneumothorax and because it is applicable only to those children with a defined consolidation.

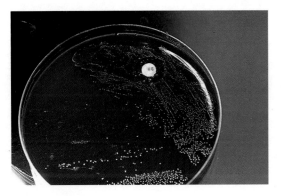

Figure 16.3

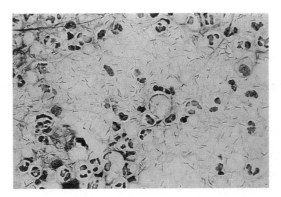

Figure 16.4   Gram stain of *Borrelia vincentii* and *Fusobacteria* from a mouth ulcer

Throat and nasal swabs

Throat and nasal swabs can be used for several diagnostic purposes. The diagnostic aim in taking a throat swab must be clearly followed if much unnecessary work is not to be performed. *Streptococcus pyogenes* and rarely *C. diphtheriae* are the bacteria most clearly associated with acute pharyngitis. Although some other corynebacteriae and *H. haemolyticus* and many viruses have been associated, diagnostic endeavour should be directed toward the isolation and grouping of beta-haemolytic streptococci. In most developed countries the prevalence of *C. diphtheriae* carriage or disease does not warrant routine culture for this organism but all laboratories must be able to isolate, identify and do toxigenicity testing so that the public health services can be alerted when sporadic cases and carriers arise (see Chapter 3).

Direct examination

A Gram-stained smear is of little value in the diagnosis of streptococcal sore throat as the normal flora and pathogens are morphologically indistinguishable. Direct immunofluorescence has been used successfully but has now been superseded by commercial antigen detection latex agglutination tests. The group-specific carbohydrate antigen is extracted from the throat swab by incubation in acid or enzyme and the solution used in a latex agglutination test.

A Gram stain may confirm the presence of *Candida* in oral thrush. It may also demonstrate the characteristic morphology of *Borrelia vincentii* which are found together with fusiform bacteria in cases of Vincent's angina (Fig. 16.4). Deep, painful ulcers are found in the mouth in this condition.

Culture

Throat swabs should be inoculated on sheep blood agar which can be made selective by the additions described above for *S. pneumoniae*. Sheep blood does not sustain the growth of *H. haemolyticus*. Incubation of plates in an anaerobic atmosphere enhances the beta-haemolysis making the selection of suspect colonies easier. Methods for the isolation of *C. diphtheriae* can be found on p. 32.

The throat and nasal swab may also be used in surveillance for organisms which are multi-drug resistant or have enhanced virulence. This is best achieved by using selective medium thus reducing the number of colonies which must be investigated. Methicillin-resistant *S. aureus* (MRSA) pose a cross-infection problem in many hospitals and swabs from one patient from multiple sites including the nose can be pooled by inoculating in a broth with a high salt content selective for staphylococci. The broth can then be subcultured on medium containing 4 mg/l methicillin. All colonies which morphologically resemble staphylococci should be investigated for coagulase and all *S. aureus* identified tested for susceptibility to antibiotics including methicillin.

Mycoplasma and ureaplasma

Classification

Mycoplasma and *Ureaplasma* are members of the Mycoplasmataceae. They have a small genome, 500 MD, the smallest amount of genetic material associated with an extracellular life cycle. Mycoplasmas lack a cell wall and are bounded only by a trilaminar membrane. These organisms are widely found in nature as saprophytes and parasites of animals, arthropods and plants. At least ten species of *Mycoplasma* as well as *Ureaplasma urealyticum* can be isolated from man. These include *M. hominis*, *M. pneumoniae*, *M. genitalium*, *M. orale*, *M. buccale*, *M. faucium*, *M. fermentans* and *M. salivarium*. Most form part of the normal flora but *M. pneumoniae* is a primary pathogen and *M. hominis*, *M. genitalium*, *M. fermentans*, and *U. urealyticum* have been associated with human infection.

Acholeplasma laidlawii* is part of the related Acholeplasmataceae and is sometimes isolated from human specimens but is not associated with disease.

Mycoplasma pneumoniae

Clinical importance

Mycoplasma pneumoniae is an important cause of primary atypical pneumonia. It is probably the second most common cause of acute community-acquired pneumonia in young adults. Infection is characterized by fever, myalgia, pleuritic chest pain, and a non-productive cough, headache is a prominent symptom. Infection can result in the development of antibodies capable of agglutinating the host's own red cells at low temperature, 'cold agglutinins'. This results in peripheral and central cyanosis after exposure to the cold. In addition, mycoplasma infection is associated with reactive (post-infective) arthritis, and neuritis. These are thought to be due to the development of cross-reacting antibodies to host tissue in the joints and the myelin in neurones.

Pathogenicity

Adhesion

Mycoplasma pneumoniae adhere to host cells by the P1-protein, a 169 kD antigen. The receptor for this molecule is not known with certainty but appears to involve sialoglyco-conjugated proteins or lipids, *N*-acetyl-*D*-glucosamine conjugated glycoproteins and glycolipids. Immunity to *M. pneumoniae* infections is short-lived and antigenic variation in the P1-protein is thought, in part, to be responsible for this.

Motility

Mycoplasma pneumoniae exhibits gliding motility, possibly under chemotactic influence, which brings the organism to the base of the cilia where it is safe from ciliary clearance. After adhesion to the ciliated epithelium has occurred ciliostasis develops. This phenomenon may be induced by secreted hydrogen peroxide which damages host membranes and interferes with superoxide dismutase and catalase.

Immune evasion

Opsonized *M. pneumoniae* is readily killed by macrophages and by the activity of the complement system. The organisms are able to overcome these problems as *M. pneumoniae* can be successfully isolated from patients after recovery or treatment of infection.

There are significant similarities between mycoplasma and host membrane glycerophospholipids and this may inhibit host responses. In addition, albumin is adsorbed to the *Mycoplasma* cell membrane. The effect of this is that alveolar macrophages have been shown to be unable to phagocytose *M. pneumoniae* in *in vitro* experiments

Laboratory diagnosis

There is no suitable method for the detection of *Mycoplasma* by direct microscopic examination of clinical specimens. In fact patients with pneumonia caused by mycoplasmas rarely produce an adequate sputum sample.

Isolation

Culture of *M. pneumoniae* is of little value clinically as the organism grows slowly in artificial media. Isolates are obtained only after the patient has recovered. Susceptibility testing is rarely clinically indicated. When culture is attempted specimens from the respiratory tract should be inoculated into PPLO agar plates together with 1/10 and 1/100 dilutions to reduce the inhibitory effect of the specimen on the growth of mycoplasmas. The medium should be between pH 6.5 and 7.5 and incubated at 37°C. Plates and broth should be inspected for up to 21 days for the presence of typical colonies which are small and can most easily be visualized with a plate microscope. Colonies typically grow in the agar with only a slight surface growth; this is described as the 'fried-egg' colony.

Broth cultures should be examined for spherule (microcolony) formation; changes in the colour of phenol red incorporated in the medium will also indicate growth. Once this colour change has occurred the broth should be immediately subcultured to another broth and agar plates for conformation that the colour change is due to the growth of a *Mycoplasma* spp.

Identification

Identification of *Mycoplasma* spp. is a complex procedure and is usually the province of a reference laboratory. Several different characteristics are used. These include the haemolysis test in which colonies are overlaid with a layer of guinea pig erythrocytes in agar and incubated overnight at 37°C. If the organism under test is haemolytic clear zones will be observed around individual colonies. Other characteristics which are used include the optimum atmosphere of growth and inhibition of colonial growth by specific anti-serum absorbed on filter paper discs.

Isolation of *Ureaplasma urealyticum*

Ureaplasma urealyticum is closely related to the mycoplasmas and has similar phenotypic and growth characteristics. It metabolizes urea in growth medium with a resulting rise in pH.

Care must be taken, therefore, as this organism dies rapidly due to exhaustion of the urea supply and the elevated pH produced. The medium should be buffered and isolation broths should be subcultured on fresh urea broth and urea agar immediately there is a change of colour in the indicator.

Serological diagnosis

The most widely used serological test for the diagnosis of *M. pneumoniae* is a complement fixation test which uses whole organisms or lipid antigen. A positive result is indicated by a fourfold rise between acute and convalescent specimens. Cross-reaction between other organisms, especially *Legionella pneumophila* and other non-infectious conditions, occur due to cross-reaction between the mycoplasma glycolipid antigens and glycolipids found in human tissues. It is essential that two serum specimens are obtained as a single high titre is not diagnostic.

An enzyme-linked immunosorbent assay (ELISA) has been described which uses protein surface antigen involved in the *Mycoplasma* – host cell interaction. This may be used for immunoglobulin class-specific antibody detection. An IgM capture ELISA is more sensitive than complement fixation tests and is capable of giving a positive result on a single acute serum.

An antigen capture ELISA has been developed for the diagnosis of *M. pneumoniae* infection, although is not as yet commercially available. The authors report some cross-reaction with *M. genitalium*, but not with the other *Mycoplasma* spp. which may be isolated from human specimens. This technique detected 90% of culture-positive specimens and 43% of culture-negative but seropositive patients.

A cDNA probe directed against specific ribosomal RNA sequences of the organism is commercially available. In comparison with culture, sensitivity and specificity of approximately 90% with a more rapid turn around time. In comparison with antigen capture ELISA, the cDNA probe had a lower limit of detection, approximately 2×10^3 colony-forming units/ml. This is between 10 and 100 times less sensitive than culture.

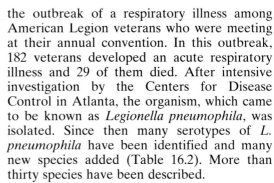

Significance of positive culture

Isolation of *M. pneumoniae* from a clinical specimen provides an aetiological diagnosis of acute lower respiratory tract infection. However, as both *M. hominis* and *U. urealyticum* are commonly found as part of the genital flora, the interpretation of isolates is more difficult. A positive culture must be interpreted in the light of clinical symptoms and examination. *Mycoplasma hominis* and *U. urealyticum* have both been associated with non-gonococcal urethritis, and isolation of one of these organisms in this clinical circumstance would provide supportive evidence of a clinical infection. They can act as opportunist pathogens especially in the female genital tract where they may be associated with salpingitis and post-partum fever. They have also been associated with male and female infertility, but their role in these circumstances cannot be clearly defined. *Mycoplasma genitalium* has been isolated from patients with acute non-gonococcal urethritis.

Antibiotic susceptibility

As they lack a cell wall these organisms are naturally resistant to beta-lactams and cephalosporins. They are sensitive to erythromycin, tetracycline, aminoglycosides, rifampicin, chloramphenicol and quinolones.

Legionella

Definition and classification

Legionella spp. are Gram-negative, aerobic, non-sporing, non-acid fast, encapsulated bacteria, 0.3–0.7 μm × 2–3 μm. The cell wall contains lipids and fatty acids and large amounts of polyisoprene ubiquinones. The catalase and oxidase reactions are variable and many species, including *L. pneumophila*, produce a beta-lactamase. All *Legionella* spp. are motile with the exception of *L. oakridgensis*. Pili have been identified on *L. pneumophila* and it also produces an extracellular acid polysaccharide layer.

Legionella pneumophila was first described as a result of the investigation which followed the outbreak of a respiratory illness among American Legion veterans who were meeting at their annual convention. In this outbreak, 182 veterans developed an acute respiratory illness and 29 of them died. After intensive investigation by the Centers for Disease Control in Atlanta, the organism, which came to be known as *Legionella pneumophila*, was isolated. Since then many serotypes of *L. pneumophila* have been identified and many new species added (Table 16.2). More than thirty species have been described.

Although *L. pneumophila* is capable of causing severe pneumonia and death it is primarily an environmental organism. Human infection usually results from the transmission, by the aerosol route, of organisms that have colonized water supplies and air-conditioning systems: person-to-person spread is rare.

Pathogenicity

In common with other Gram-negative bacteria, *Legionella* spp. express a lipopolysaccharide (LPS) which, in the case of serogroup 1, is tightly bound to the major outer membrane protein. Although distinctly different from LPS of Enterobacteriaceae cross-reactions with some salmonellas do occur.

The major outer membrane protein shares some of the antigenic characteristics with *Chlamydia*. It is made of four subunits and extensively cross-linked by disulphide bonds. The major surface protein (MSP) is a protease which has been implicated in cytotoxicity. It is thought to play a major part in the pathogenesis of Legionnaires' disease. It is a neutral exoprotease of molecular weight 39–40 kD which plays a role in the destruction of pulmonary tissue found in this disease. *L. pneumophila* and *L. micdadiae* have the capacity to survive within the cytoplasm of macrophages in vacuole lined with host ribosomes and which fails to fuse with the lysosome.

Clinical importance

The clinical picture of patients with legionellosis is similar, irrespective of the serotype of the causative organism. Serotype 1 is the organism most often associated with human

Table 16.2 Examples of biochemical reactions of *Legionella* associated with human disease

Species	Oxidase	Catalase*	β-lactamase	Hippurate hydrolytis	Gelatin
L. pneumophila	+/–	+	+	+	+
L. micdadei	+/+	+	–	–	–
L. bozemanii	+/–	+	+/–	–	+
L. long beachae	+	+	+/–	–	+
L. dumoffii	–	+	+	–	+
L. gormanii	–	+	+	–	+

* Represents peroxidase activity.

infections often in institutional or community outbreaks associated with a single source. Other serotypes or species can cause disease but usually only in patients with a compromised immune system.

Patients with legionellosis are often in an older age group and there is an association with smoking and excessive alcohol intake. The patient presents with a cough which is usually non-productive, chest pain, and fever usually above 39°C. Other associated symptoms include mental confusion, diarrhoea, nausea, and vomiting. As in other atypical pneumonias, clinical examination of the chest is often unremarkable. The chest radiograph shows patchy consolidation.

Pontiac fever is a mild form of infection caused by *L. pneumophila* serotype 1. There is no pneumonic change and patients suffer a mild influenza-like febrile illness.

Laboratory diagnosis

Specimens

Patients with legionellosis are often unable to produce a sputum sample. When it is obtained, legionella can be isolated from sputum if appropriate culture techniques are used. In many cases, however, invasive techniques, such as broncho-alveolar lavage, may be required to obtain satisfactory specimens from the lower respiratory tract.

Legionella may also be obtained from respiratory tissue, post-mortem specimens, and rarely from blood cultures and other sterile sites such as pleural effusions. Water supplies in hospitals and samples from cooling towers may be cultured for the organism.

Specimens should be transported from laboratory with minimal delay to prevent overgrowth of other bacteria. *Legionella* spp. survive readily at ambient temperatures but if inoculation is delayed, the specimen should be held in the refrigerator.

Direct examination

Microscopical examination of sputum specimens stained by Gram's method are not valuable for diagnosis as legionellas are only faintly stained. Direct fluorescent antibody methods were the first technique available for routine laboratory diagnosis but, although rapid, this is much less sensitive than culture, at best having a sensitivity of 80%. It is highly specific up to 99%, although occasional cross-reactions with non-legionella organisms do occur.

Culture

Legionella spp. have fastidious growth requirements and cysteine is required. Broncho-alveolar lavage and sputum specimens contain substances which are inhibitory to growth. To overcome this problem specimens should be diluted at least 1 : 10, and acid treatment of specimens can increase the diagnostic yield. This technique has proved to be particularly valuable in isolation of legionella from environmental specimens.

The principal isolation medium is buffered charcoal yeast extract agar, supplemented with alpha-ketoglutarate. The medium can be made selective by the addition of antibiotics (vancomycin, polymyxin B and anisomycin or cefamandole).

Legionellas grow slowly, producing colonies of 1–2 mm after three days. Colonies are round, greyish-pink and opalescent, with entire edges (Fig. 16.5). Suspect colonies are subcultured on cysteine-deficient buffered charcoal yeast extract agar (BCYE) which will confirm cysteine dependence and show that the isolate is likely to be a *Legionella* spp.

Identification

An organism can be presumptively identified as a legionella if it is Gram negative and requires cysteine for growth. Colonies of some legionella species fluoresce under long-wave u.v. light (e.g. *L. pneumophila* fluoresces yellow-green, whereas *L. gordonae* fluoresces blue-white). Many legionellas produce a brown, diffusible melanin-like pigment on media containing tyrosine and this feature can have diagnostic significance. Hydrolysis of hippurate and gelatin may be useful in differentiating the species *L. pneumophila* from others (see Table 16.2). Direct immunofluorescence can be used to identify *Legionella* spp. and to classify them according to their species and serotype. In view of the large numbers of species and serotypes, this technique is usually confined to reference laboratories.

The molecular weight of major cell wall ubiquinones can be used to distinguish *Legionella* species, as can the study of the composition of major cell wall fatty acids by gas-liquid chromatography.

Serology

Legionella pneumophila antibodies may be detected by an indirect immunofluorescence technique. A positive diagnosis may be made if a fourfold rise in titre is observed. A single value of 1 : 128 or greater in a patient with an appropriate clinical history could constitute strong supportive evidence. Serum antibody responses are often delayed in some patients; a second serum should, therefore, be obtained a month after the onset of symptoms. This technique is usually only applied to serogroup 1 *L. pneumophila* infections, as this is the most common, but the technique can be applied to other serogroups, if the appropriate antigen is used.

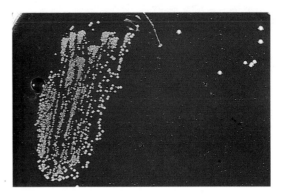

Figure 16.5 Pinkish colonies of *L. pneumophila*

A rapid microagglutination test is commercially available, which consists of stained *L. pneumophila* serogroup 1 whole bacterial antigen. The test is performed in v-bottomed microtitre plates; dilutions of patients' sera are made and antigen added, shaken and incubated for 10 minutes at room temperature followed by centrifugation in a microtitre plate carrier at 350 g. Positive results are indicated by a tight button, in contrast to negative results where bacteria are streaked down the side of the well, giving a teardrop pattern. A single titre greater than eight is suggestive of legionellosis in a patient with an appropriate clinical history. Rapid microagglutination tests should be confirmed by indirect fluorescent antibody testing.

Soluble *L. pneumophila* antigen may be detected in urine, and a commercial radio-immunoassay kit is available for this purpose. Clinical evaluation has indicated that this technique is highly specific and has a sensitivity of greater than 80%. In animal experiments, the limit of detection was shown to be 12 ng/ml of legionella LPS when a similar ELISA technique was used.

Antibiotic susceptibility

Legionellas are susceptible to erythromycin, rifampicin, 4-fluoroquinolones, and co-trimoxazole. Most species produce beta-lactamases and aminoglycosides have limited efficacy because of the intracellular location of the pathogen.

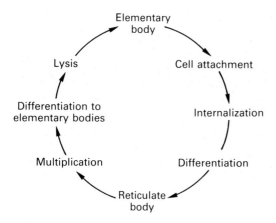

Figure 16.6 'Life cycle' of chlamydia. Elementary bodies enter host cells and differentiate into the metabolically active reticulate bodies. Before cell lysis they differentiate into elementary bodies which are adapted for extra cellular survival

Chlamydia causing respiratory infection

Classification of *Chlamydiae*

The family Chlamydiaceae has one genus, *Chlamydia* with three species: *C. trachomatis* which infects the eye and the genital tract (see Chapter 19), and the two respiratory pathogens *C. psittaci* and *C. pneumoniae*. They are all obligate intracellular bacteria which exist in two forms: the reticulate body, the non-infective intracellular vegetative form and the infective elementary body which is derived from the reticulate body by binary fission is the extracellular form (Fig. 16.6). *Chlamydia* spp. express a genus-specific antigen, the lipopolysaccharide, in addition there are species-specific antigens, polypeptide antigens and in *C. trachomatis* serotype specific antigens.

Pathogenicity

The virulence of *Chlamydia* spp. can be correlated with the *in vitro* growth characteristics but this is not understood at the molecular

level. The major outer membrane protein (MOMP) represents 60% of the OMP but is not essential for the process of cellular invasion, and may participate in mucosal cell recognition. Cysteine-rich proteins are found in elementary body OMP. Of these a 60 kD protein is thought to be associated with enhanced invasiveness and virulence. Different adhesin molecules have been recognized in *C. trachomatis* (18 and 32 kD antigens) and *C. psittaci* (17–19 kD antigen). The lipopolysaccharide of *Chlamydia* consists of lipid and ketodeoxyoctonoic acid components and is antigenically related to Re-type mutants of *Salmonellae*.

All chlamydial strains possess a small cryptic plasmid and when cured are unable to survive within cells. The function of the polypeptides coded on these plasmids is unknown.

Chlamydia psittaci

Chlamydia psittaci is a common pathogen of birds and mammals. Psittacosis is a zoonosis in which infection is transmitted to man from birds, most notably psittacine species (parrots, etc.). Human-to-human transmission does not occur. After an incubation period of 10–14 days an atypical pneumonia gradually develops characterized by fever, a dry unproductive cough, dyspnoea, headache and myalgia. Mental abnormalities including depression or agitation may be a feature. Clinical examination reveals few signs of consolidation and chest X-ray shows a patchy consolidation.

Laboratory diagnosis

Chlamydia psittaci can be cultured in cyclohexamide-treated McCoy cells in the same way as *C. trachomatis*. However, laboratory infection with *C. psittaci* has often been described and thus culture should be performed only when adequate containment facilities (category 3) are available, and isolation is clinically indicated.

Serological diagnosis

Psittacosis is usually diagnosed by serological means because the organisms grow slowly in artificial culture and is little faster than waiting for a convalescent serum. Rising or falling titres of complement-fixing antibodies indicate acute or recent infection. Species-specific micro-immunofluorescence, IgM tests, and IgM capture ELISAs have been described. With this technique, IgM antibodies may be detected early in the course of acute infection. The results correlate with whole inclusion indirect immunofluorescence and positive results are found in patients with a complement-fixation titre greater than 64. IgM antibodies rarely persist for more than six months.

Chlamydia pneumoniae

Chlamydia pneumoniae is the third and most recently recognized member of the order Chlamydiales, family Chlamydiaceae. It was previously known as the TWAR agent, a name derived by the designation of two early isolates. *Chlamydia pneumoniae* is associated with 'atypical pneumonia' but, unlike *C. psittaci*, it does not have a bird or animal reservoir, and is transmitted from human to human. It produces a pneumonia or bronchitis which is clinically mild. Infection can be associated with pharyngitis, sinusitis, sore throat, and laryngitis.

Chlamydia pneumoniae shares the genus-specific antigen, but there are no cross-reactions in the species-specific micro-immunofluorescence test with *C. psittaci* or *C. trachomatis*. Only a single serovar is recognized at present. The organism can be grown in HeLa cells where characteristic, round, dense inclusions can be seen if the cells are stained with Giemsa's stain. In contrast to *C. trachomatis* glycogen is not present and electron microscopy reveals structure and morphology distinct from other chlamydial species. The *C. pneumoniae* elementary body is typically pear-shaped, with round cytoplasmic mass and large periplasmic space.

Laboratory diagnosis

Isolation

Chlamydia pneumoniae may be isolated in HeLa cells and in the yolk sacs of embryonated chicken eggs. In contrast to other chlamydia, McCoy cells are not as sensitive as HeLa cells. Identification of *C. pneumoniae* in culture can be faciliated by fluorescence-labelled monoclonal antibody. A species-specific antibody is available, but genus-specific monoclonal antibody will stain *C. pneumoniae* but not separate it from other species.

Serological diagnosis

The genus-specific chlamydia complement fixation test will detect antibodies in *C. pneumoniae* infection. During primary infection a rise in complement-fixing antibodies takes place, but in re-infection there is no rise in complement-fixing antibody. Antibody responses are often delayed up to 21 days after the initial onset of symptoms, and thus a convalescent serum specimen should be taken at least two weeks after the acute specimen. A positive diagnosis may be made if there is a fourfold rise or fall in complement-fixing antibody.

The micro-immunofluorescence test, which is species specific, may be used to diagnose *C. pneumoniae* infection. In this type of assay IgM responses are often delayed and IgG may not reach diagnostic levels for up to eight weeks. In second infections, there may be no or only a modest rise in IgM antibody concentration.

Coxiella burnetii

Classification

The genus *Coxiella* contains a single species, *C. burnetii*, which is a small, Gram-negative, rod-shaped bacteria closely related to *Rickettsia*. It usually infects cattle, sheep and goats, localizing in the placentas of pregnant animals. It survives desiccation in the environment and although it may be found in ticks it differs from the *Rickettsia* in being transmitted predominantly by the aerosol route.

Coxiella burnetii undergo antigenic variation: phase I antigens are expressed in nature and phase II antigens after passage in tissue culture.

Clinical importance

This organism is the causative organism of Q fever which presents as an atypical pneumonia or pyrexia of uncertain origin. In about 50% of the patients the clinical picture is dominated by hepatitis and splenomegaly. In a proportion of patients infection relapses after a long latent period, taking the form of culture-negative endocarditis or granulomatous hepatitis.

Laboratory diagnosis

Q fever is usually diagnosed by a complement fixation method utilizing both phase 1 and 2 antigens. Complement-fixing antibodies to phase 2 antigens rise in the second week of infection and reach their peak two weeks later. Antibodies to phase 1 antigens remain low. However, in chronic granulomatous Q fever and endocarditis high anti-phase 1 antibody levels are found.

Examination of faeces for bacterial pathogens

Introduction

Diarrhoeal diseases are the most important cause of mortality in children under the age of five throughout the developing world and are also responsible for growth retardation and chronic ill-health. In developed countries it is rare for bacterial diarrhoea to result in a death, but it does, however, cause significant morbidity and economic loss through absence from work.

There has been an increase in food-related diarrhoeal diseases over the past 10 years. This is due to intensive methods of animal husbandry in which animals are kept in close proximity, facilitating the spread of enteric organisms. Cramped transport to market and poor slaughterhouse methods may facilitate the transfer of diarrhoea-causing organisms between animals and from one carcass to the other by implements used in slaughtering and processing. In the kitchen infection can occur when raw food contaminates cooked food which will not be heated again before eating.

The food that we eat has changed in nature with more food being purchased as 'ready to cook' chilled meals for regeneration in microwave ovens. If food is stored at too high a temperature (i.e. not in the refrigerator), enteric organisms will be able to multiply. If, while being reheated, the food is raised to an inadequate temperature or for too short a time, organisms will be able to survive.

There has been a marked increase in tropical travel over the last 20 years with the consequent increase in the likelihood of acquisition of enteric pathogens.

Our understanding of diarrhoeal diseases has been transformed over the last 10–15 years, with the discovery of many new pathogens. These include *Campylobacter* and *Helicobacter* spp. and we may expect that more bacterial and viral pathogens will be identified in the future. We also now have an improved understanding of the pathogenesis of diarrhoeal disease with the identification of toxins produced by *Escherichia coli* and *Vibrio cholerae*. The mode of action of many bacterial toxins is now understood and several have been cloned. This raises the prospect of live attenuated vaccines being developed based on organisms which have had the critical toxins genetically deleted.

A clinical microbiology laboratory must be able to isolate and identify the major human enteric pathogens, to investigate potential outbreaks of food poisoning and to examine food for the presence of diarrhoea-causing bacteria (see Chapter 22). In addition, when clinical history indicates, it is necessary to examine faeces for the presence of the more unusual organisms or their toxins: *V. cholerae*, *E. coli*, *Clostridium perfringens* and *C. difficile*.

The diverse range of pathogens which may affect the gastrointestinal tract, together with the large number of individual species that form the normal flora of the gastrointestinal tract, means that the investigation of faeces could be extremely time consuming unless selective methods are employed. Examples of some of the major bacteria and parasites infecting the gastrointestinal tract are noted in Table 17.1. This chapter concentrates individually on the major bacterial pathogens causing diarrhoeal disease.

Table 17.1 Examples of organisms found in faecal specimens or causing diarrhoeal disease

Bacteria	*Protozoa and helminths*
Salmonella spp.	*Entamoeba histolytica*
Shigella spp.	*Giardia lamblia*
Escherichia coli	*Cryptosporidium parvum*
Yersinia spp.	*Isospora belli*
Clostridium perfringens	
C. difficile	*Ascaris lumbricoides*
Vibrio cholerae	*Trichuris trichuria*
V. parahaemolyticus	*Strongyloides stercoralis*
Aeromonas spp.	*Taenia* spp.
Plesiomonas shigelloides	*Ancylostoma* spp.
Helicobacter pylori	*Enterobius vermicularis*
Campylobacter spp.	

Bacterial agents of toxic type food poisoning (see Chapter 22)
Staphylococcus aureus
Bacillus cereus
Clostridium botulinum

Direct examination

Macroscopic examination

The faecal specimen should be examined macroscopically for the presence of blood, pus, or mucous exudate, and consistency. It is obviously useful to record that a specimen submitted for the diagnosis of diarrhoea is well formed!

Microscopic examination

Microscopic examination for bacterial pathogens such as salmonellas and shigellas does not yield useful information as these organisms are morphologically identical to the normal faecal flora. In patients with AIDS mycobacteria can be demonstrated by Ziehl-Neelsen (ZN) staining. Microscopic examination is essential for the diagnosis of parasitic infections of the gastrointestinal tract. A faecal smear can be stained by the Ziehl-Neelsen or auramine techniques and examined for the presence of cysts of *Cryptosporidium parvum* and *Isospora belli*. The formol-ether concentration technique can be used to improve the quality of the specimen by clearing fat and removing faecal debris as well as concentrating

the ova and cysts before examination of an unstained preparation. For a more detailed description of methods of faecal parasitology see Chapter 11.

Bacteriological culture

Salmonella and Shigella

Classification

Salmonellae and shigellas belong to the family Enterobacteriaceae. They are Gram-negative rods, non-spore-forming facultative anaerobes which ferment glucose. *Salmonella* spp. are motile, and usually produce gas in the fermentation of sugars, one of the exceptions being *S. typhi*. Using O and H serological markers more than 2200 serotypes have been described. These serotypes conventionally take the name of the site of first isolation, e.g. *S. dublin*.

Shigellas are non-motile organisms which are divided into four species: *S. dysenteriae* (serological group A), *S. flexneri* (serological group B), *S. boydii* (serological group C) and *S. sonnei* (serological group D).

The principal source of salmonellas infecting man is the intestinal tract of cattle, pigs and hens reared by intensive methods. They are transmitted to man when cooked food which has become contaminated with raw food is eaten without further cooking, when food is contaminated by food-handlers with diarrhoea, or by person-to-person spread usually in institutions such as hospitals and old people's homes. Shigellas are transmitted from person to person via the faecal-oral route.

Clinical importance

Salmonellas usually produce a mild self-limiting intestinal infection characterized by fever and diarrhoea. Infection takes the form of an enteritis resulting in large volume stools which do not contain blood. In elderly patients and others who are immunosuppressed invasive infection with bacteraemia can occur. Acute colitis characterized by bloody diarrhoea can be caused by some salmonellas notably *S. cholera-suis* or *S. dublin*.

Infection with *S. typhi*, *S. paratyphi* A or B causes enteric fever. The incubation period is between one to three weeks and the patient presents with a fever which may rise in a stepwise fashion. The liver and spleen may be enlarged and a scanty red rash may be found on the abdomen, the 'rose spots'. Diarrhoea is often present but is not invariably found in this condition. The infection can be complicated by large bowel haemorrhage, perforation and toxic megacolon. Secondary pneumonia and meningitis may occur although this is rare. Osteomyelitis is more common especially among those predisposed by sickle cell anaemia.

Patients with defects of cell-mediated immunity have difficulty eradicating salmonella infection which is, therefore, a significant problem among those infected with HIV. Between five and ten percent of normal subjects will go on to excrete the organism in stool for an extended period. This is more likely to occur when there are abnormalities of the biliary tract or the patient has concomitant schistosomiasis.

Pathogenicity

The first phase of infection is localization to gut epithelium where the majority of salmonella infections remain. The pathogen digests the mucosal glycocalyx, penetrates the mucosal surface and is phagocytosed by the epithelial cell. Organisms localized in the mucosa result in an increase in fluid secretion, but the principal pathogenic change is in the colon where there is a defect in fluid reabsorption leading to large fluid stools.

Salmonellas possess a lipopolysaccharide (LPS) which is an endotoxin stimulating macrophages to produce lymphokines such as interleukin 1 (IL-1) and tumour necrosis factor (TNF). This antigen is also the somatic or 'O' antigen which renders the organism resistant to the bactericidal activity of serum. 'H' antigens are those found on the flagella, and they may exist in two phases: non-specific phase one, and specific phase two. In addition, some salmonellas, notably *S. typhi*, express a Vi (virulence) capsular antigen (1,4,2-deoxy-*N*-acetylgalacturonic acid). Possession of this antigen in *S. typhi* lowers the number of organisms required to initiate an infection by preventing phagocytosis and masking the O antigen.

To initiate infection *S. typhi* must survive gastric acid, and enter the small intestine where the organisms invade the intestinal wall. There they are carried to the regional lymph nodes and phagocytosed. These organisms, however, are able to resist the adverse conditions inside the macrophage and continue to multiply. The bacteria invade the blood stream but are rapidly cleared by the reticuloendothelial system where further multiplication takes place. They then re-emerge to cause bacteraemia and to re-invade the gut via the bile ducts. During the second intestinal phase the infection is located at Peyer's patches and the bowel wall becomes thinned and ulcerated, leading to perforation and haemorrhage (Fig. 17.1).

For organisms causing enteric fever the critical pathogenicity determinant appears to be the ability to survive inside macrophages. Salmonellas which have been genetically altered to be more susceptible to oxidative stress, or have a deletion in phoP locus (coding for resistance to neutrophil and macrophage cationic proteins) have reduced ability to survive inside macrophages and are non-pathogenic.

Shigellas invade the mucosa in a similar way to salmonellas but cause ulceration of the large bowel by the elaboration of toxins. In addition, there is a small excess fluid secretion from the small bowel coupled to a defect in large bowel

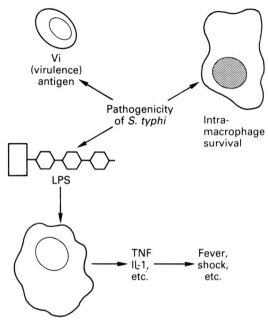

Figure 17.1 Diagram of some of the pathogenicity determinants of *S. typhi*

water reabsorption. These factors together are responsible for the characteristic clinical features of bloody diarrhoea.

Laboratory diagnosis

The isolation and identification of *Salmonella* spp. and *Shigella* spp. form an important part of enteric bacteriology. A combination of media will be required for the maximum diagnostic yield. These use bile salts or other inhibitory substances to select for enteric organisms and an indicator system to identify potential pathogens. Indicator media are used to identify salmonellas and shigellas biochemically. Some of the media used in this process are summarized in Table 17.2.

The process can be divided into a number of different phases:

1 Primary and enrichment culture
2 Screening/identification
3 Definitive identification
4 Typing.

This is summarized in Figure 17.2.

Stage one: selection and enrichment

Deoxycholate citrate agar (DCA)

This medium is highly selective for the isolation of enteric pathogens, especially salmonellas and shigellas. The growth of coliform organisms and Gram-positive bacteria is suppressed due to the presence of sodium deoxycholate and sodium citrate in the medium. Lactose is included in the medium with neutral red so that the colonies of lactose fermenting organisms will appear pink due to a colour change in the neutral-red indicator; they will also be surrounded by a zone of bile precipitated by the low pH. Non-lactose

Table 17.2 Media for selection of Salmonella and Shigella

Medium	Selection	Selective agent	Indicator
MacConkey	Low	Bile salts	Lactose/neutral red
Desoxycholate citrate	High	Bile salts, sodium citrate	Lactose/neutral red Ferric ammonium citrate (H_2S)
Xylose-lysine-desoxycholate	Medium	Bile salts	Lysine/xylose/lactose/sucrose and neutral red Ferric ammonium citrate (H_2S)
Wilson and Blair	High	Brilliant green, bismuth ammonium citrate, ferrous sulphate	Sulphite/sulphide in glucose (H_2S)
Selenite broth	Medium	Sodium selenite	None
Salmonella Shigella	High	Bile salts, brilliant green	Lactose/neutral red Ferric ammonium citrate (H_2S)

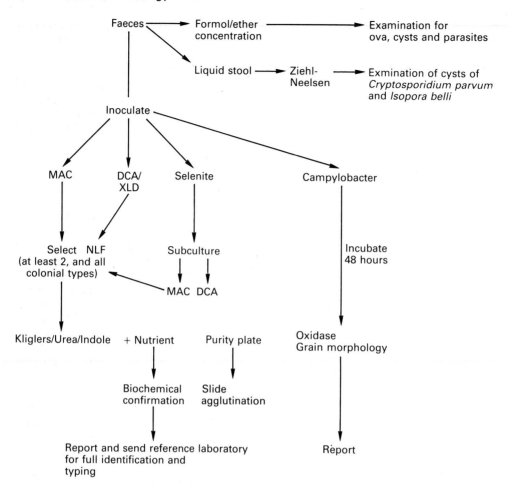

Figure 17.2   An example of a process for isolating and identifying pathogens from faeces

fermenting colonies are colourless, and organisms which produce H_2S will reduce ferric ammonium citrate to iron sulphide which gives the colonies a black centre. Thus, salmonellas produce colourless colonies which often have black centres and shigellas produce small, translucent colonies. *Proteus* and some *Citrobacter* spp. can produce similar appearances to those of salmonellas.

This medium is highly selective for *Salmonella* and *Shigella* and, thus, a heavy inoculum can be used, the only disadvantage of this is that some strains of *Shigella* are inhibited.

Xylose lysine deoxycholate agar (XLD)

XLD medium contains three sugars: lactose, xylose, and sucrose and the amino acid lysine. Colour changes in the colonies occur as the result of complex changes in the pH, depending on the balance of a falling pH caused by sugar fermentation and a rising pH when lysine is decarboxylated. Thus, organisms which ferment two or more of the sugars will cause a fall in pH, whether or not lysine is decarboxylated: coliform organisms, *E. coli* and *Klebsiella* spp. and some *Proteus* spp., will produce bright yellow colonies. Those

Table 17.3 Examples of colonial morphology on XLD medium

Species	Colour of colony
E. coli	Yellow
S. typhimurium	Red with black centres
Sh. sonnei	Red
Pr. mirabilis	Yellow +/− black centre
Providencia spp.	Red
Klebsiella spp.	Yellow

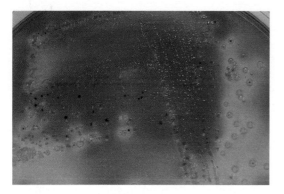

Figure 17.3 Culture of faeces on XLD

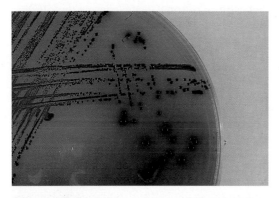

Figure 17.4 Shiny colonies of *Salmonella* on Wilson and Blair's medium

organisms which do not ferment any of the sugars or decarboxylate lysine will produce colourless colonies (e.g. shigellas and some *Proteus* spp.). Those species which decarboxylate lysine and ferment none or only one of the sugars will have red colonies. If, in addition, H$_2$S is produced, the ferric ammonium citrate in the medium will indicate H$_2$S production by the presence of a black centre to the colonies (Table 17.3 and Fig. 17.3). XLD is less selective than DCA, but does inhibit Gram-positive bacteria and favours the isolation of shigellas. A combination of XLD and DCA will optimize the isolation of *Salmonella* and *Shigella* spp.

Wilson and Blair

Wilson and Blair's medium is a modification of bismuth sulphite agar. Unlike the media described above it depends on the dye brilliant green, sodium sulphite and bismuth ammonium citrate for selection. It is highly selective for salmonellas, especially *S. typhi*, and should be used when this organism is sought in specimens of sewage. It has the advantage that salmonellas of the arizona group, which are ortho-nitrophenyl-beta-D-galactosidase-positive (ONPG) (lactose fermenters) and are often missed on conventional media, will be easily detected. Most coliforms and shigellas fail to grow on this medium but *S. typhi* produces black colonies with a characteristic silvery sheen and an adjacent brown-black zone in the agar. Some salmonellas, such as *S. typhimurium* will have a similar appearance (see Fig. 17.4), but other *Salmonella* will have black or grey colonies. *Proteus* spp. may grow as green colonies which may also have a black centre.

Selenite F broth

Selenite broth is a selective medium which is inhibitory to organisms such as *E. coli* and *Enterococcus* which are more sensitive to the toxic effects of sodium selenite than are salmonellas. The selective effect is not complete, for although the unwanted species are inhibited during the first 12 hours of incubation, they later increase rapidly. Salmonellas, in contrast, are able to multiply throughout, allowing enrichment to occur. *Proteus* and *Pseudomonas* are not inhibited, but shigellas are. Studies have shown that the maximum yield of *Salmonella* is obtained after enrichment in selenite broth and inoculation on Wilson and Blair's medium. The selective effect of selenite is most efficient under

Table 17.4   Typical reactions using Kligler's iron agar, indole and urease for screening faecal isolates

Species	Butt	Gas	Slope	H$_2$S	Indole	Urease
E. coli						
Klebsiella spp.	Acid	+	Acid	−	+	−
Enterobacter spp.						
Citrobacter freundii	Acid	+	Acid	+	−	−
Proteus vulgaris	Acid	−	Alk	+	−	+
Salmonella spp.	Acid	+/(−)	Alk	+/−	−	−
Shigella spp.	Acid	−	Alk	−	−	−
Proteus spp.	Acid	−	Alk	−	+	+

reduced oxygen tension and therefore this medium should be poured in tubes with a depth of more than 5 cm.

To obtain the maximum yield of enteric pathogens, a combination of media should be inoculated. A standard set might include a relatively non-selective medium, such as MacConkey's agar, together with XLD which has excellent characteristics with regard to shigellas, and either DCA or Wilson and Blair, which provides optimum conditions for the isolation of salmonellas. At the same time, selenite F broth should be inoculated and subcultured onto Wilson and Blair's medium (see Fig. 17.4).

Stage two: screening identification

There are three types of methods for screening potential pathogens isolated on primary inoculation: a short series of biochemical reactions in small screw-capped containers, composite media (such as triple sugar iron agar, or Kligler's iron agar), and commercial screening systems, such as the API Z.

Kligler's iron agar

When these composite media are used, it is essential to inoculate a single, well-isolated colony to ensure purity of culture. The colony should also be cultured on MacConkey's agar (to confirm purity) and a slope of nutrient agar (for serological tests). This medium permits the differentiation of bacteria on the basis of their ability to ferment glucose or lactose and to produce hydrogen sulphide. A single colony is taken with a straight wire and the surface of the

slope streaked and the butt inoculated by stabbing. This medium contains glucose, an excess of lactose, and ferric citrate, the pH indicator is phenol red. When an organism ferments glucose but not lactose, there is an initial acid production which turns the medium yellow, but under the aerobic conditions found in the slope, this reverts to alkaline. When lactose is fermented, sufficient acid is produced to change the colour of the butt and slope yellow and this does not revert. Gas-producing organisms disrupt the medium and those which produce hydrogen sulphide blacken the medium (Fig. 17.5). Kligler's iron agar can be used with additional tests, such as indole and urease for rapid screening. The reactions of some organisms are summarized in Table 17.4.

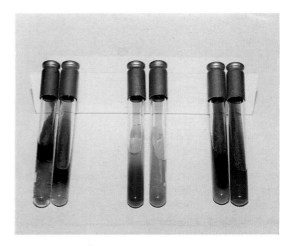

Figure 17.5   Kligler's triple sugar iron medium inoculated showing possible different reactions

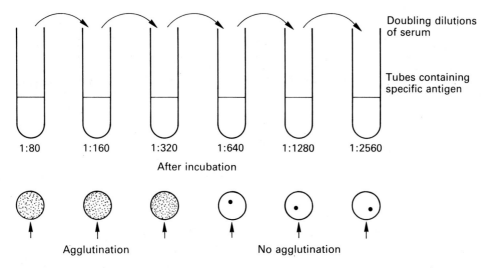

Figure 17.6 Doubling dilutions are made from an initial dilution. Where antibody binds antigen a fine mat of agglutination is seen at the bottom of the tube. Where this does not occur (because the antibodies are so dilute) a button forms as all the bacteria fall to the bottom of the tube

The API Z kit uses preformed bacterial enzymes in the colony to select for salmonellas and shigellas. It consists of two cupules, the second of which is intended to preserve the viability of the organism. The first cupule contains enzyme substrates for a number of different bacterial enzymes and the colour changes in the indicator system which occur can be interpreted by a chart provided by the manufacturers. It does not identify organisms but selects those for further study. This technique has the advantage that it may be read after two hours, effectively shortening the period of identification by 24 hours in comparison to the methods described above.

Stage three: definitive identification

Enteric pathogens such as salmonellas and shigellas should not be reported until the results of initial screening investigations are confirmed by biochemical *and* serological methods. There are many non-pathogens which share cross-reacting antigens with salmonellas and shigellas. The isolation of these organisms can have public health implications resulting in closure of restaurant premises and wards in hospitals. Premature reporting of organisms which are subsequently shown not to be pathogens results not only in inconvenience and financial loss but reduces confidence in the surveillance system. On the other hand, it is essential to initiate the appropriate infection control measures at the earliest opportunity: isolating hospital patients with diarrhoea, and closing wards to admissions when necessary.

The biochemical identification of *Salmonella* and *Shigella* utilizes the same techniques that are applied to the other Enterobacteriaceae which are described in more detail in Chapter 7.

The simplest way of performing serological identification is to use a slide agglutination technique. Slide agglutination results should be confirmed by performing tube agglutination tests (Fig. 17.6).

For salmonellas, agglutination should initially be performed with polyvalent O and specific and non-specific phase H antiserum on a colony obtained from a nutrient agar slope. Positive results should be repeated with monovalent sera. Because of the diversity of H antigens, the use of rapid diagnostic sera can speed up the testing process by the pattern of agglutinations obtained with this mixture of antisera and thus direct the investigator towards a single complex of H antigens for further testing.

(a)

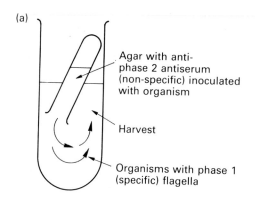

Agar with anti-phase 2 antiserum (non-specific) inoculated with organism

Harvest

Organisms with phase 1 (specific) flagella

Figure 17.7 (*a*) Craigie tube method; (*b*) Jameson filter paper strip method. In these methods antiserum is used to trap organisms with non-specific phase flagella. Those with specific phase 1 flagella retain their motility and can be harvested as shown

(b)

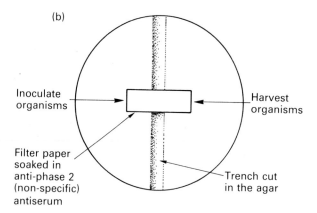

Inoculate organisms

Harvest organisms

Filter paper soaked in anti-phase 2 (non-specific) antiserum

Trench cut in the agar

In many *Salmonella* spp. flagellar antigens are diphasic, with strains varying between two phases with different sets of H antigens. Phase 1 antigens are specific, being limited to one serotype, whereas phase 2 antigens (the group antigens, or non-specific antigens) are shared between many types of salmonellas. When a salmonella is found to have flagella in the non-specific phase, variation can be induced by the Craigie tube method or the Jameson filter paper strip method. Both these techniques use antibodies against the non-specific phase antigens allowing organisms in the specific phase (and therefore lacking the non-specific antigens) to retain their motility and be harvested separately (Fig. 17.7).

Problems with serotyping salmonella

Negative O agglutination may occur if the strain is from a rare serotype not included in the polyvalent typing serum or possesses an O antigen not previously described. Negative agglutinations can also occur if the strain possesses Vi antigen, such as *S. typhi*, which acts to mask the presence of the O antigen. This latter problem can be overcome by heating a suspension of the organism at 100°C for one hour. Similarly, negative H agglutinations may occur with poorly motile strains or in non-motile species such as *S. pulorum*, which lack flagella. In the former case, motile variants can be selected by modification of the Craigie tube method, in which non-specific antiserum is added. Only fully motile variants are able to escape from the inner tube to be subcultured from the surrounding medium (see Fig. 17.7).

Serological reactions among shigellas

The identification of shigellas can be serologically confirmed using methods similar to those employed for salmonellas. As this genus is non-motile, the serotype of the organism is determined by its O antigen. The genus can be subdivided into four main serogroups: A, B, C, and D, which correspond to the four recognized *Shigella* species, *S. dysenteriae*, *S. flexneri*, *S. boydii*, *S. sonnei*, respectively. Within the serogroups, the species can be further subtyped. Cross-reactions occur between the O antigens of *Shigella* serotypes and other *Shigella* species, *E. coli* and *Plesiomonas shigelloides*. For example, *S. dysenteriae* serotype 1 is related to the *E. coli* O group 1 and Alkalescens-Dispar group 1.

Some strains of *Shigella* spp. carry K antigens, which are capsule-like structures which will render them non-agglutinable with the relevant O antiserum. The K antigens are specific for individual serotypes and unrelated to all the other serotypes. Cultures possessing the K antigen can be rendered agglutinable by heating to 100°C for one hour.

Typing

For *S. flexneri*, *S. dysenteriae*, and *S. boydii*, the determination of serotype is usually sufficient to investigate the sources of an outbreak. *Shigella flexneri* can be further subdivided by phage typing. *Shigella sonnei* is serologically homogeneous and phage typing has not been found useful as it gives variable results. The most usual method for subdivision of this species is colicine typing. Many bacteria produce colicines which are protein antibiotics which assist bacteria to establish itself against the competition from other closely related organisms. Colicine production is a relatively stable characteristic and typing is performed by determining the pattern of inhibition in a standard set of indicator strains by the colicine produced from the test strain.

Antibiotic susceptibility

Salmonellas are usually susceptible to chloramphenicol, ampicillin, trimethoprim, fluoroquinolones and aminoglycosides. Chloramphenicol has for many years been the treatment of choice despite the rare idiosyncratic reaction which results in aplastic anaemia. There is increasing evidence that fluoroquinolones are at least equally effective both in producing clinical cure and treating patients with chronic carriage.

Shigellas readily develop antimicrobial resistance by acquisition of resistance plasmids.

Diagnosis of typhoid

Culture

The organisms causing enteric fevers (*S. typhi* and *S. paratyphi* A and B) may be cultured by the techniques described above. The organism can be isolated from stool, urine, blood, bone marrow, duodenal string capsule, or even from the characteristic skin lesions found on the abdomen, the rose spots.

Early in the course of infection, culture of the stool is relatively insensitive, being negative in up to 50% of the cases in the first week. After the beginning of the second week, culture of the stool is likely to be positive, and since 5–10% of patients may become chronic typhoid excreters, the isolation of this organism in stool cannot be considered diagnostic in the absence of the characteristic clinical features of enteric fever.

A definitive diagnosis is made by isolating *S. typhi* from blood. In studies from developing countries in the early phase of infection, blood cultures have a variable sensitivity of between 45 and 77%. The sensitivity of blood culture is enhanced when a large volume of blood is cultured and there is a dilution factor of >1 : 10. In conventional systems, media containing ox bile was found to be superior to simple enrichment media. In laboratories utilizing automated techniques, such as the BACTEC, the sensitivity of blood culture in typhoid fever is over 90%. This compares well with bone marrow aspirate culture, which has consistently been shown to be positive in approximately 90% of cases. Bone marrow aspirate has the added advantage that cultures remain positive after antibiotics have been commenced. Clot culture is a system in which blood is allowed to clot, the serum is taken for a Widal agglutination test, and the clot minced or lysed by streptokinase and cultured. It is now largely a historical curiosity as it is much less sensitive than the techniques described above. *Salmonella typhi* can be found in the urine and this may provide a diagnosis in some cases.

Duodenal string capsule cultures have similar sensitivity to blood culture: patients swallow a duodenal string capsule which is kept in place for at least 4 hours. It is then removed and the duodenal juice obtained is cultured. This technique is also useful for the diagnosis of giardiasis and strongyloidiasis (see Chapter 11).

Serological techniques

Widal test

The Widal test is a bacterial agglutination test which utilizes O and H antigens from enteric organisms. There are a number of problems with Widal agglutinations, most notably their low sensitivity and specificity. This has led many laboratories in developed countries to discard the technique altogether. However, in many cases in developing countries, the Widal agglutination is the only way in which a positive laboratory diagnosis of typhoid can be made. Interpretation of the results in light of knowledge of the patient's background and vaccination history can solve many of the difficulties associated with this technique. Acute and convalescent sera should be used but often only one serum is obtained. A diagnosis can be made only on a single serum if a high value is obtained. The value which is considered significant will vary depending on the population from which the patient comes. Thus, in endemic countries, a background titre of 160 is the norm in healthy subjects and values of 320+ might provide evidence of acute infection. In contrast, patients from developed countries with a titre of 160 might be considered to be positive. Rising titres are also difficult to demonstrate, as often patients from endemic countries have high antibody levels at presentation. Other confounding variables include the patient's vaccination history or previous experience of salmonella infection. To some extent, this position is simplified as more patients are vaccinated with the monovalent typhoid vaccine. However, in response to vaccination, H agglutinations persist for many months, whereas O agglutination titres fall, usually within six months.

Enzyme-linked immunosorbent assay (ELISA) techniques for determination of IgM and IgG antibodies to *S. typhi* LPS have been evaluated and are suprior to Widal agglutination techniques.

Antigen detection

O, H, and Vi antigens may be detected in blood and urine by CIE coagglutination and ELISA. Sensitivities of over 90% and specificity of over 80% have been reported. These techniques cannot replace culture, however, and are currently the subject of research; they are not commercially available.

Yersinia

The genus *Yersinia* is described in more detail in Chapter 7. This organism is found as a common cause of terminal ileitis, acute gastroenteritis, and mesenteric enteritis in some Nordic countries and may be associated with reactive arthritis or erythema nodosum. It is not as commonly reported in other countries and this may reflect, in part, differences in the epidemiology of the organism and also the diligence with which it is sought.

Faeces should be cultured for *Yersinia* when the clinical details are suggestive or when specifically requested by the clinician. The organism grows slowly on MacConkey agar, producing pinpoint red colonies after 48 hours' incubation. Yersinia-selective medium yields more rapid growth, enabling culture to go hand in hand with conventional media. A medium incorporating the selective agents cefsulodin, irgasan, and novobiocin is employed. This medium also contains mannitol and neutral red as *Y. enterocolitica* ferments mannitol, appearing as dark pink colonies after overnight incubation. This species can be further identified by methods suitable for other Enterobacteriaceae.

Escherichia coli

Introduction

This organism poses many difficulties for the microbiologist: to isolate salmonellas, shigellas, and other enteric pathogens selective agents are included to inhibit the growth of *E. coli* without inhibiting the pathogens. Over recent years, however, strains of *E. coli* have been recognized as important primary pathogens in their own right. A microbiologist is, therefore, faced with the problem of selecting pathogenic *E. coli* from the faecal flora.

Several different types of *E. coli* are capable of causing diarrhoeal diseases, such as enteropathogenic (EPEC), enterotoxigenic (ETEC), enteroinvasive (EIEC), enterohaemorrhagic (EHEC). Enteroadherent (EAEC) *E. coli* is the most recent addition.

Pathogenicity determinants and clinical importance

Attachment

Some strains of *E. coli* elaborate a polysaccharide capsule. Strains expressing a K88 antigen are responsible for scour (an acute diarrhoeal disease in pigs), and others with a K1 capsule are most frequently associated with neonatal *E. coli* meningitis and septicaemia. The capsule may act to facilitate adherence as in the case of K88 or as an antigen which mimics host antigens as in the case of K1.

Fimbria play a major role in attachment in the gastrointestinal and urinary tract. Among ETEC a number of families of colonizing factors have been described each of which relates to a different type of fimbrium. CFA/I are 6–7 nm rigid fimbria, and CFA/II are 2–3 nm fibrillar fimbria.

EPEC are capable of causing outbreaks of gastroenteritis in neonatal nurseries and paediatric wards. Electron microscope studies show that they cause destruction of the intestinal microvilli without evidence of invasion. They have been shown to adhere strongly to Hep-2 cells, and this property has been correlated with virulence. Hep-2 adherence is determined by possession of an enteroadherence factor EAF which is a 94 kD protein coded on a plasmid.

The enteroadherent EAEC do not belong to the EPEC serotypes and do not express the EAF plasmid.

Toxins

ETEC make two main toxins, the heat-labile (LT) toxin and the heat-stable (ST) toxin. The LT toxin consists of a single A subunit and five B subunits. As its structure suggests it is biologically and immunologically closely related to cholera toxin acting via stimulation of adenyl cyclase. The ST mediates its activity via the guanylate cylase pathway.

Escherichia coli O157 serotypes have been implicated in the haemolytic-uraemic syndrome, and they have been shown to produce a verotoxin analogous to the shiga toxin of *S. dysenteriae*.

Laboratory diagnosis

Enteropathogenic E. coli (EPEC)

Specimens coming from patients under the age of three years with suspected gastroenteritis should be inoculated on a selective medium such as MacConkey's agar and blood agar. After overnight incubation, coliform colonies can be tested with polyvalent antisera to EPEC strains by slide agglutination. Isolates which are positive with polyvalent antisera should be retested with monovalent antisera and full biochemical identification performed.

Enterotoxigenic E. coli (ETEC)

These strains are important causes of diarrhoeal diseases, especially in those travelling to tropical countries. Identification of strains producing enterotoxin either heat labile (LT) or heat stable (ST) is necessary for confirmation of this diagnosis. ST production can be diagnosed by a DNA hybridization method, but this is likely to be beyond the means of many routine diagnostic laboratories. Demonstrating LT production is more straightforward and uses a reversed passive latex agglutination or coagglutination assays. If large numbers of specimens are being examined, a tissue culture assay can be performed which utilizes a cell monolayer of Y1 mouse adrenal cells.

Enterohaemorrhagic E. coli (EHEC)

These strains of *E. coli* are associated with the haemolytic uraemic syndrome. This is a febrile illness typically occurring in children infected with EHEC which results in a haemorrhagic colitis complicated by intravascular haemolysis and acute renal failure. This has been most frequently associated with serotype 0157:H7, although other serotypes have been implicated. As most of these strains do not ferment sorbitol, a modified MacConkey medium containing 10 g/l of sorbitol in place of lactose can be used to select for them. Suspect

Table 17.5 Campylobacter genus

Catalase negative	*C. sputorum*	
	subsp. *sputorum*	Mouth commensal
	subsp. *bulbulus*	Commensal bovine genital tract
	subsp. *mucosalis*	Intestinal adenomatosis of pigs
Catalase positive Non-thermophilic	*C. fetus*	
	subsp. *venerealis*	Cattle infertility
	subsp. *fetus*	Abortion in sheep and cattle; occasional opportunist
Catalase positive thermophilic	*C. jejuni*	Acute enterocolitis (see text)
	C. coli	Commensals birds and animals
	C. laridis	Commensal seagulls; occasional infection in man

colonies can then be identified with antiserum to 0157 and H7 and confirmed by conventional biochemical testing.

Campylobacter

Introduction

Campylobacter were first recognized in 1915 as a cause of abortion in cattle and sheep. There were later anecdotal reports of human disease caused by 'vibrio-like organisms'. In 1972, Dekeyser developed a membrane filtration method, permitting the isolation of *Campylobacter* spp. from stools for the first time. However, it was only when Skirrow developed a selective medium that it became feasible to isolate *Campylobacter* by faecal culture in the routine laboratory and their role in human infections was firmly established.

Classification

The genus is divided into two groups depending on the presence of catalase. The catalase-negative group are usually not pathogenic to humans but are commensals and pathogens of animals. Included in this group is *C. sputorum* which has been found in up to 2% of faecal samples from healthy subjects, but a pathogenic role for this organism has not been found. *Campylobacter mucosalis* is thought to be associated with intestinal adenomatosis in

pigs. Human infection has not been reported.

The catalase-positive group includes species which are pathogens and commensals of animals and humans. This group can be subdivided into thermophilic and non-thermophilic species. The non-thermophilic species *C. fetus* ssp. *fetus* and *C. fetus* ssp. *venerealis* are mainly animal pathogens. *Campylobacter fetus* ssp. *fetus* is associated with spontaneous abortion in cattle and sheep and can occasionally cause septicaemia and meningitis in patients predisposed to infection. It can also be found in the human intestine and may be responsible for some cases of diarrhoea. *Campylobacter fetus* ssp. *venerealis* is a commensal of animals, but human infection has only rarely been reported.

The thermophilic *Campylobacter* spp. are responsible for most human infections: the species implicated are *C. jejuni*, *C. coli*, and *C. laridis*. Campylobacter infection is essentially a zoonosis although person-to-person and institutional infections have been reported. These organisms are found in the intestine of poultry and cattle. Infection is transmitted to humans through eating inadequately cooked meat or drinking contaminated milk. It can also be transmitted by water if it becomes contaminated with faecal material from infected animals (Table 17.5).

Clinical importance

An acute enterocolitis with prodromal symptoms of malaise, headache, myalgia, abdominal pain, and fever is typical. This is followed by acute crampy abdominal pain and diarrhoea, which may be blood stained. The illness is usually short-lived (three to five days) and long-term carriage is unusual. Serious complications are also unusual, but septicaemia may occur, and, in some cases, acute campylobacter infection may be mistaken for an acute abdomen or in infants for intussusception prompting unnecessary surgery. Campylobacter enterocolitis has also been postulated as one of the causes of reactive arthritis.

Pathogenicity determinants

Campylobacters are readily killed at low pH and therefore infection is more likely if milk is the vehicle or patients have low gastric acidity.

They possess flagella and are actively motile which may assist the organism in initiating infection. Campylobacters are thought to adhere to intestinal mucosa via L-fucose receptors. *Campylobacter jejuni* elaborates an enterotoxin which causes fluid accumulation in rabbit ileal loops. It has a similar mode of action to that of cholera toxin. A cytotoxin may also be implicated in the pathogenesis of enteritis. *Campylobacter* spp. express a low molecular weight lipopolysaccharide which is similar in structure to that of *Haemophilus* and *Neisseria* in which there is marked antigenic diversity between isolates.

Isolation

Campylobacters can be isolated from human faeces by culture on selective media and the correct conditions of atmosphere and temperature. Media are made selective for these organisms by inclusion of a mixture of antibiotics, examples of these media are shown in Table 17.6. Inoculated plates should be incubated at 43°C as this increases the selection, but if *C. fetus* is suspected, additional sets of plates should be incubated at 37°C as this species is inhibited by the higher temperature. A micro-aerophilic atmosphere must be provided with 5–6% oxygen, 10% carbon dioxide, and 85% nitrogen. Although candle jars may be used, this atmosphere is most usually generated by a micro-aerophilic gas generating kit, similar in principle to that employed for anaerobic isolation.

Table 17.6　Selective agents for *Campylobacter* isolation

Skirrow	Vancomycin, polymixin B, trimethoprim
Butzler	Bacitracin, novobiocin, cyclohexamide, colistin, cefazolin
Blaser	Vancomycin, polymixin B, trimethoprim, cephalothin, ampotericin B

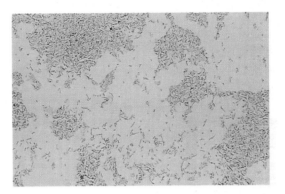

Figure 17.8　Gram stain of *Campylobacter*

Identification

After 48 hours' incubation campylobacter colonies appear as grey, flat droplets. A Gram stain will demonstrate small, curved or spiral, Gram-negative bacteria with a 'gull wing' morphology (Fig. 17.8). If the organism is oxidase positive it may be presumptively reported as *Campylobacter* spp. If species identification is required the organism should be tested for catalase production, its growth temperature requirements and its nalidixic acid sensitivity determined. Hippurate hydrolysis will distinguish between *C. jejuni* and *C. coli*. The usual reactions of campylobacter in these tests are set out in Table 17.7.

Helicobacter pylori

This is one of the 'new' pathogens first described in 1983 and identified as a pathogen in gastritis and duodenal ulcer. It was originally classified as a *Campylobacter* but phylogenic studies have indicated that they are not

Table 17.7 Identification of *Campylobacter*

	Growth 25°C	Growth 43°C	Nalidixic acid	Hippurate hydrolysis
C. fetus	+	−	R	−
C. jejuni	−	+	S	+
C. coli	−	+	S	−
C. laridis	−	+	R	−

related to this group and have been classified as a new genus *Helicobacter*.

Pathogenicity

This organism is the subject of intensive research and some of the potential pathogenicity determinants have been identified. The organism produces copious amounts of urease which may protect the organism from the effects of gastric acid. Other toxins which have been described include a mucinase and several cytotoxins, but the role of these proteins has not been established. The organism agglutinates red cells via a fibrillar haemagglutinin which may bind a glycolipid found on red cells and in the stomach.

Laboratory diagnosis

Many of the tests to diagnose patients suffering from helicobacter infection are clinical and include a ^{14}C urea breath test. Specimens of gastric antrum can be obtained at endoscopy. The simplest diagnostic test is to place such a biopsy specimen in a urease medium and observe for a rapid colour change. Commercial examples of this approach (e.g. CLO-test) are cheap and accurate and do not require microbiological culture. Histological examination of biopsy specimens is an effective way of making the diagnosis.

Helicobacter pylori can be cultivated from biopsy specimens which have been homogenized and inoculated on fresh medium. Media which have been successfully employed include chocolate agar, Skirrow's, and Marshall's brain heart infusion agars. The antibiotic supplement should contain vancomycin 6 mg/l, nalidixic acid 20 mg/l, and amphotericin B 2 mg/l and plates should be incubated in increased humidity in a microaerophilic atmosphere. Translucent colonies 1–2 mm can be seen after three days, but may be delayed until seven days. The organism can be identified on the basis of the Gram morphology, positive oxidase and catalase and rapid urease reactions. Individual isolates can be typed by chromosomal DNA restriction endonuclease digest analysis.

An ELISA can be used for serological diagnosis. The antigen used in the solid phase of this test is crude extract of a mixture of *Helicobacter* strains.

Antibiotic susceptibility

Helicobacter pylori is susceptible to a wide range of antibiotics including erythromycin, tetracycline, gentamicin, fluoroquinolones, and clindamycin. It is resistant to trimethoprim, sulphonamides, and nalidixic acid. The role of these agents in the treatment of disease is not established, however, and there is therefore no indication for antimicrobial susceptibility testing in routine diagnosis.

Vibrionaceae

Classification

There are more than 30 species of vibrios and they are classified together with three other genera: *Photobacterium*, *Aeromonas*, and *Plesiomonas* in the family Vibrionaceae. The genus has been simplified by recent taxonomic changes which have removed genera such as *Campylobacter*, *Pseudomonas*, *Altermonas*, and *Wolinella*.

Vibrios are natural inhabitants of aquatic environments. They are Gram-negative, curved bacilli (the comma bacillus), which are motile by virtue of a single polar flagellum. They are facultative anaerobes, are fermentative and not nutritionally demanding. They do not form spores and are catalase and usually oxidase positive.

Only a few vibrios are associated with human diarrhoeal disease, principally *V. cholerae* and *V. parahaemolyticis*. *Vibrio mimicus* is a species which has been associated with diarrhoea following consumption of seafood. *Vibrio vulnificus* is a lactose-positive halophilic vibrio found in marine environments on the coasts of North America. It is associated with wound infections and primary septicaemia in patients predisposed by liver disease. Primary septicaemia may have a high mortality.

Vibrio cholerae

Clinical importance and pathogenesis

Vibrio cholerae is responsible for pandemics of severe diarrhoeal disease, characterized by acute, severe, watery diarrhoea which rapidly leads to severe fluid depletion, shock and death. Infection is transmitted to man via water contaminated by human faeces. The principal pathogenicity determinant of this organism is cholera toxin. This is a membrane-acting cellular deregulating toxin consisting of five B subunits responsible for attachment to intestinal epithelial cells and a single A subunit which is responsible for toxin activity. The toxin acts by interfering with the regulation of adenyl cyclase within the cell resulting in a massive efflux of water and sodium into the intestinal lumen. It also possesses minor toxins which were identified when human volunteers were given genetically engineered cholera toxin-free mutants but still suffered a mild diarrhoeal illness. All strains possess a lipopolysaccharide and more than 80 serovars have been described. Only *V. cholerae*, however, possessing the 01 LPS, gives rise to cholera, an exception is an outbreak in Bangladesh caused by 0139 *V. cholerae*. *Vibrio cholerae* is motile by virtue of a polar flagellum, and all possess a common H antigen. The 01 *V. cholerae* strains can be divided into three subtypes by absorbed serum: Ogawa, Inaba, and Hikojima. It may also be divided into two biotypes: the El-tor and the classical strain. El-tor is responsible for a lower attack rate and symptomless excreters are more common, the illness is milder with a lower mortality. The strain survives more easily in the environment and these factors facilitate its spread. The non-01 vibrios are biochemically similar to classical and El-tor strains, and have considerable DNA homology. They can cause enteritis or secretory diarrhoea and occasional isolates possess cholera toxin and give rise to a cholera-like disease.

Vibrio parahaemolyticus is an important cause of food poisoning, especially in the Far East, and is associated with the consumption of raw or undercooked fish or other seafood.

Specimens

Fresh faecal specimens should be collected from cases or carriers. When these are obtained, direct microscopy with dark ground illumination may detect the presence of vibrios by their characteristic darting motion which is immobilized when specific antiserum is added. Properly taken rectal swabs can also be used, and vomitus should be cultured if available. Vibrios survive well in liquid stool but are very susceptible to drying. If there is delay in transport Cary-Blair's medium or taurocholate peptone transport medium, both of which contain a high salt content at pH 8.4, will preserve viability for many weeks.

Isolation

Media
The medium recommended for the growth of vibrios including *V. cholerae* and *V. parahaemolyticus* is thiosulphate citrate bile sucrose agar (TCBS) as it inhibits most enterobacteria and Gram-positive organisms. It is rather inhibitory, with a high pH and containing bile salts. However, some *Proteus* and *Enterococcus* spp. may grow and form small colonies. As some of these species ferment sucrose they will appear as yellow colonies. Some *Proteus* spp. produce H_2S resulting in colonies with black centres. *Vibrio cholerae* forms large, yellow colonies that are 2–5 cm after 24 hours' incubation. *V. parahaemolyticus*, in contrast, has green or blue colonies.

An alternative medium is Monsur's tellurite taurocholate gelatin agar. This medium is more sensitive than TCBS, especially for classical strains of *V. cholerae*. The high pH and potassium tellurite inhibit most enterobacteria and Gram-positive organisms, but as in the case of TCBS some *Proteus* spp. may grow. *Vibrio cholerae* produce 1–2 mm colonies with a grey-black centre, with an opalescent halo, which is caused by a gelatinase possessed by the bacterium.

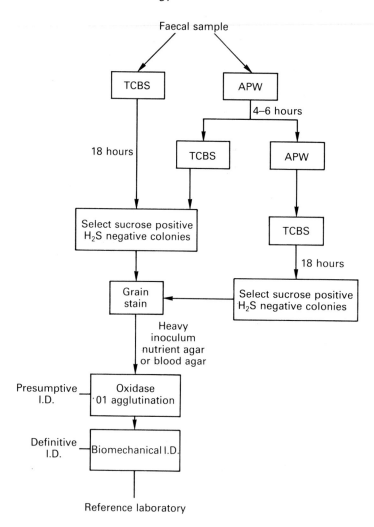

Figure 17.9 An example of a protocol for the isolation and identification of *Vibrio cholerae* from stools

Alkaline peptone water

Alkaline peptone water (APW) is an efficient enrichment media for *V. cholerae* in faecal specimens. Its high salt concentration and pH are inhibitory to other organisms. This inhibition is relatively short-lived, however, so subcultures should be made between five and eight hours after inoculation. In addition, the dilution factor is important in the selective enrichment effect. In consequence, 2 g of faeces should be placed into 20 ml of APW in a 30 ml screw-capped container.

Procedure

A specimen of faeces should be inoculated on primary isolation medium, such as TCBS, and 2 g added to alkaline peptone water. This should be subcultured after five to eight hours onto a second TCBS and alkaline peptone water to be incubated overnight which is again subcultured onto TCBS.

Suspect large, yellow colonies should be selected by the oxidase reaction and Gram stain. Agglutination with 01 antiserum should be performed immediately: suspicious colonies should be cultured with a heavy inoculum on a non-selective medium such as blood agar and incubated for five to eight hours and a standard bacterial agglutination performed. An organism which grows on TCBS, ferments sucrose, is oxidase positive and agglutinates with 01 antiserum can be presumptively reported as *V. cholerae*, enabling the appropriate public health control measures to be initiated without delay.

Table 17.8 Differentiation of classical and El-tor
V. cholerae

Test	Classical	El-tor
Haemolysis	–	+
Chick cell agglutination	–	+
Polymyxin 50 IU	S	R
Vokes-Proskauer	–	+
Classical phage IV	S	R
El-tor phage V	R	S

Biochemical tests employed in the identification of vibrios include sodium requirement, nitrate reduction, arginine dehydrolase, lysine decarboxylase, and ornithine decarboxylase, indole production, Voges-Proskaüer reaction and fermentation tests (Fig. 17.9). Commercial identification kits for enterobacteraceae can be used; however, they do not work well for halophilic vibrios, which require a higher salt content for accurate results. The classical and El-tor biotypes can be differentiated using the characteristics shown in Table 17.8. Two and possibly three subtypes of 01 *V. cholerae* can be differentiated by agglutination with absorbed antiserum: the Ogawa and Inaba subtypes. Strains which agglutinate both antisera fall into the Hikojima subtype. Classical and El-tor biotypes can be phage typed using separate sets of phages.

Aeromonas hydrophila and *Plesiomonas shigelloides*

These organisms are facultative, anaerobic, Gram-negative rod-shaped bacteria which are classified in the family Vibrionaceae, although it has recently been proposed that *Plesiomonas* be moved to the genus *Proteus* on the basis of molecular genetic evidence.

Aeromonas

Aeromonas are part of the family Vibrionaceae. They are Gram-negative, facultative anaerobes which ferment glucose, and are oxidase and catalase positive. Most are motile by virtue of a polar flagellum. There are four main species in the genus: *A. hydrophila*, *A. caviae*, *A. sobria*, and *A. salmonicida* and recently a further four have been added, *A. media*, *A. veronii*, *A. schubertii*, and *A. eucrenophilia*.

Their natural habitat is fresh and salt water and they can be isolated from soil and food such as vegetables and seafood. *Aeromonas* spp. are pathogens of fish and reptiles. Human infection usually takes the form of diarrhoeal disease and outbreaks have been reported. In addition they may infect wounds after water exposure, and cause primary septicaemia in patients predisposed by malignancy or liver disease. Each of the four main species has been shown to cause human disease but *A. hydrophila* is most common. A number of toxins and adhesins have been described but not all strains of *A. hydrophila* carry these putative pathogenicity determinants. Thus, the isolation of this species does not necessarily provide an aetiological diagnosis.

Isolation and identification

Aeromonas hydrophila is most easily isolated by cultivating faeces on sheep blood agar containing 15 mg/l of ampicillin. On this medium *Aeromonas* spp. produce beta-haemolytic colonies which become greener on prolonged incubation. Suspect colonies can be screened by Gram staining and oxidase testing. Identification can be confirmed by standard methods using Kligler's iron agar, etc. (see above).

Most *Aeromonas* spp. are resistant to beta-lactam antibiotics by virtue of beta-lactamase production. They are usually susceptible to aminoglycosides, chloramphenicol, trimethoprim, tetracyclines and fluoroquinolones.

Plesiomonas shigelloides

This organism gained its name because it grows on MacConkey's agar with pale colonies and is agglutinated by *S. sonnei* antiserum with which it shares an antigen. It is found in fresh and estuarine waters, and is more common in tropical areas. It is a cause of enterocolitis associated with the consumption of seafood, or ingestion of untreated water. A number of putative pathogenicity determinants have been reported including heat-labile and heat-stable

Table 17.9   Examples of biochemical reactions of vibrios

| Species | Colonies on TCBS | VP | Growth in nutrient broth with NaCl | | | Indole | Arabinose | Cellobiose |
			0%	6%	10%			
V. cholerae	Yellow	+/–	+	+/–	–	+	–	–
V. parahaemolyticus	Green	–	–	+/–	+/–	+	+/–	–
V. mimicus	Yellow	–	+	+/–	–	+	–	–
V. vulnificus	Green	–	–	+	–	+	–	+
Aeromonas spp.	Yellow/–	+/–	+	–	–	+	v	v/–
P. shigelloides	–	–	+	–	–	+	–	–

enterotoxins. *Plesiomonas shigelloides* can be isolated on MacConkey's agar or DCA where most of these strains are non-lactose fermenters. It is oxidase positive and can be identified using conventional biochemical techniques. It has similar susceptibilities to *Aeromonas* spp., although ampicillin sensitivity is more common.

Examples of biochemical reactions of some vibrios are summarized in Table 17.9.

18

Examination of urine and pus

Urine

Introduction

The microbiological examination of urine is one of the most frequent procedures performed in the microbiological laboratory. The difficulties of obtaining an adequate specimen and transporting it to the laboratory pose a number of technical problems which must be solved by the microbiologist if misleading reports are to be avoided.

The renal pelvis, ureters, and bladder are sterile but the lower urethra is colonized with a wide range of organisms (Table 18.1).

Specimens

Suprapubic aspiration

Urine obtained directly from the bladder should, in the absence of infection, be sterile. In young children the bladder rises out of the

Table 18.1 Organisms found in the normal urethra

Coagulase-negative staphylococci
α and non-haemolytic streptococci
Lactobacillus spp.
Neisseria spp. (other than *N. gonorrhoeae*)
Corynebacterium spp.
Enterobacteraceae
Mycoplasma hominis
Candida spp.
Proprionobacterium spp.
Mycobacterium spp. (other than tuberculosis)

pelvis when full, and can be aspirated when serious sepsis is suspected. A specimen obtained by suprapubic aspiration should be processed like other sterile fluids (see Chapter 15).

Intermittent catheterization

Specimens can also be obtained by intermittent catheterization, but it is possible both to introduce pathogens and to contaminate the specimens.

Mid-stream specimen (MSU)

Most urines submitted for microbiological examination are in the form of a mid-stream specimen, where it is hoped that the flushing action of urine will cleanse the urethra and limit contamination by urethral commensals. Such contamination is inevitable; thus, if the glans or the vulva are not adequately cleaned and the specimen carefully taken in mid-stream, heavy contamination with organisms from these sites will occur. This is a special problem as the organisms forming the normal flora are also implicated in urinary tract infections and therefore cannot easily be disregarded if isolated.

Non-cultural screening methods

A wide range of screening techniques has been developed for detection of urinary tract infection. These have evolved in two ways: the first for general practitioners and hospital clinicians who in their outpatient practice wish to make a rapid diagnosis so that treatment can be initiated before culture results are obtained. These techniques typically use 'dip sticks'. Glucose can be measured in overnight fasting urine as most patients have a trace of glucose present but this will be metabolized by bacteria or white cells. If glucose is absent it may indicate active urinary infection. A protein exudate is made at the epithelial surface as a result of an inflammatory process and may give a positive reading on a protein strip. Many urinary pathogens catalyse the reduction of nitrate to nitrite: detection of nitrite in the urine may also indicate urinary infection.

Microscopy

Microscopy is a valuable adjunct in the diagnosis of urinary infections. The presence of red cells, crystals or casts may indicate systemic diseases such as glomerulonephritis. Detection of epithelial cells helps in establishing the quality of the specimen and, indirectly, the clinical significance of any isolate. Epithelial cells have their origin in the skin of the perineum or the vagina and when they are present it indicates that organisms normally resident in the perineum or vagina are likely to have contaminated the specimen.

The presence of large numbers of white cells provides indirect evidence of infection. It must be remembered that white cells are normally found in urine and it is only an excess which is clinically relevant ($>8/mm^3$). Many conditions may bring about a rise in the number of white cells in the urine other than infection (e.g. high fever) and the absence of white cells does not exclude infection as they die rapidly in acid urine and may only indicate a specimen which has been delayed in transit to the laboratory.

The presence of bacteria detected by direct microscopy of unstained, uncentrifuged samples of urine can be correlated with infection. The limit of detection of bacteria in the urine by microscopy is between 10^4 and 10^5 which is close to the number typically found in infection. Bacteria which enter the urine as contaminants are usually firmly attached to epithelial cells and therefore not easily seen.

Microscopic examination of urine is a highly individual technique and most laboratories have their own methods. These include examination of uncentrifuged, well-mixed urine deposits in commercially prepared plastic counting chambers, conventional glass Neubauer or Fuch-Rosenthal counting chambers, or examination of Gram-stained smear centrifuged deposits. Each of these techniques has its own advantages but the methods are relatively time consuming and expensive in materials. With the desire to reduce the use of glass materials in examining patient specimens alternative techniques should be sought. One simple method is to use an inverted microscope and flat-bottomed micro-titre plates to perform cell counts. This method has the advantage that a large number of urines can be screened rapidly and it also reduces manipulation of the specimen.

Other non-culture techniques

In the laboratory, tests have evolved to determine those specimens which are most suitable for full microbiological investigation by culture and sensitivity testing. Microscopy may be used in this way, but it is inevitable that some specimens where white cells have lysed, or where bacteria may not be seen (i.e. cocci are small and more difficult to identify than Gram-negative rods) will be missed. More 'high tech' solutions to this problem have included enzyme-linked immunosorbent assay (ELISA) techniques to detect secretory IgA and techniques which utilize limulus amoebocyte lysate reaction to detect Gram-negative lipopolysaccharide, although initial results with these techniques have been disappointing. Computer-driven automated culture methods have also been employed, whereby urine specimens are cultured for a short period (e.g. three hours) and the multiplication of bacteria detected automically, usually by optical density reading. Those specimens which show bacterial multiplication are selected for culture.

The diversity of techniques which have been employed and the continuing active research in this area is indicative that none have succeeded in establishing themselves in a pre-eminent place.

Quantitative techniques

Bacteria which infect the bladder or upper urinary tract will be present in large numbers, having had the opportunity to multiply in those sites whereas commensal organisms introduced during micturition will be present only in low numbers. This idea was developed by Kass who stated that an organism with more than 100 000 cfu/ml isolated in pure culture was likely to be participating in an infection. These criteria related to pregnant women submitting an early morning specimen as organisms in the bladder would have had the opportunity to multiply overnight. This approach has now been generalized to include all types of MSU. Multiplication of organisms in the specimen during transit will affect this interpretation. Moreover, urine is a variable sample: urine volume depends on the patient's fluid intake, a higher fluid intake could easily reduce the apparent numbers of cfu/ml in an infected patient to a degree that the urine obtained would not fulfil these criteria. Early morning urine, which contains concentrated urine, and in which organisms have been able to multiply in the bladder during the hours of sleep should be obtained if possible.

Urine provides a rich culture medium, and if specimens are not examined soon after being taken, or are refrigerated, bacterial multiplication will take place, introducing another confounding variable.

Urinary infection in antenatal patients is often asymptomatic, 'asymptomatic bacilluria'. To detect it urine specimens must be cultured in the absence of clinical symptoms. This generates a large number of specimens and means that rapid screening techniques must be used.

Culture

Most culture methods for urine centre around the need to provide a simple method for enumerating the organisms. This can be achieved by using a standard bacteriological loop which inoculates a constant amount of urine (10 µl) on the culture medium. The number of colonies which grow can be counted and an estimate of the viable count made by simple multiplication. An alternative technique is to use the filter paper strip method in which an L-shaped piece of filter paper forming a foot 6 × 12 mm can be used for a

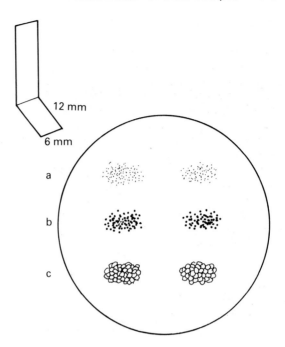

Figure 18.1 Liegh and Williams method. A sterile filter paper 6 × 12 mm is dipped into fresh urine and planted on CLED agar in duplicate

standardized inoculum. In this latter method, the foot is dipped into urine and excess urine tapped off against the side of the jar. The foot is then touched on the surface of well-dried culture medium, this should be done in duplicate. The advantage of this technique is that a large number of individual urine specimens can be cultured on a single Petri dish (Fig. 18.1). Subculture is facilitated if the duplicate inoculation is smeared over the medium. The dipslide is an alternative which uses a paddle which is coated with agar. This method is particularly suitable for general practice when organisms will be delayed in transit and this is described below (p. 215).

Media

As discrete colonies are required for accurate enumeration of bactrial count, media used in the primary isolation of urinary pathogens from MSU and CSU must contain a method of inhibiting the swarming of *Proteus* spp., which

Table 18.2 Example of an MSU reporting protocol

Reporting	
MSU (and bag urines)	
Culture result	*Report*
No bacterial growth	No significant growth
Single organism	
1 $<10^4$ CFU/ml	No significant growth
2 10^4–10^5 CFU/ml	10 000–100 000 CFU/ml of (isolate 1); report no sensitivities; ? significance; sens. available
3 $>10^5$ CFU/ml	$>100 000$ CFU/ml of (isolate 1); report 1st line sensitivities; release any resistance plus any extra antibiotics according to clinical details
Two organisms	
1 Both $<10^5$ CFU/ml	No significant growth; please repeat if appropriate
2 One $>10^5$ CFU/ml	Mixed growth including $>100 000$ CFU/ml of (isolate 1)
If no epithelial cells	please repeat if appropriate
3 Both $>10^5$ CFU/ml	$>100 000$ CFU/ml of (isolate 1)
If no epithelial cells	$>100 000$ CFU/ml of (isolate 2); report sensitivities available; ? significance
$>$+Epithelial cells	Specimen contaminated; please repeat
More than two organisms	No significant growth
$>10^5$ CFU/ml	
Pseudomonas aeruginosa	$>100 000$ CFU/ml of *Pseudomonas aeruginosa*; ? significance; sens. available

are frequent urinary pathogens. Although MacConkey's agar is satisfactory for this purpose, it is inhibitory to some urinary pathogens. Cystine lactose electrolyte-deficient medium (CLED) supports the growth of a wide range of pathogens, but inhibits the swarming of *Proteus* spp.

Anaerobes cause less than 1% of all urinary tract infections and these usually occur in patients with malignancy of the urinary tract. If such a condition is suspected attempts should be made to obtain urine uncontaminated by urethral flora.

Some authors consider that micro-aerophilic organisms, including *Lactobacillus* and *Haemophilus,* may be important in some cases of urinary tract infection. It would be inappropriate to investigate all urines in this way, but where urinary tract infection is strongly suspected, where white cells are present in excess, and the specimen is correctly collected and transported, the specimen could be inoculated on chocolate agar and incubated in a micro-aerophilic atmosphere.

Reporting

The results of urine examination must be carefully reported. Guidance must be given to the clinician about the significance of individual isolates and appropriate antibiotics, if any to be prescribed. When reporting the delay in transport of the specimen must be taken into account when deciding the clinical relevance of each isolate. Numerical criteria have been set up to establish significance but are not the sole determinant. The purity of the culture is also important as a pure culture of *E. coli* of 10^4/ml may be significant whereas isolation of $>10^5$ *E. coli* in mixed culture and where epithelial cells have been seen on the direct microscopy may not. Mid-stream specimens in which more than one organism is cultured are likely to have been contaminated by urethral flora. When a specimen is suspected of being unsuitable by virtue of contamination or delay in transport a repeat specimen should be requested. An example of a reporting protocol is set out in Table 18.2.

Catheter specimens of urine

Urinary catheters, which may be inserted in patients with neurological defects of bladder function, bladder outflow obstruction, or the chronically incontinent, are inevitably colonized with micro-organisms. However, a dynamic balance between host defences and pathogens is rapidly set up so that these organisms are often cultured in high numbers without any evidence of invasive infection. Laboratory protocols and reporting strategies must be modified if unnecessary antibiotic therapy is to be avoided.

Patients with long-term indwelling urinary catheters are at risk of recurrent bouts of bacterial invasion. Organisms are able to multiply rapidly in the catheter bag and therefore the numeric criteria applied to MSUs do not apply. Urine should be sent only from patients who are febrile and in whom a diagnosis is sought. In asymptomatic patients colonizing strains may be identified and their antimicrobial susceptibility pattern determined so that early appropriate treatment can be initiated if, later, there is clinical indication of infection. The validity of this second approach has not been established.

Direct microscopy is of little value as bacteria will usually be seen and a high white cell count can be predicted because of the presence of the catheter acting as a foreign body. A semi-quantitative count should be performed as in the case of MSU and all colonial types (up to a maximum of three) should be followed up with identification and susceptibility testing performed. As most patients are unlikely to require antibiotic therapy for their colonization, susceptibility results should not be reported unless it is clinically indicated.

General practice

In the primary health care setting it is difficult for clinics to ensure that urine specimens are transported to the laboratory with sufficient speed to prevent bacterial overgrowth with commensal species. This can be overcome by using a non-culture approach, selecting patients for treatment on the basis of sideroom examination or biochemical testing of the urine (see above). This approach has the virtue of speed but does not provide an aetiological diagnosis. Although the majority of infections are caused by *E. coli*, *Proteus* spp. or *Enterococcus*, less common and unexpected pathogens can occur and the susceptibility pattern of these organisms may be less predictable. Some patients have recurrent urinary infection and are more likely to carry resistant strains as a result of previous antimicrobial therapy.

There is a need to continue to culture urine and there are several methods for overcoming the difficulties stated above. A dipslide culture method can be used: in this technique, an agar-coated slide is dipped into urine, excess fluid is drained off, and the slide placed in a screw-capped container to maintain the moisture while it is being transported to the laboratory where it is incubated. Commercial dipslide preparations often have two types of agar on the slide, MacConkey's and CLED (see Fig. 1.2). This technique is semi-quantitative; the approximate viable count is estimated by comparison with illustrations provided by the manufacturer. Subcultures can be made and individual colonies picked off for full identification and susceptibility testing.

Other techniques depend on inhibition of multiplication in the urine specimen by the addition of inhibitors to the urine collection container. By inhibiting multiplication of organisms in the urine, it is hoped to preserve the colony count at the level of urine as it is passed. However, this may result in false-negative results being obtained if viability is reduced and, if inhibition is not complete, false-positive results also.

Prostatic massage

The diagnosis of chronic bacterial prostatitis is complicated by the difficulty of obtaining a satisfactory specimen but segmented culture can be helpful. Four specimens are collected: the first 10 ml; the next 200 ml, the MSU; prostatic massage is then carried out and the secretions collected; finally, a 10 ml sample is collected. All of these specimens are subjected to quantitative culture. In bacterial prostatitis higher bacterial counts are obtained in the prostatic secretions and the last 10 ml collected than in the MSU.

Antibiotic susceptibility

Rapid turn around of urine results is essential if they are to have any value to the majority of patients in the primary health care setting. Primary susceptibility plates may be set up by inoculating urine directly on sensitivity testing agar and placing six susceptibility discs on the surface (see Chapter 20). Urine which has a significant number of pathogens provides a suitable inoculum. It would be wasteful of resources to process all urines in this way so selection criteria, such as the visualization of bacteria on an uncentrifuged urine, should be agreed. The antibiotics chosen for this screen should be applicable to a wide range of patients (including pregnant women), and be active against the major urinary pathogens. One typical set might include ampicillin, co-trimoxazole, a fluoroquinolone, nitrofurantoin, nalidixic acid and gentamicin.

With primary isolates different groups of agents can be tested for different patients and pathogens. The 'set' for outpatients will differ from that for inpatients because of the need to use orally active agents. Similarly the different resistance patterns of, for example, *Pseudomonas* or *Staphylococcus* isolates will mean separate batteries are set up to take account of each group.

Examination of pus

Specimens

The microbiological examination of pus poses a significant challenge to the routine laboratory as the range of pathogens which may be present is very wide (Table 18.3). When an abscess is formed the only correct specimen to receive is pus, if it is available. Much time and effort is wasted in examination of minute specimens of pus, sent to the laboratory on swabs which have been delayed in transit and are completely desiccated. The diagnostic yield from these specimens is very poor.

Pus should be aspirated by aseptic technique and sent to the laboratory with minimal delay, preferably in the syringe in which it was obtained. It should be properly secured to prevent needlestick injury. It is best to minimize the amount of air in the syringe as this can reduce the survival of strict anaerobes. Ideally, in serious cases, the laboratory should be notified in advance so that it may be ready to receive the specimen and process it immediately on arrival (see Chapter 1).

The likely pathogens will vary, depending on the clinical condition of the patient and this

Table 18.3   Organisms commonly isolated from pus

Staphylococcus aureus
Streptococcus pyogenes
Strep. milleri
Mycoaerophilic streptococci
E. coli
Proteus spp.
other Enterobacteriaceae
Pseudomonas aeruginosa
Bacteroides spp.
Porphyromonas spp.
Prevotella spp.
Fusobacteria spp.
Clostridium spp.
Peptostreptococcus spp.
Actinomyces spp.
Nocardia asteroides
Mycobacterium spp.
Candida albicans

will influence the choice of media and processing of the specimen. In specimens from brain abscess, *Staphylococcus*, *Streptococcus*, *Peptostreptococcus*, and *Porphyromonas* spp. are the most likely pathogens. In abscesses arising from the gastrointestinal tract, *Bacteroides*, Enterobacteraceae and *Enterococcus* are the most likely invading organisms. Abscesses from the bone are likely to yield Staphylcocci or Streptococci. An abscess with a long incubation period, perhaps with a history of tropical travel of residence overseas might suggest a diagnosis of amoebic abscess or tuberculosis. A chronic discharging lesion might suggest actinomycosis if located in the cervical facial region, or Madura foot if located in the foot.

The underlying condition of the patient should be taken into consideration as, for example, invasive fungal infections are likely to occur in severely neutropenic patients, e.g. those undergoing bone marrow transplantation.

Rapid diagnosis

Microscopy

A simple Gram's stain provides much valuable information about the likely pathogens

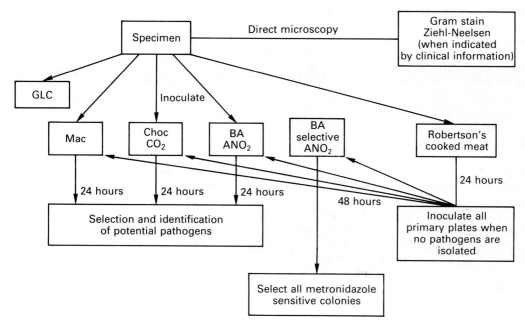

Figure 18.2   An example of a protocol for isolation and identification of pathogens from pus

present. As well as indicating the presence of staphylococci, streptococci, and Gram-negative rods it may indicate unexpected findings, such as the presence of *Nocardia*, *Actinomyces* or fungal elements. The Gram stain also provides some quality control for the subsequent cultures. The presence of Gram-negative bacilli and Gram-positive cocci which are not subsequently cultured, might indicate inadequate anaerobic technique. Additional staining techniques may be used when clinically indicated (e.g. Ziehl-Neelsen) to demonstrate mycobacteria or a weak Ziehl-Neelsen to demonstrate the partial acid-fastness of *Nocardia* species.

Gas-liquid chromatography

Anaerobes in a specimen of pus can be detected rapidly by gas-liquid chromatography (GLC), which detects the end products of metabolism. This technique can produce valuable information in expert hands, although the value of the investment of time and technology might be doubted as in most circumstances the presence of anaerobes could

be predicted on the basis of the specimen type and condition of the patient.

Antigen detection

Antigen detection is of limited value in making an aetiological diagnosis in a pyogenic abscess. This is mainly due to the diversity of microbiological pathogens which may be present. In the future, any methods which are likely to be used are more likely to detect broad groups of pathogens and therefore are subject to the same criticisms as for the use of GLC.

Culture

A wide range of pathogens are found in pus and, thus, a combination of enrichment and selective media must be employed. Such a scheme of investigation is set out in Figure 18.2. Chocolate agar incubated in CO_2 is used to support the growth of fastidious capnophilic organisms. MacConkey's agar will aid the selection and identification of Gram-negative pathogens and a 24-hour culture in blood agar

Table 18.4 Organisms commonly found on the skin

Bacteria

Streptococcus pyogenes	*Pseudomonas aeruginosa*
Streptococcal species (e.g. Gp C)	*Peptostreptococcus* spp.
Staphylococcus aureus	*Bacteroides* spp.
Corynebacterium diphtheriae	*Fusobacterium* spp.
Erysipelothrix rusiopathiae	*Fusobacterium ulcerans*
Mycobacterium tuberculosis	*Treponema pallidum**
M. marinum, M. ulcerans	*C. perfringens*
M. leprae*	*Actinomyces* spp.
Bacillus anthracis	*Nocardia* + related species

Fungi

Microsporum spp.	*Madurella* spp.
Trichophyton spp.	*Malassezia furfur*
	Trichosporon beigelii
	Peidraia hortae

Protozoa
Leishmania spp. (see Chapter 11)

* Non-cultivatable

in an anaerobic atmosphere will allow the isolation and identification of beta-haemolytic streptococci and rapidly growing anaerobic species. A pair of selective and non-selective anaerobic blood agar plates incubated for 48 hours will help to obtain the maximum yield of more oxygen-sensitive anaerobes. An enrichment broth should be inoculated where viable organisms are scanty. Robertson's cooked meat medium will support the growth of most organisms found in pus. When the primary plates are negative the broth should be subcultured onto all the media used in primary isolation.

When tuberculosis or fungal infection is likely, the pus should also be inoculated into appropriate media. Moreover, if slow-growing organisms such as *Actinomyces* are suggested, for example by the history of chronic discharging abscess with sinus formation, prolonged incubation in an anaerobic atmosphere is indicated.

Miscellaneous sterile fluid specimens

A wide range of fluid specimens are submitted from sterile sites including ascites, pleural or joint fluid. As a normally sterile site a Gram stain, a cell count and differential should be performed. The fluid should be inoculated into a fluid enrichment medium such as Robertson's cooked meat, blood and MacConkey agar aerobically, chocolate agar in CO_2 and unselective blood agar anaerobically. The fluid enrichment medium should be subcultured the next day if the primary plates are negative. Peritoneal dialysis fluid is treated slightly differently. The specimen is received as a dialysis bag and an aliquot is aseptically removed. A cell count should be performed on an aliquot, and a portion centrifuged and the pellet resuspended in sterile distilled water and shaken. This releases cell-associated organisms. The specimen is then centrifuged and the deposit inoculated onto blood agar and incubated aerobically. The plates are read after 24 and 48 hours.

Skin

A wide range of pathogens and commensal organisms can be found on skin (Table 18.4).

Clinical syndromes

There are four main ways in which specimens from the skin are submitted to the microbiological laboratory for investigation, as follows:

1 Acute infections
2 Burns, wounds, and ulcers
3 Blistering eruptions
4 Establishing carrier status

Acute infections

Infections of the skin may present with a variety of clinical syndromes such as erysipelas, cellulitis, impetigo, furunculosis, and toxic epidermal necrolysis usually caused by *Staph. aureus* or *Strep. pyogenes*. Specimens from acute infections of the skin can also contain other primary pathogens rare in this country, such as *Corynebacterium diphtheriae*, or anthrax, in patients who are exposed to infected animal products. In addition, there are a number of clinical syndromes, such as erysipelothrix or erythrasma, which are chronic skin infections caused by *Erysipelothrix rusiopathiae* and *C. minitissimum* respectively. Rarely the skin may also be infected by mycobacteria including *Mycobacteria chelonei* and *M. marinum* (see Chapter 4).

Burns, wounds, and ulcers

These skin conditions have a tendency to chronicity. Colonization and infection with a wide range of pathogens is common.

Burns often become colonized with *S. aureus* and *Pseudomonas aeruginosa*. In many instances, these organisms do not cause problems but septicaemia may develop. *S. pyogenes* is an important pathogen in burns, as its presence may cause the failure of skin grafts and it readily causes septicaemia.

The interpretation of isolates from post-operative wounds is more difficult. In many instances the organisms found in wounds are not acting as pathogens and antimicrobial treatment is not indicated. Pathogens such as *S. pyogenes* pose a serious risk to the patient because of their propensity to cause serious skin sepsis and life-threatening septicaemia. *S. pyogenes* is readily transmitted in the hospital environment causing epidemics of wound infection if not controlled. For most other isolates the role is less clear-cut. *S. aureus* can cause serious wound sepsis or may be only a colonizer. The outcome of colonization is dependent in part on the immunity of the host and the virulence of the organism. Several *S. aureus* phage types have been shown to be more invasive or transmissible than others. *Escherichia coli* may colonize or rarely infect abdominal wounds. Full interpretation of the clinical significance of isolates can only be made by inspection of the wound.

Venous ulcers are, by their nature, chronic and have their own bacterial flora including staphylococci and anaerobic species. Thus, the isolation of organisms other than primary pathogens such as *S. pyogenes* does not indicate a need for treatment. The results of culture should be interpreted in the light of clinical examination. Chronic ulcers can be a reservoir of multi-drug-resistant or virulent staphylococci.

Blistering eruptions

Many conditions, such as pemphigus or dermatitis herpetiformis, are of the non-infectious nature. Herpes virus infections are usually diagnosed on the characteristic clinical pattern of the blistering. However, when there is doubt, examination of blister fluid by electron microscopy can clarify the diagnosis. Toxin-producing strains of *S. aureus* may cause blistering eruptions and in some cases this may be severe as in the staphylococcal scalded skin syndrome.

Establishment of carrier status

Examination of skin swabs is often performed to define a patient's carrier status with respect to organisms such as *S. pyogenes* and staphylococci-carrying methicillin or other important resistance (see Chapter 2).

Microscopic examination

Direct microscopic examination, other than electron microscopy of blister fluid, is of little value for bacterial infections, as the infecting species are morphologically similar to the commensal organisms.

Culture

Routine screening skin swabs can be inoculated on blood and MacConkey's agar, which should be incubated aerobically. Additional

Table 18.5   Organisms associated with infection of the eye

	Organism	Typical syndrome
Helminths		
	Toxocara canis	Endophthalmitis, uveitis
	Onchocerca volvulus	'River blindness'
	Loa loa	Usually asymptomatic
Protozoa		
	Toxoplasma gondii	Chorioretinitis
	Acanthamoeba	Keratitis
Fungi		
	Candida albicans	Endophthalmitis
	Aspergillus spp.	Orbital infection
Bacteria		
	Neisseria gonorrhoeae	
	Chlamydia trachomatis	Neonatal conjunctivitis
	Streptococcus pneumoniae	Conjunctivitis
	Haemophilus influenzae	
	Staphylococcus aureus	
	Moraxella lacunata	
	Pseudomonas aeruginosa	Postoperative endophthalmitis
	S. aureus	

media for the isolation of other pathogens, such as Sabouraud's and Lowenstein-Jensen are appropriate when fungal or mycobacterial infection is suspected. Similarly, Hoyle's medium would be required where *C. diphtheriae* was suspected.

In swabs from burn sites for skin grafting, a selective media such as crystal violet blood agar might be used in addition to enhance the recovery of beta-haemolytic streptococci. Recent work has indicated the importance of anaerobic species in cutaneous ulcers which form an important part of the flora. However, the clinical utility of isolating and reporting these organisms is not clear.

A new species, *Fusobacterium ulcerans*, has recently been identified from cases of tropical ulcer.

When skin swabs are examined to identify carriers of multiresistant organisms, appropriate selective indicator media should be used. For the diagnosis of methicillin-resistant *S. aureus* (MRSA) carriers, skin swabs from multiple sites should be placed in a salt-broth medium and subcultured onto nutrient agar containing 4 mg/l methicillin. This means that the only organisms to be identified are those able to tolerate high salt and resistance to methicillin, predominantly methicillin-resistant *S. aureus* and some strains of coagulase-negative staphylcocci. Identification and susceptibility testing can then definitively identify MRSA. It is essential that screening systems which may bring in large numbers of specimens are carefully designed to optimize the use of resources and maximize diagnostic yield.

Diagnosis of ocular infection

Infection

When ocular infection is being investigated, two conjunctival swabs should be taken: one should be used for Gram stain and inoculation on conventional media and the other used for the diagnosis of chlamydia infection. Chlamydia diagnosis can be performed by culture in McCoy cells or by enzyme-linked immunosorbent assay (ELISA) antigen detection (see Chapter 21).

Conjunctivitis

The conjunctiva can become infected at the time of birth by pathogens in the maternal

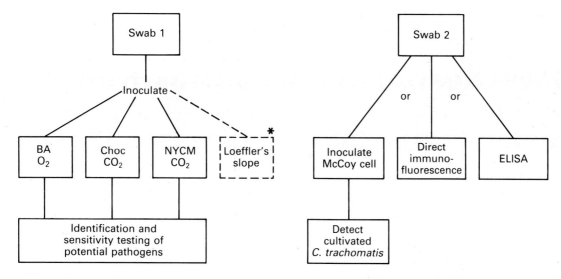

* When clinically indicated

Figure 18.3   Example of a protocol for investigating swabs

genital tract. Infections commencing shortly after birth may be caused by *N. gonorrhoeae*, *C. trachomatis*, *S. aureus* or *S. pneumoniae*. In children the main causes of bacterial conjunctivitis are *H. influenzae*, *S. pneumoniae* and *S. aureus*. In developing countries infection with *C. trachomatis* leads to a severe scarring infection of the eye which often results in blindness. Other bacteria which may infect the eye include *H. influenzae* subsp. *aegyptius* and *C. diphtheriae*. *Moraxella lacunata* produces an acute angular conjunctivitis and many other pathogens are capable of initiating infection (Table 18.5).

Laboratory diagnosis

Microscopy

Direct examination by Gram's stain is useful, especially if gonococcal infection is suspected as the Gram-negative intracellular diplococci are readily seen providing a rapid presumptive diagnosis. Small numbers of diphtheroids and Gram-positive cocci seen in the smear are not helpful as these organisms form part of the normal flora.

Direct immunofluorescence examination of the conjunctival swab can bring a rapid diagnosis for *Chlamydia trachomatis* infection.

Culture

The organisms causing conjunctivitis are readily grown on conventional media and conjunctival swabs should be inoculated onto blood agar, incubated aerobically, and chocolate agar incubated in CO_2. After 24 hours' incubation colonies resembling the organisms on the pathogen list should be selected (Fig. 18.3).

Endophthalmitis

Endophthalmitis can have a multiplicity of infective causes as can be seen from Table 18.5. Infection is more likely to occur in intravenous drug abusers and in patients who have undergone open eye surgery with the insertion of a prosthetic device. The immunocompromised are at particular risk of fungal infection. Parasites such as *Toxoplasma* cause a chorioretinitis while *Toxocara* usually produces a retinal granuloma but may affect any of the structures of the eye.

19

Investigation of specimens from the genital tract and diagnosis of sexually transmitted diseases (STDs)

Many organisms are implicated in disease of the genital tract, and some of these are summarized in Table 19.1.

Syphilis

Introduction

Treponema pallidum is a spirochaete which is capable of infecting all of the body systems. It is transmitted by sexual contact, by direct inoculation (a risk for medical attendants), and blood transfusion. It crosses the placenta to cause congenital infection. Syphilis is, to a large extent, controlled in developed countries following the introduction of open access venereal disease clinics, the availability of penicillin and antenatal serological screening. It still remains a problem in high-risk populations with multiple sexual partners, and in some developing countries.

Treponema pallidum

Classification

The non-cultivatable treponomal pathogens were previously divided into four species but recent DNA homology studies demonstrate a close relationship between three which are now classified as subspecies of *T. pallidum*.

Table 19.1 Pathogens implicated in infections of the genital tract

	Organism	Typical syndrome
Protozoa		
	Trichomonas vaginalis	Vaginal discharge
Fungi		
	Candida albicans	Vaginal discharge
Bacteria		
	Neisseria gonorrhoeae	Vaginal discharge (often asymptomatic)
	Chlamydia trachomatis	Discharge, pelvic inflammatory disease
	Mycoplasma hominis	Pelvic inflammatory disease, post-partum fever
	Ureaplasma urealyticum	
	Gardnerella vaginalis	Vaginal discharge
	Mobiluncus spp.	
	Haemophilus ducreyi	Genital ulcer
	Treponema pallidum	Syphilis (not cultivatable)
	Calymmatobacterium donovani	Genital ulcer disease (not cultivatable)

Thus, the causative organism of syphilis is *T. pallidum* subsp. *pallidum*, of yaws is *T. pallidum* subsp. *pertenue* and *T. endemicum* is now *T. pallidum* subsp. *endemicum*. *Treponema carateum*, the causative organism of pinta, retains its previous classification.

Treponema pallidum is a Gram-negative micro-aerophilic bacterium, 6–20 µm long, 0.1–0.2 µm wide and tightly coiled. The treponemes are motile by three flagella (axial filaments) that wrap around the surface of the organism and are covered by the outer membrane which contains lipopolysaccharide. They impart the characteristic rapid axial rotation and bending around the centre. There is a central peptidoglycan layer, and plasma membrane. The treponemes are coated with an amorphous layer of glycosaminoglycans which can be stained by ruthenium red. It cannot be cultivated *in vitro* but can be maintained in laboratory animals.

Clinical features

Infecting organisms are capable of invading through intact skin and rapidly disseminate to all the organs of the body. The duration of the incubation period is directly related to the size of the initial inoculum. Four phases of the natural history of this disease are recognized and it is important to understand these phases as different diagnostic tests are appropriate in each.

The characteristic pathological lesion process is the gumma which consists of an area with a centre of necrosis, obliterative endarteritis with fibroblastic proliferation and lymphocyte infiltration. It can be found in all the organs of the body.

Primary infection

This period immediately follows infection with an incubation period of nine days to one month. The initial lesion is a painless ulcer, usually in the genital tract, which has a rubbery edge and is associated with regional lymphadenopathy. Serum can be expressed from the ulcer crater. This lesion is known as the primary chancre and is self-healing. In some countries endemic syphilis can be transmitted by direct non-sexual contact.

Secondary phase

A proportion of patients completely eradicate infection at each of the stages but the majority go on to secondary syphilis six weeks or more later. This is characterized by an acute febrile illness with a generalized non-itchy scaling rash, which is also found on the palms and soles, and generalized lymphadenopathy develops.

Latent phase

After the secondary phase the infection enters a latent period during which the disease becomes quiescent. Some patients may cure their infection spontaneously whereas others may suffer an episode of acute meningoencephalitis. The latent phase may last from five to more than 20 years.

Tertiary syphilis

This is the final stage of the disease and is now very rare in developed countries. It is associated with several syndromes as the systemic pathogenic process can leave multiple lesions in the cardiovascular and neurological system. Syphilitic aortitis can produce an aneurysm of the ascending aorta and consequent aortic valve incompetence. Neurological involvement can give rise to destruction of the posterior columns in the spinal cord producing tabes dorsalis. In this syndrome the patient has diminished vibration and joint position sense resulting in the characteristic 'stamping gait'. Destruction of neural tissue in the cerebral cortex gives rise to a dementia which can be associated with psychiatric disturbance including delusions and megalomania known as general paralysis of the insane.

Congenital infection

Transmission of infection to the unborn child results in the congenital syphilis syndrome. There may be no abnormal signs or children may suffer an acute syndrome with rhinitis, rash and osteochondritis and hepatosplenomegaly. Later complications may arise with neurosyphilis, cranial nerve palsies, and the results of the infection on the developing bone and cartilage.

Laboratory diagnosis

Dark ground microscopy

Patients with primary chancre may be diagnosed rapidly by detecting *T. pallidum* by dark ground illumination microscopy from the primary chancre. When sampling, the operator should wear gloves as *T. pallidum* may invade through intact skin. The genital ulcer should be cleaned with sterile saline and exudated serum from the base of the lesion placed on a glass slide. After firmly pressing a coverslip, the preparation is examined by dark ground illumination and the oil immersion objective. *Treponema pallidum* has a corkscrew motility and a characteristic undulation about its midpoint. A lesion may only be considered non-syphilitic after three satisfactory negative specimens have been examined. Mouth lesions cannot be examined by this method since many non-pathogenic treponemes are found in this site. A more definitive result may be obtained by direct immunofluorescence staining. Fixed material is stained with fluorescence-labelled *T. pallidum*-specific antibody and examined under u.v. illumination.

Serological tests for syphilis

Serological tests for syphilis may be divided into two groups: tests which detect non-specific antibodies (reagin tests) and tests which detect antibodies specific to *T. pallidum*. Examples of results and their interpretation can be found in Table 19.2.

'Reagin' tests

The first of these tests was described by Wassermann, who reported the use of a complement fixation test (CFT) based on a ethanolic extract of heart muscle. The classical Wassermann CFT is now rarely used as more modern developments of this basic technique, such as the venereal disease reference laboratory test (VDRL) or the rapid plasmin reagent card test (RPR), are more technically simple to perform and provide an accurate diagnosis.

The VDRL antigen uses a defined mixture of cardiolipin lecithin and cholesterol which is mixed with patients' serum. Positive results are indicated by flocculation and should be titred. The rapid plasma reagent card test is a modification of this basic technique, in which VDRL antigen is mixed with finely divided carbon particles. Serum and reagents are mixed on a card and positive results are indicated by agglutination (Fig. 19.1). Both of these techniques may be used for routine diagnosis and mass screening. These tests become positive approximately two weeks after the primary chancre appears. In latent syphilis, reagin tests are often negative and the titre diminishes to become negative after successful treatment is initiated.

VDRL and RPR are the most sensitive early serological tests. The disadvantage of cardiolipin-based tests is the biological false/positive, which is a non-specific positive result which occurs in other non-treponemal diseases. Examples of causes of biological false-positive results are recorded in Table 19.3.

Specific tests

The antigen utilized in specific treponemal tests is derived from Nichol's strain of *T. pallidum*. These tests are more specific (i.e. there are few biological false-positive results) and remain positive after successful

Table 19.2 Investigation of luetic disease

	VDRL/RPR	*TPHA*	*FTA-ABS*	*FTA-IgM*
Congenital syphilis	+	+	+	+
Primary syphilis	+	–/+	–/+	+
Untreated secondary	+	+	+	+
Treated or late	–	+	+/–	–

VDRL: venereal disease reference laboratory test; RPR: rapid plasmin reagent card test; TPHA: *Treponema pallidum* haemagglutination test; FTA-ABS: fluorescent antibody absorbed test; FTA-IgM: fluorescent IgM test.

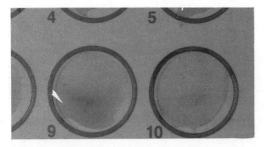

Figure 19.1   VDRL test with negative test on the left and positive (agglutinated) on the right

Table 19.3   Examples of diseases causing biological false-positive results in cardiolipin (reagin) serological tests for syphilis

Connective tissue diseases
  Rheumatoid arthritis
  Systemic lupus erythematosus
  Rheumatic fever
Pregnancy
Bacterial endocarditis
Malaria, leishmaniasis, trypanosomiasis
Leptospirosis, Lyme disease, relapsing fever
Old age

chemotherapy. They may therefore be used to confirm positive cardiolipin tests, and to screen antenatal patients.

Treponema pallidum haemagglutination test (TPHA)   The TPHA is a simple, specific test which is suitable for routine screening purposes. It may be negative in primary infection and typically remains positive for life, even after successful therapy. Sheep or turkey red cells coated with extracts of *T. pallidum* are mixed with the patient's serum which has previously been absorbed with Reiter's treponemes to remove group specific antibody. The patient's serum is screened at an initial dilution of 1 : 80 and a positive should be titred. Controls which should be included in this test are illustrated in Table 19.4.

Fluorescent antibody absorbed test (FTA-ABS)
This is an indirect fluorescent antibody test which is highly specific. Serum is absorbed with sonicated Reiter's treponemes to remove group specific antigens. Serum is applied to treponemal antigen fixed to a glass slide, and specific antigen-antibody binding detected by fluorescein-labelled anti-human globulin. False-positive reactions are rare but can occur in patients with systemic lupus erythematosis, South American trypanosomiasis, and toxoplasmosis. Specific IgM immunoglobulin may be detected by using an anti-human IgM conjugate. This is usually present in untreated primary or secondary syphilis and persists for up to six months after treatment of primary disease. The interpretation of the FTA-IgM in late syphilis is less clear-cut and a positive result may reflect persisting antigen. This technique is, of course, valuable for the diagnosis of congenital infection as it distinguishes between maternal IgG and treponemal specific IgM which must have been produced by the infected infant as IgM does not cross the placenta.

Treponema pallidum immobilization test   The *Treponema pallidum* immobilization test (TPI) has the reputation of being the most specific serological test for syphilis. Because of the requirement for cultured live treponemes, it is available only in reference centres. In this test,

Table 19.4   Controls required in *Treponema pallidum* haemagglutination assay

Control	*Expected result*
Diluted test serum and unsensitized cells	No agglutination
Absorbing diluent and sensitized cells	No agglutination
Absorbing diluent and unsensitized cells	No agglutination
Positive control serum and sensitized cells	Agglutination

live treponemes are mixed with heat-inactivated serum. The mixture is then inspected under the microscope and the presence of more than 50% of treponemes immobilized indicates a positive response. The expense and technical difficulty of this test means that it is largely used for research purposes.

Enzyme-linked immunoabsorbent assay (ELISA) Although ELISA tests were first described in 1975, they are now only just entering routine service. The advantages of these techniques are that they readily lend themselves to automation and are thus most applicable for screening purposes. IgG and IgM ELISA systems have been described for the diagnosis of syphilis and have similar sensitivity and specificity as VDRL and TPHA. IgM antibody capture ELISAs have proven valuable in the diagnosis of congenital syphilis.

Diagnosis of the late stages
In patients with syphilis, CSF tests should be performed to detect early CNS involvement. Cell count and total protein should be measured and specific treponemal serology performed, including VDRL, TPHA and FTA-ABS. The VDRL is negative in up to 70% of patients with active neurosyphilis. Negative TPHA results are very uncommon. A positive result should be related to the CSF albumin content, which will detect false positive results caused by transudation of serum proteins. The demonstration of specific IgM in the CSF would indicate active neurosyphilis.

Neisseria gonorrhoeae

Neisseria gonorrhoeae is one of the most important sexually transmitted diseases in developed countries. The clinical features and detailed methods for isolation and identification of *N. gonorrhoeae* can be found in Chapter 5.

As *N. gonorrhoeae* is a delicate pathogen which dies readily outside the body, it is essential that appropriate laboratory investigations are taken and processed in side rooms in the clinic. Table 5.1 sets out the specimens which are required for the diagnosis of gonococcal sepsis.

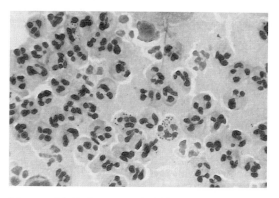

Figure 19.2 Gonococci visible inside polymorphs

Laboratory diagnosis

Direct microscopy

Direct microscopy of urethral pus in males is highly sensitive and specific in the diagnosis of gonorrhoea; 95% of patients subsequently shown to be culture positive will have a positive Gram smear. In females this percentage is much lower, usually less than 50%. Thus, two specimens must be taken and culture must be performed. Direct microscopy should not be performed on throat swabs in the diagnosis of orogenital gonorrhoea because of the presence of normal flora which are morphologically similar. Direct examination of pus from abscesses is valuable. Gonococci are characteristically seen inside the polymorphs (Fig. 19.2).

Direct immunofluorescence techniques have been described but have failed to find a place in routine diagnosis.

Isolation

Neisseria gonorrhoeae is a fastidious organism which must be isolated from sites which are heavily contaminated with other organisms. The media which are used for the isolation of the gonococcus are rich and usually supplemented with yeast extract or Iso-vitalex and blood, which may be lysed as in New York City medium or 'chocolated' as in Thayer Martin. Several cocktails of antibiotic inhibitors are used. One such is vancomycin, nystatin, colistin and trimethoprim. A small proportion of

Table 19.5 Specimens required for diagnosis of *C. trachomatis* infection

Male	Urethra	Pus swab, 3–4 cm and rotate gently before removal
Female	Cervix	Clean cervix, sample squamo-columnar junction
Trachoma		Scrapings from upper tarsal conjunctiva
Ophthalmia neonatorum		Swabs from lower tarsal conjunctiva
Lymphogranuloma venerum		Aspirate of fluctuant nodes
Salpingitis		Aspirated fluid
Rectal mucosa		
Nasopharynx		Only suitable for culture methods
Throat		

gonococci are inhibited by vancomycin and a mixture of lincomycin, colistin, amphotericin, and trimethoprim is used in New York City medium (see Table 5.2).

Chlamydia trachomatis infection

Taxonomy

Chlamydia are found in the order Chlamydiales with a single family Chlamydiaceae which has a single genus *Chlamydia*. There are now three recognized species: *C. trachomatis*, *C. psittaci*, and *C. pneumoniae*. *Chlamydia psittaci* is transmitted from birds to man and causes an atypical pneumoniae syndrome and occasionally culture negative endocarditis (see Chapter 16). *Chlamydia pneumoniae* has recently been discovered as a cause of acute community-acquired pneumonia (see Chapter 16).

Clinical importance

Chlamydia trachomatis is an important pathogen of the genital tract in both men and women. Infection can result in 'non-specific' or non-gonococcal urethritis, cervicitis or acute pelvic inflammatory disease, which may subsequently compromise fertility or predispose to ectopic pregnancy.

Some serotypes of *C. trachomatis* are responsible for lymphogranuloma venereum (LGV). This infection begins with an initial papule which develops into a chronic ulcerative lesion on the genital tract with associated regional lymphoadenopathy. *Chlamydia*

trachomatis can be transmitted to the fetus, resulting in neonatal conjunctivitis, otitis media, pharyngitis, or pneumonia.

Laboratory diagnosis

Specimens

Specimens for the diagnosis of chlamydial infection should be taken according to the schedule in Table 19.5. The type of swab used must be chosen according to the laboratory technique which will be employed for diagnosis. For example when culture is to be used, swabs provided for commercial antigen detection techniques should not be taken as they reduce viability. Dacron swabs may produce artifacts in cell culture and alginate swabs produce non-specific fluorescence in direct immunofluorescence tests. When sampling the cervix, the whole area should be wiped clean with sterile saline and the squamo-columnar junction sampled. Alternative methods of specimen collection include using cervical brush specimens but may be associated with an increase in false-positive results.

Specimens for direct immunofluorescence examination should be rolled or rubbed gently on a glass slide and fixed with methanol for four minutes. Specimens for culture should be transported in a tube of sucrose phosphate, supplemented with fetal calf serum. When specimens are not inoculated directly, they should be stored at –70°C. This results in the least reduction in viability, and higher temperatures of storage result in significant losses.

Specimens for commercial enzyme immunoassay methods will utilize sample systems provided by the manufacturers.

Direct examination

Direct examination of smears with fluorescein-conjugated monoclonal antibodies can be performed and kits are commercially available for this purpose. These use a standard direct immunofluorescence protocol with a monoclonal antibody. Two monoclonal antibodies are available: one is directed at the outer membrane protein (which is species specific), and another directed against genus-specific lipopolysaccharide. This latter antibody will detect all *Chlamydia* spp. but will be unable to distinguish between them.

The results of direct immunofluorescence compare well with cell cultures but the main disadvantage with this technique is that like all immunofluorescence methods it is subjective. In consequence, false-positive results can occur, especially if this technique is applied in low prevalence populations. It does have the advantage, however, of enabling the quality of the specimen provided to be checked. Direct immunofluorescence is most suitable when only small numbers of specimens will be tested or where rapid results are required (e.g. an outpatient clinic).

Culture

Chlamydia spp. can be isolated with cell culture using McCoy's cells which have been treated with cyclohexamide. The specimen is centrifuged onto the cell monolayer and incubated for 72 hours. Cultured *Chlamydia* may be detected by staining with Giemsa, iodine or fluorescein-labelled monoclonal antibody. Blind passage may increase diagnostic yield but results in excessive delay in obtaining results. However, blind passage should be performed when the specimen contains detritis which makes reading of the culture difficult or when lymphogranuloma venereum is suspected. The estimated sensitivity of cell culture is 75–80%.

Antigen detection

Enzyme-linked immunoabsorbent assays for the diagnosis of *Chlamydia* infections usually use polyclonal and monoclonal antibodies directed against chlamydial LPS and are, thus,

genus specific. Sensitivity of 97% and specificity of 92.5%, in comparison with single cycle cell culture, have been reported. False-positive results occur with ELISA methods as a result of cross-reactivity with other bacterial species. For this reason, antigen detection by ELISA should not be performed on specimens obtained from the mouth or from stool which are likely to be heavily contaminated with other Gram-negative bacteria. The use of blocking tests improves the specificity of results. In patients with positive or borderline results which are not confirmed by the blocking assay a further specimen should be requested and tested. False positives are a particular problem in low-risk populations when only a small number of specimens are likely to be from patients with infection. In cases with medico-legal implications, antigen detection techniques with ELISA methods should not be used.

Nucleic acid probes

DNA hybridization methods have been developed for the diagnosis of chlamydial infections. These tests are highly specific but lack the sensitivity of other currently available techniques.

Serology

The serological diagnosis of chlamydial infection is difficult. Complement fixation tests (CFT) are relatively insensitive and, as genus-specific antigens are used, it is impossible to differentiate between the different species or serotypes. When the clinical features of a case support the diagnosis LGV may be diagnosed by single antibody titre of 32 or greater. The CFT is not useful in diagnosing trachoma inclusion conjunctivitis, genital tract infection, or neonatal infections. It can be valuable in the diagnosis of psittacosis and *C. pneumoniae* infection in which there may be shown a fourfold rise in the titre in 10 days following the onset of symptoms.

A micro-immunofluorescence (IF) test has been described which is species and serovar specific. This is an indirect immunofluorescence technique which may be used to detect either specific IgG or IgM. Rising titres of IgG antibody may be demonstrated in psittacosis.

In LGV, rising titres are usually not found due to the acute nature of the infection, but single-point IgM antibodies and very high levels of IgG antibodies may be detected. In highly sexually active populations, levels of anti-chlamydial antibodies make serological diagnosis by micro-IF difficult. However, if timed, paired, acute and convalescence sera are obtained, this technique may be successful.

Genital mycoplasmas

There are at least 10 species of *Mycoplasma* which may be isolated from human material. These include *Ureaplasma urealyticum*, *Acholeplasma laidlawii*, and eight species of the genus *Mycoplasma*. *Mycoplasma pneumoniae* is a major cause of primary atypical pneumonia (see p. 184). Four species are found in the oral cavity: *M. salivarium*, *M. oralae*, *M. faucium*, and *M. buccale* and appear to have no pathogenic significance. The pathogenic role of mycoplasmas in the genital tract is more complex as up to 60% of women carry *U. urealyticum*, and 30% carry *M. hominis*. The incidence of these species is higher in sexually active populations. *Mycoplasma hominis* and *U. urealyticum* may have a role in pelvic inflammatory disease. Other species which may have a role include *M. fermentens* and *M. genitalia*. This latter organism, recently characterized, shows significant cross-reactivity with *M. pneumoniae*. Mycoplasma are described in more detail in Chapter 16.

Ahtough these organisms are associated with non-gonococcal urethritis, female/male infertility, pelvic inflammatory disease, etc., they do form part of the normal flora in a large proportion of healthy adults. In consequence, their isolation from the genital tract does not imply disease. It is therefore of little value for routine microbiology laboratories to culture them. Details of methods for culture and identification of mycoplasmas can be found in Chapter 16.

Chancroid

Infection with *Haemophilus ducreyi* results in development of genital ulcers and associated acute suppurative regional lymphadenitis. Clinical disease begins three to five days after contact when a painful ulcer develops at the site of infection which breaks down to form a non-indurated ulcer, which is very painful, the base of which is friable and bleeds easily. Inguinal lymphadenopathy develops and abscess formation occurs with discharge through the skin. Chancroid is thought to facilitate the transmission of HIV because of the presence of open ulcers.

Chancroid may be diagnosed by culture of *H. ducreyi* from the ulcer. The ulcer should be cleaned thoroughly with a sterile saline and material from the base or aspirates from inguinal buboes should be inoculated directly on chocolate agar and enriched gonococcal agar. (For a detailed description of this species, see Chapter 6.)

Enzyme-linked immunoassays have been developed for the detection of *H. ducreyi* antibody. These techniques are currently being evaluated. Elevated antibody concentrations develop in 55–86% of patients with chancroid and up to 20% of non-infected controls.

Donovanosis or granuloma inguinale

Granuloma inguinale is an uncommon infection which is largely confined to Papua New Guinea and the Kerala coast of India. It is caused by *Calymmatobacterium granulomatis*. It is a pleomorphic Gram-negative bacillus surrounded by a well-defined capsule. It is usually intracellular and has a characteristic safety pin morphology. It shares several antigens with *Klebsiella* spp.

Clinical infection begins as a papule which develops into a subcutaneous nodular ulcer that may spread and involve a larger area. Ulcers are painless unless secondary infection occurs. The ulcer has a pink, velvety serpiginous edge and may be hypertropic. Regional lymph nodes are not enlarged and the infection remains active for up to eight months. Donovanosis is complicated by fibrosis of the lymphatics in up to 20% of patients. Sclerosis and stenosis of the vulva or urethra may develop.

The diagnosis of granuloma inguinale is usually made on the basis of the characteristic clinical features. Giemsa staining of ulcer

Table 19.6   Pathogens implicated in vaginal discharge

Pathogen	Diagnostic methods	
Trichomonas vaginalis	Direct microscopy	Wet preparation (stained Giemsa/Papanicolaou immunofluorescence)
	Culture	
Candida albicans	Direct microscopy	Gram stain
	Culture	Sabouraud's medium
Bacterial vaginosis:	Clue cells, pH, odour, Gram stain	
Gardnerella vaginalis	Culture	Human blood agar with gentamicin, nalidixic acid and amphotericin B supplement
Mobiluncus spp.	Culture	Anaerobically or blood-containing media
Gonorrhoea	(see p. 226)	
Chlamydia trachomatis	(see p. 228)	

scrapings enables the detection of typical 'Donovan bodies'. These organisms appear in clusters within the cytoplasm of mononuclear cells and show marked and bipolaris staining. *Calymmatobacterium granulomatis* may be cultured in embryonated hen's eggs, but this technique is of unknown sensitivity in comparison with direct examination. Culture of this organism is technically difficult.

Vaginal discharge

Vaginal discharge is a common clinical problem for which a microbiological diagnosis is sought. Bacterial, fungal, and protozoan pathogens are implicated as summarized in Table 19.6. The other classical STDs described above may cause mucopurulent cervicitis and vaginal discharge.

Trichomonas vaginalis

Trichomonas vaginalis is a protozoan pathogen which is found only in its tropozoite stage (see Figure 19.3). It is up to 23 μm by 12 μm with a central axostyle, an undulating membrane and four flagella and divides by binary fission.

It is found in the human vagina and prostate gland and may be seen in the urine. Male infection is typically asymptomatic, but urethritis, epidydimitis and prostatitis can develop. Female infection may also be asymp-

tomatic in up to 50% of patients. In the remainder it causes vaginal discharge which often has a very offensive odour and may be yellow/green and frothy. The vagina may be inflamed with the result that patients complain of vaginal and vulval pruritis. Cervical erosions may be present.

Laboratory diagnosis

Microscopy

Trichomoniasis is most readily diagnosed in vaginal discharge by direct microscopic

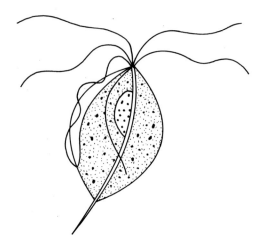

Figure 19.3   *Trichomonas vaginalis*

examination of clinical material in a saline-wet preparation in the clinic. Motile *T. vaginalis* are seen with characteristic morphology and motility. A lower yield is obtained if swabs are sent to the laboratory and fixed stained preparations examined. Giemsa and Papanicolaou stains have been used, although greater sensitivity can be obtained by use of direct immunofluorescent methods.

Culture

Improved sensitivity is obtained by culturing giving an improvement in the yield of up to 30%. Solid or semi-solid media (e.g. Diamond's medium) can be inoculated with a high vaginal swab at the clinic. The cultures are then incubated for 37°C and examined microscopically. The incorporation of an indicator dye to show acid production simplifies the processing of large numbers of specimens.

Many antibody detection techniques have been used in *T. vaginalis* infections and, in general, agree with the results obtained by other methods. However, as antibody responses only return to baseline some time after acute infection and antibody concentrations may be low in mild infections, false-positive and false-negative results are common.

An enzyme immunoassay for detection of *T. vaginalis* antigen in vaginal swabs has been described with sensitivity of 93.2%, specificity of 97.5%, the predictive value of a positive result 82%, and predictive value of a negative result 99.3%. However, these antigen detection methods are not yet commercially available. A rapid antigen detection test using latex agglutination has also recently been described.

Candida albicans

Candida albicans is an important cause of vaginal discharge which is characteristically white, and resembles milk curds. If one of the white patches is removed a point of bleeding is left behind. Candidal vaginitis is easily diagnosed by direct microscopy of a high vaginal swab stained by Gram's method. Additional sensitivity can be obtained by

inoculating the vaginal swab onto Sabouraud's agar. (For detailed methods for the isolation and identification of *Candida albicans*, see Chapter 10.)

Bacterial vaginosis

Bacterial vaginosis, which goes under a number of names, e.g. anaerobic vaginosis and non-specific vaginosis, is a common condition. It is characterized by increased vaginal discharge which may have an offensive odour. Symptoms such as dysuria or dyspareunia are rare. This diagnosis can sometimes only be made when *Trichomonas vaginalis* or *Candida* infection have been excluded.

Pathogenesis

Bacterial vaginosis is thought to be of mixed bacterial aetiology without signs of inflammation in the vaginal mucosa. No individual organism has been shown to have a direct pathogenic role in this syndrome, but isolation of *Gardnerella vaginalis* from the vagina has been associated. More recently, *Mobiluncus* species has also been implicated in bacterial vaginosis and other anaerobes are thought to be important (Fig. 19.4).

The way in which these organisms interact to produce bacterial vaginosis is not clear. *Gardnerella* has a pH optimum of 6–6.5 and the growth of *Mobiluncus* is favoured when the pH is greater than 5.0. The vaginal pH is usually kept very low due to acid production by commensal lactobacilli. It is thought that amine produced by the metabolism of *Bacteroides* raises the pH of the vagina sufficiently for *Gardnerella* and *Mobiluncus* to grow and cause symptoms (Fig. 19.4).

Laboratory diagnosis of bacterial vaginosis

Because of the polymicrobial nature of bacterial vaginosis, the association of individual species with this syndrome is less clear. The laboratory diagnosis can be aided by simple tests:

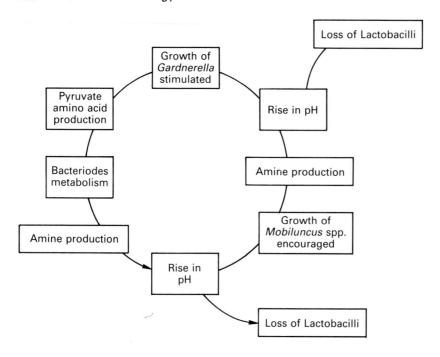

Figure 19.4
Production of amines by *Bacteroides* spp. lowers the pH stimulating growth of *Mobiluncus* spp. (pH >5.0) and *Gardnerella vaginalis* (pH >6.5). Amino acids and pyruvate produced by *Gardnerella* are metabolized by *Bacteroides* to amines

1 The demonstration of clue cells, which are vaginal epithelial cells with edges darkened by the presence of numerous small bacteria adhering to their surface
2 An amine test. Vaginal discharge is placed on a slide and a few drops of KOH is added. The presence of amines determined by the characteristic fishy smell which is generated
3 Vaginal pH. In patients with bacterial vaginosis, the vaginal pH is >4.5
4 Bacteriological culture for *Gardnerella vaginalis* and *Mobiluncus* spp.

Demonstration of these laboratory features will enable a diagnosis of bacterial vaginosis to be made with confidence.

Mobiluncus *spp.*

Mobiluncus is an anaerobic, Gram-variable, curved bacillus. The genus is divided into two species: *M. curtisii* and *M. mulieris*. Their characteristics are set out in Table 19.7. They are fastidious and slow growing, typically motile, catalase, oxidase and indole negative. *Mobiluncus* can be isolated in up to 50% of patients with bacterial vaginosis. Clear, colourless colonies 2 mm in diameter develop after five days' incubation. Gas-liquid chromatography of the metabolic products can distinguish the species. Detection of enzyme activity notably proline aminopeptidase and alpha-*D*-glucosidase is useful and commercial kits are available.

Gardnerella vaginalis

Gardnerella vaginalis is a slow-growing, Gram-variable bacillus which has been previously classified as a *Haemophilus* and *Corynebacterium*. It has now been assigned to its own genus. It is aerobic, non-motile, does not require X or V factors and it is catalase and oxidase negative. It produces beta-haemolysis on human blood agar, but none

Table 19.7 Features of *Mobiluncus* spp.

Characteristic	M. curtisii	M. mulieris
Morphology	Short curved	Long curved
Gram reaction	Variable	Negative
Saccharolytic	–	+
Growth enhancement by arginine	+	–
Metabolic products	A, S	A, (L) S
Nitrate	+/–	–
G+C	51–52%	49–50%

A: acetic; S: succinic; L: lactic.

Table 19.8 Characteristics of *Gardnerella vaginalis*

Test	Result
Gram stain	Small pleomorphic Gram variable coccobacilli or short rods
Colonial morphology	β-haemolysis on human blood agar
Catalase	Negative
Oxidase	Negative
Hippurate hydrolysis	Positive
Starch fermentation	Positive
Metronizadole 50 µg disc	Sensitive
Sulphonamide 1000 µg disc	Resistant

on sheep blood agar. Blood agar can be made selective by the addition of gentamicin, nalidixic acid and amphotericin B. It may be identified by testing for hippurate and starch hydrolysis (positive) and by using high concentration metronidazole (50 µg), sulphonamide (1000 µg), trimethoprim (5 µg) discs (Table 19.8).

20

Antimicrobial susceptibility

Introduction

The rapid matching of a patient with an antibiotic has been seen by some as the *raison d'être* of the microbiology laboratory, and therefore susceptibility testing is of immediate importance to the patient. In many cases the choice of antibiotic therapy must be made before the results of culture are available. In these circumstances it is the knowledge of the likely pathogens in a given clinical situation and the susceptibility pattern which is the most important consideration in planning an empirical antimicrobial regimen.

When culture results are available accurate identification to genus or species level is central to the decision-making process as the susceptibility pattern of many organisms is often predictable, e.g. *Streptococcus pyogenes* is invariably sensitive to penicillin. Not all organisms have predictable resistance patterns, the use of antibiotics in a hospital environment and in the community has led to increasing resistance in many important human pathogens, e.g. *Staphylococcus aureus* and *Neisseria gonorrhoeae*. These cannot be predicted in advance, and *in vitro* testing is required.

This is a simplification of a complex situation, but it remains a central task of the laboratory to generate reproducible susceptibility results which will provide a guide to therapy. A multiplicity of methods has been evolved to fulfil this need and the more important of these are described in this chapter.

Clinicians who interpret laboratory tests will not have access to raw data from which the test result was derived; thus, a definition of the meaning of the terms used in susceptibility testing must be agreed. Three categories of results are conventionally used: susceptible, moderately susceptible (or intermediate), and resistant. A patient infected with an organism that is reported as sensitive to a given antibiotic can be expected to respond to conventional doses of that drug. A patient infected with an organism designated resistant to a given antibiotic would not be expected to respond to that antibiotic. Intermediate, or moderate, susceptibility means that a positive response could be expected if higher than conventional doses can be safely given or the antimicrobial agent was concentrated at the site of the infection (e.g. in the urine).

It is facile to suggest that the behaviour of an *in vitro* bacterial culture exposed to antimicrobial agents incorporated in a paper disc can predict the outcome of the interaction between pathogen, host immune system and underlying disease. It is essential, therefore, to remember the empiric nature of susceptibility testing. The results are of value only as part of the overall process of antibiotic selection. Antibiotic choice will be influenced by the site of the infection, the ability of antibiotics to penetrate that site, the dose that is achievable, the immune response of the host and the presence of indwelling prosthetic devices. It is only together with these factors that the susceptibility of the pathogen is considered.

Susceptibility testing can be divided into two broad categories: the qualitative tests (which include the disc susceptibility and break point methods) and the quantitative methods (which provide an absolute value for the minimum bacteriostatic and bactericidal concentration of an agent which will inhibit or kill the organism respectively).

Media

Composition

The composition of the medium is important, as it must support the growth of a wide range of pathogens in a reproducible way. Bacteriological media are variable in their characteristics both between different formulations, between the same formulation made by different manufacturers and between batches of the same formulation from the same manufacturer. This happens because of variation in the composition of the natural components which make up a complex medium. Defined media have a more reproducible performance. The International Collaborative Study of Susceptibility Testing (ICSST) reported that an ideal susceptibility testing medium would be defined to the level of the production details for crude components. It should support the growth of the majority of human pathogens without supplementation and should not be antagonistic to commonly used antibacterials. It should be isotonic, not subject to significant pH changes as a result of bacterial multiplication and agar and broth formulations should be the same. The ICSST recommended the use of diagnostic susceptibility test agar (DST). The NCCLS recommended Mueller-Hinton for use in the Kirby-Bauer method and the report of the British Society of Antimicrobial Chemotherapy recommended Isosensitest agar (Table 20.1). The Stokes method (see below) does not specify a particular medium, and it is this in part which makes it popular in British laboratories.

Individual components of culture media may affect the results of susceptibility tests. Bacteriological agars are highly variable in their composition and their suitability for susceptibility testing. They contain differing concentrations of, for example, divalent cations, and trace elements. Agar with increased concentrations of sulphate groups have increased binding of peptide antibiotics and basic antibiotics such as aminoglycosides.

Table 20.1 Disc potency for sensitivity testing

	Stokes	*Kirby-Bauer*
Penicillin G		
staphylococcus	2 IU	
pneumococcus/		
meningococcus	0.25 IU	10 IU
Ampicillin		10 µg
Enterobacteriaceae		
and enterococci	10 µg	
Haemophilus,		
moraxella	2 µg	10 µg
Piperacillin	30 µg	
Cephalexin	30 µg	
Cefotaxime	30 µg	30 µg
Ceftazidime	30 µg	30 µg
Methicillin	5 µg	5 µg
Imipenem	10 µg	10 µg
Gentamicin	10 µg	10 µg
Netilmicin	10 µg	30 µg
Amikacin	30 µg	30 µg
Erythromycin	5 µg	15 µg
Clindamycin	2 µg	2 µg
Tetracycline	10 µg	30 µg
Fusidic acid	10 µg	
Ciprofloxacin	1 µg	5 µg
Trimethoprim	2.5 µg	5 µg
Co-trimoxazole	1.2/23.75 µg	1.25/23.75 µg
Spectinomycin	100 µg	
Vancomycin	30 µg	
Rifampicin	2 µg	

The concentration of cations, such as Mg^{2+} and Ca^{2+}, will alter the results of susceptibility testing, e.g. zone sizes for aminoglycosides for *P. aeruginosa* are reduced with increasing concentrations.

Specific inhibitors

As sulphonamides and trimethoprim act by interfering with bacterial folate metabolism, media which incorporate intermediate and end products of these pathways such as thymidine or purines may antagonize these drugs and lead to reports of false resistance. Susceptibility media should therefore have low levels of thymidine and thiamine and levels can be reduced further by the addition of 5% lysed horse blood.

Supplements

For some organisms, the media may require supplementation because of their intrinsic fastidiousness. Some streptococci are pyridoxine dependent as are some *S. aureus* and *E. coli*. Lysed blood must be added to ensure adequate growth of *Neisseria* spp. and streptococci.

The pH

The pH of the medium should remain constant during incubation as the activity of many antibiotics is affected. The activity of aminoglycosides, macrolides, lincomycin and some cephalosporins is increased at alkaline pH. The activity of tetracycline, methicillin, fusidic acid and novobiocin and pyrazinamide is increased at acid pH. In most situations the zwitterionic effect of the peptides in the medium is adequate to maintain pH around 7.4.

Wherever possible susceptibility plates should not be incubated in an atmosphere with increased CO_2 as this reduces the pH causing both false susceptibility and resistance. When a medium contains glucose to encourage growth it should be carefully buffered because of the decrease in pH caused by the metabolism of these organisms.

Protein concentration

The protein concentration of susceptibility testing media may affect the results for antibiotics, such as fusidic acid which are highly protein bound.

Selection of anaerobic media

For anaerobic susceptibility testing, Wilkins-Chalgren medium is widely recommended. Although many laboratories use DST batch-to-batch variation is thought to be responsible for the variation in results obtained with this media in one study. When broth media are required brain heart infusion supplemented with haemin, menadione and yeast extract is satisfactory.

Disc diffusion tests

Introduction

Disc susceptibility methods utilize a filter paper disc in which an antibiotic has been incorporated and dried. When placed on the surface of an agar plate, the antibiotic diffuses into the agar at a rate which is dependent on the molecular weight and chemistry of the antibiotic and the characteristics of the medium. At increasing distances from the disc, the concentration of antibiotic in the agar falls. Where the agar has a high concentration of antibiotics, inoculated organisms fail to grow. Further away from the disc, where concentrations are lower, the bacteria are able to grow normally. At a distance intermediate to this, a line of demarcation is formed where, on one side, no growth is found and, on the other side, bacteria are able to grow. The position of this zone, which is measured by the zone radius, may be related to the minimal inhibitory concentration (MIC) of the antibiotic for that organism (Fig. 20.1).

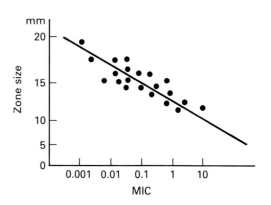

Figure 20.1   A regression line describes the relationship between zone size and logMIC. Measurements of the zone size are an indirect measure of the MIC

It has been shown that there is an approximately linear relationship between the zone size and the log of the minimal inhibitory concentration. This relationship forms the basis of the Kirby-Bauer (NCCLS) method.

Variation in zone size

Conditions of incubation

Susceptibility tests should be incubated at a temperature of 35–37°C in an aerobic atmosphere. There are exceptions to this such as *S. aureus* where methicillin susceptibility is more reproducible when incubated at 30°. Incubator temperatures should be controlled with a maximum/minimum thermometer, which should be regularly monitored.

Inoculum

Variation in inoculum density makes the result of disc diffusion tests difficult to interpret. The size of zone decreases with increasingly heavy inocula.

It is UK practice to use an inoculum which will produce semi-confluent growth after overnight incubation. This method has the advantage that variation from the standard is easily detected visually (Fig. 20.2). For the NCCLS (Kirby-Bauer) methods, a confluent growth is recommended. Inocula can be standardized by the use of a barium sulphate standard (Fig. 20.3).

The inoculum can be placed on the plate by flooding with a bacterial suspension and drying before the discs are applied. A swab can be dipped in a bacterial suspension, the excess fluid squeezed out by pressing against the side of the container the swab before it is used to spread the inoculum evenly over the plate. Plates inoculated with control organisms can be prepared in advance and stored at 4°C.

Prediffusion and preincubation

If organisms are planted on the medium and allowed to multiply (preincubation) before the antibiotics discs are placed the zone sizes will be reduced. This has the same effect as having too heavy an inoculum. If discs are placed on the medium and diffusion (prediffusion) takes place before the organisms have a chance to grow zone sizes will be increased.

To limit these effects a standardized inoculum should be inoculated within 15 minutes of preparation and the discs should be applied within 15 minutes and the plates incubated within 15 minutes of applying the discs.

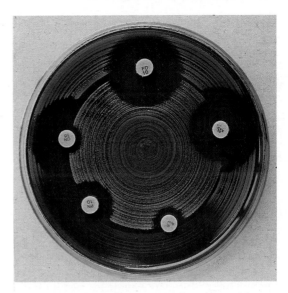

Figure 20.2 Stokes sensitivity plate with semi-confluent growth

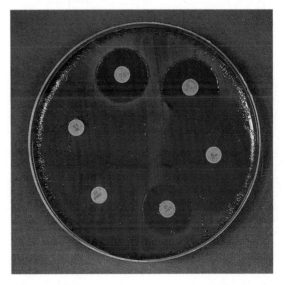

Figure 20.3 Confluent growth of Kirby-Bauer technique

Depth of agar

The depth of agar will affect the zone size. Shallow agar results in increased diffusion and, therefore, zone size. An optimal depth of agar is 4 mm, but this requires 25 ml of agar per plate and is expensive in reagents. More typically, 18 ml is used, giving a more shallow agar, which may be more susceptible to variation.

Antibiotic discs

Selection of antibiotics to test

The selection of antibiotics for susceptibility testing should be based on the local antimicrobial policy if such is in place, or local prescribing policies or as a result of epidemiological surveys of antimicrobial resistance. The group selected in each 'set' should aim to give a range of alternatives which could enable clinicians to choose between oral and parenteral preparations and have a choice in cases of allergy.

As there is a very wide range of available antibiotics numbers of agents tested can be limited by picking individual representatives of antibiotic classes. For example, methicillin susceptibility is used as a guide for susceptibility to the other members of the group (i.e. flucloxacillin and oxacillin). In the choice of agents as group representatives, the least active member of the group should be chosen. Although some cases false resistance will result, this is preferable to a false susceptibility report.

The potency of discs selected is dependent on the site of the specimen being tested and the method used. As higher concentrations of antibiotics are usually achieved in urine, higher content discs can be used. The disc contents for the Kirby-Bauer method (NCCLS) are laid down and quality assurance standards are regulated by the Food and Drugs Administration of the US Department of Health. This is essential because the interpretation of the results is dependent on strict adherence to protocols and extrapolation of results from regression lines. Examples of disc contents for use in the Kirby-Bauer and Stokes methods are found in Table 20.1.

Handling

Discs and disc dispensers should be stored in sealed containers in the dark in a refrigerator. Discs should then be warmed to room temperature before use and refrigerated overnight when they are not in use. Before use, plates should be dried and discs should be applied so that a firm, even contact is made with the medium. A 90 mm plate will accommodate no more than six antibiotic discs without the risk of overlapping zones. The labelling of individual discs is controlled by the WHO Expert Committee on Biological Standardization.

Methicillin susceptibility

The expression of resistance among *S. aureus* is markedly influenced by the conditions by which susceptibility testing is performed. Tests should be incubated at 30°C or, alternatively, at 37°C if the medium contains 5% NaCl. This medium may, however, inhibit a minority of strains. Resistance may be detected by the presence of a reduced zone diameter, a reducing size of colony up the disc, or isolated colonies within the zone of inhibition.

Kirby-Bauer method

This method is laid down as the standard technique by the NCCLS in the USA. The medium used is Mueller-Hinton, and the inoculum is standardized against a barium sulphate standard. Plates are inoculated using a swab dipped into a standardized broth and streaked across the medium to give a confluent growth after overnight incubation (see Fig. 20.3). The disc contents are specified, and examples are shown in Table 20.1. Organisms are classified as susceptible, moderately susceptible and resistant by comparing with interpretation tables. These have been prepared by performing MICs of many hundreds of isolates and comparing zone sizes in a regression plot (see Fig. 20.1). Controls with defined standard strains must be set up daily until defined performance criteria are met after which tests are required weekly.

Comparative methods

In comparative methods susceptibility and resistance are determined in comparison with organisms of known susceptibility. In the comparative method these organisms are on separate plates. In the Stokes method test and control organism are placed on the same plate. This is achieved by applying the bacteria on a swab with a rotary plater (Fig. 20.4). The advantages of this method is that minor variations in the medium and conditions of incubation apply to both the test and control

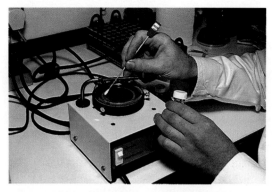

Figure 20.4 Circular platers may be used to inoculate Stokes sensitivity plates

Table 20.2 Control organisms for comparative and Stokes method

Control strain	Organisms tested
Staphylococcus aureus NCTC 6571	Aerobic organisms
Haemophilus influenzae NCTC 11931	*Haemophilus* spp.
Neisseria gonorrhoeae (sensitive strain)	*N. gonorrhoeae*
Escherichia coli NCTC 10418	Enterobacteriaciae
Pseudomonas aeruginosa NCTC 10662	*Pseudomonas* spp.
Clostridium perfringens NCTC 11229	*Clostridium* spp.
Bacillus fragilis NCTC 9343	Other anaerobes

organism. It is not necessary to define the medium for use in comparative methods. Thus, it is hoped that results will be more reproducible but this is dependent on the reproducibility of the inocula as differences between test and control inoculum will make the interpretation of this test impossible. Susceptible, moderately susceptible and resistant isolates can be defined as shown in Figure 20.5.

As this technique has developed a range of different control organisms have been used, these include the 'Oxford' strain of *S. aureus* NCTC 6571, *E. coli* NCTC 10418 and *P. aeruginosa* NCTC 10662. Control strains for fastidious organisms are also defined (Table 20.2).

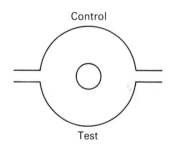

a. Sensitive: the zone radius of the test strain is not more than 3 mm less than the control zone.

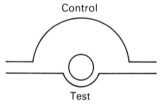

b. Resistant: the zone radius of the test strain is < 3 mm.

Figure 20.5 Definitions of sensitive, intermediate and resistant using Stokes criteria

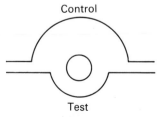

c. Intermediate: The zone radius of the test strain is >3 mm but is more than 3 mm smaller than the control zone.

Primary susceptibility

A patient's specimen can be used as the inoculum and this is known as primary susceptibility testing. This provides a rapid indication of susceptibility but has a number of disadvantages. If more than one organism is present in the specimen, it may be difficult to measure the individual zone sizes. Moreover, the inoculum is uncontrolled, which may result in variability in zone size. A low inoculum results in a larger zone size and apparent susceptibility; a higher inoculum, a lower zone size and apparent resistance. Primary susceptibility testing is frequently used in examination of urinary infections, where approximately 10^5 organisms/ml are found in patients. Primary susceptibility testing is wasteful of resources, as many specimens will have no organisms present. Thus, if this method is employed it should be restricted to urine specimens in which organisms are seen under direct microscopy.

Reading zones

Any plates which have incorrect inocula (either test or control) must be rejected. The radius of the control zone is measured with callipers, the most accurate method, with a clear millimetre rule or with a ruled template. The plate can be accepted for reading if the control zones fall inside the limits set by the laboratory. The test zone size is measured in the same way and the value obtained subtracted from the control value. A test with a zone size not less than 3 mm smaller is considered susceptible. A zone size less than 3 mm is considered resistant with values falling in between considered moderately susceptible (see Fig. 20.5).

The zone edge can sometimes be heaped up for organisms which produce a beta-lactamase. These isolates should be considered resistant. Some *Proteus* strains may swarm beyond the zone edge but this should be disregarded as it does not indicate resistance. When nitrofurantoin is being tested against *Proteus*, large zones can be obtained, but because the drug is not active at the alkaline pH normally found in the urine of patients with *Proteus* infection, resistance should be reported.

Quality control

In comparative methods quality control for each test is in theory built into the test. Variation in the size of control zones should, of course, prompt an investigation. Control organisms should be stored on agar slopes and subcultured fortnightly. These working slopes should be replaced from freeze-dried cultures frozen in glycerol at $-70°C$ every two months or when contamination is suspected. The performance of disc susceptibility testing should be reviewed by recording control zone sizes regularly. Limits for zone sizes should be set to provide 95% confidence.

Before a new batch of susceptibility testing agar is used routinely, control strains should be tested against the main antibiotic agents used in the laboratory.

Incorrect zone sizes may indicate that the antibiotic within the disc has become inactive due to poor handling technique. Individual workers may use the incorrect inoculum or measure incorrectly, resulting in aberrant zone sizes. Variation in the composition of the medium will also be indicated by changes in the zone sizes for control organisms.

For the Kirby-Bauer, standards of variation of control zones are defined by NCCLS. A single test should give a result with defined limits. If more than one in twenty results is outside a given range corrective action is necessary (95% confidence). Control zones must not be more than four standard deviations above or below the mid-point of the range and the mean control zone size should be close to the mid-point of the range.

Breakpoints

Definition

A breakpoint is an antibiotic concentration which may be used to discriminate sensitive from resistant organisms in a susceptibility testing method. Most organisms with a MIC lower than the breakpoint should be successfully treated with that antibiotic. Similarly, in those with an MIC above the breakpoint, therapy with that antibiotic would be expected to fail. This definition depends on the assumption that *in vitro* susceptibility can be correlated with *in vivo* activity. In order to make the correlate correct the breakpoint must be carefully chosen taking into account the pharmacokinetics of the antibiotic including protein binding, penetration into special sites, absorption, metabolism and excretion.

Setting the breakpoint

The MIC provides the firmest reference point for predicting the outcome in clinical infection. Breakpoint determinations work best if there is a clear difference in the MIC between organisms which are considered sensitive from those that are resistant. In other words the breakpoint falls in the trough between peaks of MIC in a bimodal distribution (see Fig. 20.6). In these circumstances organisms which are below the breakpoint are obviously sensitive and those above are clearly resistant. Not all organisms have this tidy pattern. Moreover, a breakpoint must be chosen for a number of different species and their 'troughs' may not lie close together. It must therefore be chosen to accommodate the majority of clinical isolates from the group of organisms tested. A system of MIC monitoring must also be built in so that

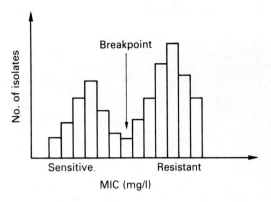

Figure 20.6 Sensitive and resistant strains fall into two separate populations (bimodal distribution) enabling strains to be readily differentiated using a breakpoint concentration

the laboratory can be assured that the breakpoints chosen have relevance to the population of bacteria isolated by that laboratory.

Two breakpoints are usually defined. Isolates which fail to grow on the lower concentration are fully susceptible (see above for definition); those growing at the lower

Table 20.3 Examples of breakpoint concentrations (mg/l) recommended by BSAC (see Further Reading)

| | Group I (staphylococci, streptococci H. influenzae, M. catarrhalis) | | Group II Enterobacteriaciae, Pseudomonas, et al. | |
	Low	High	Low	High
Pentamycin	1	4	1	4
Amikacin	4	16	4	16
Penicillin G	0.12			
Methicillin	4			
Ampicillin	1		8	
Mezlocillin	2		16	64
Cephradine	2	8	2	8
Cefotaxime	1	8	1	
Ceftazidime	2	8	2	
Imipenem	4		4	
Aztreonam			8	
Ciprofloxacin	1	4	1	4
Erythromycin	0.5			
Clindamycin	0.5			
Vancomycin	4			
Chloramphenicol	2	8		
Tetracycline	1		1	
Fusidic acid	1			
Trimethoprim	0.5	2	0.5	2

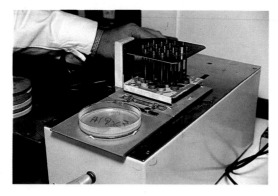

Figure 20.7   Multi-point inoculator is used to inoculate plates in the agar incorporation MIC method

breakpoint but failing to grow on the higher concentration are classified as intermediate, or moderately susceptible, and those which grow at both concentrations are fully resistant (Table 20.3).

Application

Breakpoint methods have the advantage of the large number of isolates that can be tested using an agar incorporation technique with a multi-point inoculator (Fig. 20.7). Most multi-point inoculation devices deliver 20–36 spots per 90 mm petri dish. Rectangular plates accommodating more than 100 spots can be used. As there is a simple endpoint, reading can be automated using computer image analysers. A disadvantage is that the method will have poor reproducibility for organisms with MIC values close to the breakpoint.

The breakpoint method is most suitable for laboratories with a moderate to high throughput and is most effectively applied to Enterobacteraceae, pseudomonads, other Gram-negative rods, staphylococci and streptococci. Slow-growing, fastidious, or unusual organisms are more successfully tested by conventional methods.

Media and agents

The choice of agent to test and considerations of media are similar to those for disc susceptibility testing. A mechanism to prevent the swarming of *Proteus* must be used by incorpo-

rating 15 mg/l *p*-nitrophenylglycerol (PNPG) in the medium or by increasing the agar content to 2%. Medium should be prepared weekly and stored in the plastic sleeves in the refrigerator.

Inoculum

The inoculum should be standardized and applied by a multi-point inoculator (see Fig. 20.7). For breakpoint and MIC methods, 10^4 cfu per spot are used. However, for the testing of sulphonamides, 10^3 cfu per spot must be used, as there is a significant inoculum effect. When testing organisms which produce an extracellular beta-lactamase, high inocula (10^6 cfu per spot) give more reproducible results.

An inoculum of 10^4 cfu per spot can be achieved by a multi-point inoculator which delivers one microlitre of a broth with 10^7 cfu/ml. When staphylococci are being tested against beta-lactams, an inoculum of 10^6 cfu per spot is required. Otherwise, weak penicillinase producers may appear susceptible. An opposite effect is found if pseudomonads are being tested against anti-pseudomonal beta-lactam antibiotics.

Quality control

The MICs of the standard quality control strains are usually not close to the breakpoints chosen for routine testing, and thus these organisms are of little value. Control strains with MICs above and below each of the breakpoints must be chosen but not so close that normal day-to-day variation in the results of the test will bring about rejection of the batch.

The number of controls required will limit the number of tests which can be performed, and therefore a batch control method may be adopted. A range of control organisms should be applied to a set of plates from the beginning of the batch and another set tested at the end. Discrepant results can then be investigated.

Minimal inhibitory and bactericidal concentrations

Definition

The minimum inhibitory concentration (MIC) is defined as the lowest concentration that completely inhibits growth of a micro-organism. Although the relationship between MIC and successful outcome of antimicrobial chemotherapy cannot be clearly established, it is considered the most useful guide to the efficacy of antimicrobial therapy. The minimal bactericidal concentration (MBC) is defined as the lowest concentration that prevents growth after subculture to antibiotic-free medium. This is conventionally defined as a 99.9% kill.

Indications for use

MICs can be measured in the routine clinical laboratory to aid the interpretation of disc susceptibility testing, to confirm susceptibility in unexpected treatment failures, and together with the MBC as part of the laboratory control of endocarditis. They are often also used in patients who are severely immunocompromised and whose antimicrobial therapy must be optimized. MICs are used to study new drugs so that their likely clinical value can be determined.

Medium

Iso-sensitest or Mueller-Hinton agar can be used for the agar incorporation technique, and broth versions can be used as required.

Antimicrobial agents

The choice of antibiotics for MIC/MBC testing is usually defined by the clinical situation as the patient is already on therapy before an MIC becomes necessary. The drugs should be obtained as pure substances, together with the manufacturer's statement of potency. Oral preparations are unsuitable and some intravenous preparations are also unsuitable, e.g. choramphenicol, clindamycin and pro-drug esters. Antimicrobial powders should be stored in the dark at 4°C with silica gel. Stock solutions can usually be stored at –70°C for several months at concentrations in excess of 1000 mg/l but potency can be lost if the solutions are subject to repeated freeze/thaw cycles.

Stock solutions should be prepared so that MIC values can be based on doubling dilutions based on the unit of 1 mg/l, e.g. 16, 8, 4, 2, 1, 0.5, 0.25, 0.125 mg/l. Commercially prepared antibiotic tablets for incorporation into agar are available. The ranges which are used in determining MIC will vary, depending on the organism being tested.

Methods

Several methods of determining MIC are available. The agar incorporation dilution technique uses varying concentrations of antibiotic incorporated into the agar. The organisms are inoculated, as in the breakpoint method, with a multi-point inoculator. This technique is valuable for processing a large number of individual isolates quickly. It may also be automated (see above), both in reading and in data handling. With careful attention to the quality control of media, the technique can be highly accurate but it suffers the disadvantage that MICs cannot be readily turned into MBCs. With a velvet pad technique, however, MBCs can be obtained, although this technique is too cumbersome for routine use.

MICs can be set up by having different concentrations of an antibiotic in a broth medium. After overnight incubation, the MIC is recorded as the lowest concentration of antibiotic in which growth is inhibited. All negative tubes are subcultured and the lowest concentration which prevents regrowth on subculture on antibiotic-free medium is reported as the MBC. In practice, this represents the 99.9% kill.

A variation of this method uses micro-titre plates but great care must be taken due to the small volumes involved and the influence of inoculum on the result. Commercial modifications of the micro-titre method have been developed in which pre-prepared microtitre plates are provided and the inoculum is standardized by measuring its optical density.

A simpler approach suitable for laboratories performing occasional tests are commercially manufactured plastic cupules containing differing concentrations of test antibiotic. A standardized inoculum is made up and put in each cupule. It is then read as in the standard tube method. A novel technique uses a paper strip in which antibiotic has been incorporated. The concentration of antibiotic incorporated falls throughout the length of the strip which

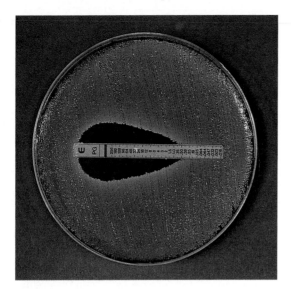

Figure 20.8   The E-test is a method of obtaining an MIC result. The point at which the elipse meets the strip approximates to the MIC

means that when it is placed on a suitable agar medium with a lawn inoculum of the test organism differing concentration gradients are set up along the length of the strip. The point at which growth meets the paper strip corresponds to the MIC which can be read from a scale (Fig. 20.8).

Quality control

Control strains should be tested in parallel with the test strains (see Table 20.5). The MIC of the control strain must fall inside the range of the dilution series tested (Table 20.4). The MIC for this strain should be established and the results in each assay should not be more than one dilution up or down from the published value if the test result is to be accepted as valid. An antibiotic-free control must be included in each test to prove that the organism is capable of growing in the test medium. After incubation the purity of the inoculum should be confirmed by subculture.

Tests for synergy

Indications for use

Combination chemotherapy is indicated when the identity and therefore the susceptibility of the infecting pathogen is unknown. Two or more antibiotics are used to ensure that all of the likely pathogens are fully treated. The same considerations apply when infection is mixed in, for example, an abdominal abscess. Combinations are also required to prevent the emergence of resistance. The best example of this is in the therapy of tuberculosis where treatment with a single agent rapidly results in the development of resistance. In patients with diminished immunity a combination is often prescribed to attempt to achieve optimum bactericidal activity when little help can be expected from the immune system. A second drug may be given so that the dose of a toxic one may be reduced to lower levels. The dose of amphotericin B can be reduced when given in combination with 5-fluocytosine for the treatment of *Cryptococcus neoformans* infection. Some antibiotics are given together with another drug which inhibits degradative enzymes. These may be bacterial in origin as in the case of beta-lactamases, or of host origin as in the case of renal dihydropeptidase which breaks down imipenem. Finally a combination can be given to obtain synergy which is defined as an effect which exceeds that of either agent alone. When combinations of drugs are used they may inhibit

Table 20.4   Examples of MIC ranges

	Enterobacteriacieae	Pseudomonads	*Staphylococci*	*Streptococci*	Neisseria	*H. influenzae*
Penicillin G	–	–	0.12–128	0.008–8	0.004–32	–
Ampicillin	0.25–128	–	0.03–128	0.008–8	0.004–32	0.06–128
Gentamicin	0.03–128	0.06–128	0.008–128	1–128	0.5–16	0.12–16
Cefotaxime	0.004–128	0.5–512	0.5–128	0.004–128	0.004–128	0.004–0.06
Imipenem	0.12–32	0.25–128	0.004–1	0.004–16	0.004–1	0.06–4
Vancomycin	–	–	0.03–8	0.12–16	–	–

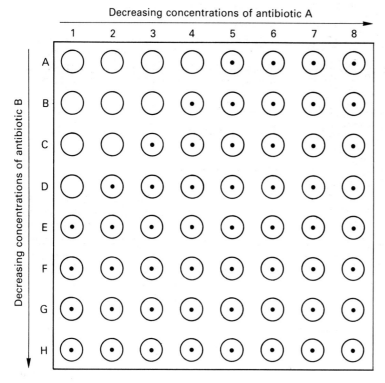

Figure 20.9 In a chequerboard concentrations of two antibiotics are diluted in two dimensions. This diagram shows no synergy, i.e. there is no increased effect by having a combination

each other's action (antagonism) or there may be no interaction (indifference).

In the clinical laboratory the value of synergy testing is limited as it is very rare for therapeutic decisions to be altered by the results of synergy tests.

Methods

Synergy is determined in the laboratory by use of checkerboard titrations, in effect a two-dimensional MIC (Fig. 20.9). The considerations of antibiotics, medium and inoculum, etc. also apply to synergy testing. The test can be performed in large tubes or more conveniently in micro-titre trays. When a large number of strains are to be tested the agar incorporation technique can be modified.

A row of discs can be set at right angles to a row of discs of a different antibiotic on a lawn inoculum. After overnight growth evidence of synergy or antagonism can be seen (Fig. 20.10).

Results

The fractional inhibitory concentration (FIC) can be calculated by dividing the MIC of the drugs acting together by the MIC of one of the drugs acting alone. This calculation is repeated for the second drug and the results added. If this value is less than one it indicates synergy, a value of one: indifference and greater than one: antagonism.

Antibiotic assays

Indications

The most important reason for antibiotic assay in the serum is to monitor the concentrations of drugs with a narrow therapeutic index. Chief among these are the aminoglycosides such as gentamicin and netilmicin and the glycopeptide vancomycin, all of which may cause renal failure. Assays should be performed regularly in all patients but more frequent monitoring is required in the elderly, in those taking potentially renal toxic drugs. Other patients predisposed to aminoglycoside toxicity in whom monitoring should be more frequent include patients who have received aminoglycosides in the last month, have evidence of impaired renal function or in whom renal function is changing rapidly because of sepsis or other coexistent conditions.

The concentration of antibiotics can be measured in body fluids to ensure that dosage is adequate. Assays can confirm that oral therapy is achieving therapeutic concentrations in the blood if a shift to oral therapy has occurred. Antibiotic concentrations can be measured in body fluids where drug penetration may be a problem (e.g. CSF). In cases where there is unexpected therapeutic failure measurement of serum antibiotic levels will form part of the investigation of this problem.

Samples and interpretation

Serum should be collected immediately before and one hour after the dose. Some authors suggest that different sample times be chosen for i.v. and i.m. administration but this is likely to result in confusion for the person taking the specimen. Such confusion will reduce the value of the test as the most important part of the interpretation of the result is the timing of the samples. It is essential to ensure that when the patient has an indwelling line that the assay is taken from a peripheral site or that the canula is thoroughly flushed. Examples of therapeutic ranges are found in Table 20.5.

Methods

Microbiological assays

Until recently microbiological assay was the main means of measuring the concentration of antibiotics. A lawn inoculum of a strain susceptible to the antibiotic under test was poured onto a large, square plate. Wells were then cut in the agar and standard concentrations of antibiotic placed in the wells in triplicate. Unknown samples were placed in wells in

Table 20.5 Examples of peak and trough antibiotic concentrations

	Trough (mg/l)	*Peak (mg/l)*
Gentamicin	<2.0	4–8
Netilmicin	<4	8–12
Amikacin	<5	25–30
Chloramphenicol	10–20	<25
Vancomycin	5–10	25

the same way and the zones of inhibition carefully measured after 4–18 hours' incubation. The concentration of the unknown specimens could be determined by comparison with the standard curve plotted on semi-logarithmic graph paper. The reading and data interpretation of these plates can be facilitated by image analysis and computer.

The advantage of this technique is that it is cheap and can be performed without sophisticated equipment but results are often too late to influence therapy. Results are also influenced by undeclared antibiotics present in the serum.

Automated methods

Serological techniques have been harnessed to assay antibiotics. Immunoassay methods using the techniques of polarizing fluorescence immunoassay, and enzyme immunoassays (EMIT), and substrate-labelled fluoroimmunoassay have all been used with success. Unknown samples are all measured in comparison with a calibration curve derived from the measurement of standard concentrations.

EMIT depends on the inhibition of an enzyme drug conjugate by an antibody. The enzyme used is glucose-6-phosphate. The higher the amount of aminoglycoside in the specimen the less antibody is available to bind to the enzyme drug conjugate, and thus more substrate will be converted.

Polarizing fluorescence immunoassay works because antigen linked to a fluorophor will be preferentially excited if the molecules are parallel to the light. If antibody is present complexes are formed which rotate slowly so much of the emitted light is polarized. The more free drug the less antibody will be present, complexes will not form and less polarized light is emitted.

In the substrate-labelled fluoroimmunoassay the antibiotic is labelled with a fluorogenic compound which is also an enzyme-releasing fluorescein. When antibody binds to labelled drug the substrate cannot be acted on by the enzyme and there is less fluorescence. The more free drug in the sample the more fluorescence will be detected.

These techniques are commercially available from manufacturers who provide equipment, standards and controls. The process of measurement and data handling is automated.

The advantages of these techniques are that large numbers of specimens can be handled at one time and the results are available sufficiently quickly to enable the next dose to be altered. Undeclared antibiotics do not interfere with the results. The disadvantages are the expense of the equipment and of the reagents.

High performance liquid chromatography (HPLC)

If an antibiotic-containing solution is injected on a HPLC column the identity of the antibiotic can be determined by the elution time. The concentration can be calculated by comparing the peak heights or area with those of solutions of known concentration. This technique is largely confined to research laboratories. It can be applied to a wide range of antimicrobials and can be used to measure concentrations in patients on combination chemotherapy.

Although parts of the process can be automated it remains a largely manual procedure.

Serum bactericidal levels

This test measures the ability of a patient's serum to kill the organism isolated from that patient. It is performed in a similar way to the MIC determination. Specimens of serum are taken before antibiotic therapy and one hour afterwards. Doubling dilutions are made in broth and organisms are added to each tube. A non-serum-containing control is also inoculated, together with a tube of broth without inoculation. The highest dilution which completely inhibits growth is the bacteriostatic titration. All tubes are then subcultured and the highest dilution which produces a greater than 99.9% kill is the bactericidal titre.

Indications for use

Serum bactericidal concentrations are traditionally performed in the management of infective endocarditis, and other situations where the effectiveness of the prescribed regimen is in doubt. It has the advantage that serum from a patient receiving more than one antibiotic can be tested. There is experimental evidence to suggest a relationship between bactericidal titre and success in the therapy of endocarditis. The correlation between bactericidal titre and clinical outcome in human infection remains unproved.

Beta-lactamase testing

For some organisms, rapid testing of beta-lactamase is very helpful, e.g. *H. influenzae* and *N. gonorrhoeae*. Individual colonies may be applied to paper discs containing the chromogenic cephalosporin nitrocefin, which, when broken down by beta-lactamases, changes colour from red to yellow. Alternatively, a less sensitive method is to culture the organism in the medium containing the beta-lactam antibiotic, the acid produced in this reaction being detected by a simple indicator. Control strains which do and do not produce beta-lactamase should be tested in parallel.

21

Serological techniques

Introduction

Serological methods have always been at the forefront of developments in microbiology and will play an increasing role in diagnosis in most routine microbiology departments in the future. Central to all serological techniques is the interaction between antigens and antibodies. It is the specificity and sensitivity of this reaction which gives serological diagnosis its attraction.

Antigen–antibody interactions

At the molecular level this interaction takes place between antigenic determinants (or epitopes) on the antigen and antigen-binding sites (paratopes) on the antibody. Epitopes are short amino acid sequences, five to seven amino acids long, or short chains of sugar residues. Antigens usually contain many different epitopes, on average one epitope for every 40–80 amino acids. Antibody binding takes place through binding sites in the variable Fab portion of the immunoglobulin molecule. The immunoglobulin molecule is made up of two major regions the Fab, antigen binding, and the Fc, constant region molecules. They are made up of two heavy and two light chains: the light chains contain two domains, and the heavy chains three to five depending on the isotype. The domains are described as being variable or constant (Fig. 21.1). The variable domains have framework residues in which the amino acid sequence is conserved and hypervariable regions which are responsible for diversity of

antigen binding. The constant regions are made up of domains in which the amino acid sequence is conserved. It is the Fc portion which is responsible for the secondary interactions of immunoglobulin molecules, e.g. complement fixation (Fig. 21.2).

The interactions between antibodies and antigen are non-covalent and depend upon electrostatic interactions, van der Waals forces, hydrogen bonds and hydrophobic interactions. All of these forces are weak and operate only over a short distance. It is essential, therefore, that the antigen and antibody make a 'good fit', like a key in a lock, so that these forces are able

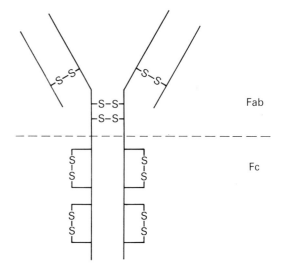

Figure 21.1 Schematic diagram of immunoglobulin molecule (IgG). The Fab portion is responsible for specific antigen binding

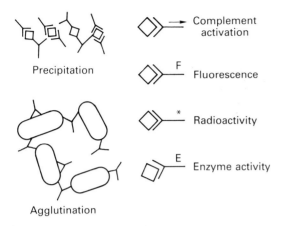

Figure 21.2 Primary interactions concern the specific binding of antigen and antibody. The secondary interactions are the way in which we recognize antigen–antibody binding has occurred. This may occur as a result of altering the immunoglobulin molecule by labelling (e.g. with fluoroscein)

to operate. The corollary of this is that antibodies which have a poor fit will bind to an antigen only weakly.

Primary activity

The binding of an antigen and antibody is described as the *primary interaction*. This occurs as a result of a good fit between the antigen-binding site on the Fab portion of the immunoglobulin molecule and the epitope present in the antigen. As a consequence of this binding many secondary phenomena occur, the precise nature of these depending on the isotype of antibody involved in the binding process. These *secondary interactions* include precipitation, agglutination and complement fixation. It is these secondary phenomena which can be used as a means of detecting antigen–antibody binding.

Secondary activities

Precipitation is the formation of an insoluble complex from antibody and antigen in a

solution. Agglutination is the formation of a lattice of clumps and aggregates of a particulate antigen, for example a sensitized red blood cell or a whole organism, with antibody. Complement fixation is the activation of the classical complement cascade initiated by the interaction of antigen and antibody.

Some methods use only the primary interaction between antigen and antibody, the secondary phenomenon used to detect the primary interaction occurs as a result of manipulation of antigen and antibody by labelling. In direct immunofluorescence an antigen present in patient material is detected by the binding of a fluorescein-labelled antibody. Under u.v. light the target organism will fluoresce apple green. Indirect immunofluorescence uses a similar approach, except that known antigen is applied to the slide and binds to specific antibody in patient serum. Binding is detected by a fluoroscein-labelled anti-human immunoglobulin raised in another species. Radioimmunoassay and enzyme-linked immunosorbent assay (ELISA) techniques also depend only on natural primary interaction, the secondary phenomena are proved by laboratory manipulation of the reagents; in the former case by isotopic labelling and in the latter by enzyme labelling (see Fig. 21.2).

Antibodies

Two types of antibody are used in immunoassays, polyclonal or monoclonal. Polyclonal antibodies are produced by immunization of experimental animals. They contain a mixture of antibody species with different isotype and subclass (and thus secondary activity) and will bind to several epitopes on one antigen. In contrast, a monoclonal antibody is produced as the result of a fusion of a B cell from an immunized animal and a myeloma cell line. The antibodies which are subsequently produced will bind to a single epitope and will be of a single isotype (and thus have uniform secondary activity).

Definition of terms

A number of terms are used in serology and are used loosely to form an impenetrable jargon.

Detectability

This refers to the ability of an assay to detect a defined amount of target antigen or antibody.

Sensitivity

The sensitivity of an assay may be defined as the ability to identify correctly all of those patients suffering from a disease. It depends partly on level of detection and the accuracy of the assay. Thus an assay with low detectability will miss many positive subjects, i.e. it is insensitive.

Specificity

The specificity may be defined as the ability to identify correctly all of those patients not suffering from the disease investigated. Specificity is determined by the uniqueness of the antigen–antibody interaction. In an assay with low specificity many subjects who do not have the target antigen/antibody will be positive, i.e. it will have poor specificity.

Accuracy

This may be defined as the conformity of a result to an agreed standard value (e.g. an international reference standard serum). The accuracy of methods which depend on titres can be low because of the subjectivity of such tests which can mean that the result could vary by a factor of two or more.

Titre

The titre is the integer representing the greatest dilution in which there is a positive reaction. Thus if the greatest dilution at which agglutination was found in a standard Brucella agglutination assay was 1 : 320, the titre would be 320 (not 1/320).

Some indications for serological investigation

Serological techniques may be applied in many circumstances, for organizational reasons, cost or because no other means of diagnosis is readily available.

Screening

Most serological techniques are made up of several very simple activities which may readily be automated, thus serology may provide the ability to make microbiological observations in a large number of specimens at relatively low cost. Taken together with the fact that in most instances screening investigations are not seeking evidence of acute infection, serological methods are most appropriate when such programmes are planned.

Rapid diagnosis

Serology can provide rapid diagnosis, long before the results of cultural methods are available. This can be achieved by detecting the presence of antigens specific to the pathogen sought (e.g. meningococcal group C polysaccharide in the CSF) or detecting the presence of pathogen-specific IgM (e.g. the diagnosis of neonatal toxoplasmosis).

Non-cultivatible pathogens

When organisms are difficult or dangerous to cultivate, serology may be the only means available for the resources of a routine diagnostic laboratory. *Treponema pallidum* may be maintained in whole animal culture (rabbit testes) but this facility is only available at the national reference laboratory or in commercial companies who manufacture antigen.

In some infections diagnosis by culture is available, but clinicians need to confirm the diagnosis as soon as possible so that appropriate treatment can be initiated. Typhoid fever and brucellosis exemplify a number of these points. Both organisms are easily cultivatable but are relatively slow to grow. Clinicians may wish to confirm or exclude these diagnoses as part of their overall differential diagnosis and thus a serological technique which gives the answer in a few hours can speed the diagnostic process.

Serology has much to offer when organisms are difficult to detect by direct examination or slow to grow in culture, e.g. *Mycobacterium tuberculosis*. No serological method has ever established itself to fill this niche, but the large number of different techniques which have been investigated are evidence of the need.

Evaluation of immunization

Serological techniques are used in establishing immunity to infectious diseases, e.g. rubella. Response to vaccination can also be evaluated by serological means, and the concentration of antibody achieved may be determined. For some vaccines there is an agreed antibody concentration which should be achieved after vaccination to result in immunity. In hepatitis B, subjects should have >10 IU anti-hepatitis B surface antigen antibody to be considered immune.

Identification of organisms

Serological techniques are used frequently in the identification of organisms isolated in culture. Here the ability of antibodies to bind specific antigens is used to identify organisms such as salmonellas or shigellas to species and serotype (see Chapter 17).

Antibiotic assays

Antibody detection systems have been harnessed to provide antibiotic assays; antibody modulation (EMIT) assay methods, fluorescence polarization, and ELISA have all been used in antimicrobial assay. These methods are discussed in more detail in Chapter 20.

Precipitation and agglutination techniques

The principle of precipitation is exhibited in double diffusion, crossed immunoelectrophoresis, and countercurrent immunoelectrophoresis (CIE). Agglutination can be used in direct agglutination either in tubes (e.g. Brucella standard agglutination titre), or on slides (e.g. direct agglutination of salmonellas

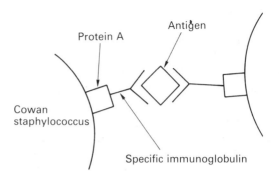

Figure 21.3 Specific immunoglobulin is bound to Protein A-coated *Staphylococcus aureus*. When antigen is present in the specimen many staphylococci can be linked to form visible agglutination

by specific antisera). Artificial particles can be sensitized with specific antibody or antigen. Particles which have been used include sheep red cells (*Treponema pallidum* haemagglutination assay, TPHA), latex beads (pneumococcal capsular polysaccharide antigen detection) or Cowan Type I strain of *Staphylococcus aureus* (streptococcal grouping) (Fig. 21.3).

A number of infectious diseases may be diagnosed by complement fixation (see below). Although these are the secondary phenomena most frequently used as detector systems a number of others are used: virus neutralization where specific antibody in patient serum inhibits infection and cytopathic effect of a virus; *T. pallidum* immobilization where specific anti-*T. pallidum* antibodies will inhibit the movement of live organisms; haemagglutination inhibition where the natural haemagglutinating activity of a virus is inhibited by specific antibody.

Precipitation

Precipitation occurs as a result of the interaction of antibody and antigen in solution. The amount of antigen precipitated is dependent on the proportions of antigen and antibody present in the reaction. When antigen is in excess all antibody binding titres have bound antigen, there is free antigen in solution and large aggregates do not form as there are no

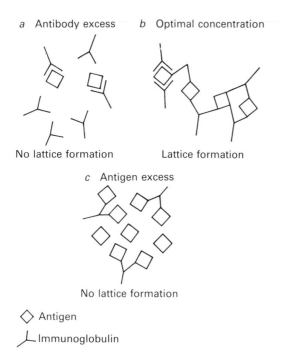

a Antibody excess   *b* Optimal concentration

No lattice formation   Lattice formation

c Antigen excess

No lattice formation

◇ Antigen

⅃ Immunoglobulin

Figure 21.4 When there is an excess of antibody or antigen a lattice does not form and precipitation will not occur

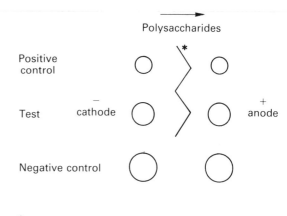

Polysaccharides

Positive control

Test   cathode   —   +   anode

Negative control

*Line of identity

Figure 21.5 Schematic diagram of a counter-current immunoelectrophoresis. At pH 8.2 polysaccharides move toward the anode and neutral immunoglobins are swept toward the cathode on a stream of buffer ions

free antibody binding sites to cross link into larger aggregates. In antibody excess large aggregates are similarly unable to form because all the binding sites are saturated by antibody and there is only a small chance of an antibody molecule being able to bind two antigen molecules to form a lattice. This is illustrated in Figure 21.4. At optimal concentrations of antigen and antibody free binding sites remain. There is a good chance that antibody will be bound to antigen which has already bound another antibody molecule enabling a lattice to form.

Precipitation techniques can be performed in tubes or in agar, but the latter is more common. The latter technique is known as double diffusion. Wells are cut in a layer of agar in a small Petri dish. Antigen and antibody are placed in wells opposite each other. Both antigen and antibody slowly diffuse in the plate, a process which can take up to 48 hours. At a point between the two wells optimal conditions for precipitation will occur and a precipitin line will form. Several

unknown sera or antigens can be discriminated using this technique, when the antigen and antibody are the same a line of identity is formed. When there is partial cross-reactivity a line of partial identity forms, and when both antigen and antibody are participating in the reaction different lines of non-identity form (Fig. 21.5). As can be seen this method is most suitable for the analysis of complex mixtures of antigens. The basic concepts, however, are applied in important microbiological investigations. Perhaps the simplest use is the Elek plate (see p. 35).

Countercurrent immunoelectrophoresis

Double diffusion is a cumbersome technique not least because it is slow. The technique which has gained widest use is a variation of double diffusion where antiserum is placed in one well and antigen in another. The gel is made in a buffer at pH 8.2 at which bacterial polysaccharides will move towards the anode when placed in an electric field. The immunoglobulin molecules which are neutral at this pH are swept along towards the cathode in a stream of buffer ions, a process known as endosmosis. A precipitation line will be formed when optimum concentrations of antigen and antibody develop. The major advantage of this technique over simple immunodiffusion is the speed at which a precipitation line is formed – usually one hour. In addition, in comparison with other serological techniques, very small quantities of reagents are used (see Fig. 21.5).

The formation of precipitin bands can be encouraged by running CIE on a cooling platen as the electrical field applied generates heat which acts to disperse the precipitin band. Once the gel has been run it may be placed overnight at +4°C when additional weak bands may develop. Weak bands may be visualized more easily if the gel is stained with Coomassie blue.

Countercurrent immunoelectrophoresis (CIE) has been used in the diagnosis of bacterial meningitis, the typing of pneumococci and the diagnosis of systemic mycoses.

Specimens for CIE

Any body fluid can be examined by CIE, but CSF, urine and serum are most commonly submitted. Bacterial polysaccharide antigens are degraded and slowly excreted over a prolonged period during acute infection.

Serum is ready for CIE directly but CSF should be centrifuged. Sputum should be homogenized by adding an equal volume of dithiothreitol, vortex mixed and shaken at room temperature for 15 minutes.

If urine specimens are cloudy they should be centrifuged and the supernatant fluid should be concentrated by ethanol precipitation or ultrafiltration. Ethanol precipitation is achieved by making an 80% ethanol mixture with urine by the addition of absolute ethanol and cooling to +4°C. The precipitate should be resuspended in physiological saline. Ultrafiltration can be easily performed with one of the commercially available kits (e.g. Minicon Amicon).

Non-specific lines in CIE

There is often a hazy zone around the antigen or antibody wells. This non-specific precipitation will be removed by washing the gel, whereas a precipitin line will remain. Non-specific precipitation lines may develop to a number of different antisera due to the presence of rheumatoid factor or C1q but these lines are not removed by washing. To prevent it developing the specimen can be treated by heating to 100°C for three to five minutes, mixing with equal volumes of 0.003M DTT and incubating for 1 hour. Serum can also be treated by mixing with equal volumes of 0.1M EDTA and heating to 100°C for three to five minutes.

Difficulties with CIE

CIE is unable to detect neutral polysaccharides (*S. pneumoniae* type 7 or 14) unless a buffer containing a sulphonate derivative of phenyloronic acid is used. Group B *N. meningitidis* is a poor immunogen and good antiserum suitable for use in CIE is not available.

Agglutination

Agglutination occurs as a result of the interaction between antibodies and a particulate antigen. The particulate antigen can be a whole organism, as in a slide agglutination test, or a particle which has been sensitized with an antibody or antigen, as in a latex agglutination test. Artificial particles which have been used include red blood cells, uniform latex beads, and Cowan type I *Staphylococcus aureus*. In some infections IgM antibodies capable of agglutinating normal human red cells at +4°C develop (cold agglutinins). These diseases include mycoplasmosis, malaria, trypanosomiasis and syphilis.

Agglutination reactions are subject to the same considerations of antigen or antibody excess as in precipitation. Thus in high titre positive serum the first tubes of the solution series may be negative due to initial antibody excess (the prozone phenomenon). Further in the dilution series antibody concentration is reduced so that optimal conditions develop and agglutination takes place. The titre is the point at which antigen excess arises and where no visible agglutination occurs.

Agglutination occurs as a result of the activity of several antibody isotypes including IgM. If an agglutination titre is performed with or without the addition of 2-mercaptoethanol

(2ME), which destroys IgM, and shows a lower titre in the 2ME tubes greater than fourfold it would indicate the presence of specific IgM. This technique has been applied to the diagnosis of acute brucellosis.

Slide agglutination

Slide agglutination is carried out on a microscope slide or black tile. A drop of physiological saline is placed on the slide, a portion of colony for identification is placed nearby. The bacteria are then emulsified by thorough mixing with a wire loop. The suspension should be carefully inspected to ensure that clumping (auto-agglutination) has not occurred. A drop of antiserum is placed next to the bacterial suspension and gently mixed into it until the suspension is smooth once again. The slide is gently rocked backwards and forwards for not more than three minutes. Significant agglutination will occur rapidly and should be easily visible to the naked eye. The negative control should be one drop of saline added to the bacterial suspension. This method is mainly used in the identification and typing of bacterial cultures.

The standard tube agglutination test for antibodies to brucella has been modified using stained brucella antigen as a slide agglutination test. This has the virtue of rapid results and small volumes of reagents being used. When equivocal results are obtained in any slide agglutination it should be repeated using a quantitative tube agglutination technique.

Coagglutination

Most strains of *S. aureus* have an immunoglobulin-binding protein, protein A, on the surface; the Cowan type I strain produces large quantities and it is this strain which is usually used in coagglutination tests. Protein A has the ability to bind to the Fc portion of IgG leaving the Fab region available for antigen binding.

Coagglutination is performed in a similar manner to a slide agglutination test. One drop of COAG reagent and one drop of clinical specimen is applied to a grease-free microscope slide. The drops are mixed thoroughly with a wooden applicator stick and the slide rocked back and forwards for two to three minutes. Each specimen should be investigated with non-immune control reagent to detect a non-specific positive result.

Latex agglutination

Latex agglutination is a similar technique, where antibody or antigen is passively applied to the surface of uniform latex beads.

The simplicity and stability of latex agglutination has meant that these reagents are gaining wide acceptance for bacterial antigen detection in body fluids, and in serotyping. In addition test kits to serotype streptococci straight from a throat swab have been developed. Latex agglutination has also been applied for the screening detection of antibodies to *Toxoplasma gondii*.

Sheep red cells have traditionally been an important carrier in passive haemagglutination tests. The most widely applied of these being the TPHA (see Chapter 19).

Tube agglutination

This may be performed in simple round-bottomed test tubes or round-bottomed wells in a Perspex plate. Doubling dilutions of patient serum are made and a constant amount of antigen is added. The tubes are then incubated at 37°C for a number of hours. When antibody and antigen combine a lattice is formed which falls to the bottom of the tube in a fine mat, unagglutinated antigen falls to the bottom in a button. The dilution of the last tube in which visible agglutination is present is the titre. (Some methods use a 50% agglutination endpoint but this adds to the subjectivity of the test.) It is essential that a suitable initial dilution is chosen, and the dilution series is of sufficient length so that the prozone phenomenon can be detected in very high titre serum.

Complement fixation

In complement fixation tests the secondary phenomenon of activation of the classical complement pathway is used as an indicator of antigen–antibody interaction. In this technique an unknown inactivated serum is added to test

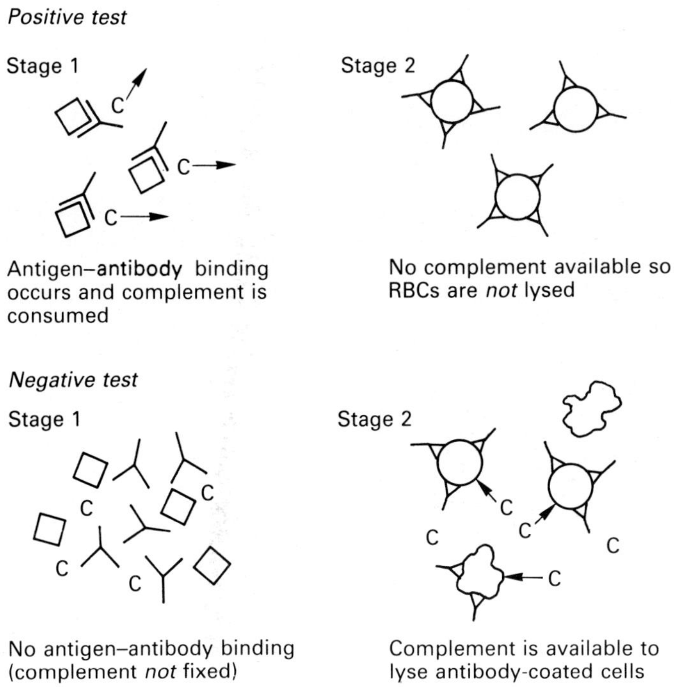

Positive test

Stage 1

Antigen–antibody binding
occurs and complement is
consumed

Stage 2

No complement available so
RBCs are *not* lysed

Negative test

Stage 1

No antigen–antibody binding
(complement *not* fixed)

Stage 2

Complement is available to
lyse antibody-coated cells

Figure 21.6 Diagram of a
positive complement fixation
test (no lysis) and negative
complement fixation test
(lysis)

antigen and guinea pig complement. After
a period of incubation if a specific
antigen–antibody interaction has taken place
the classical complement pathway will have
been activated and the complement consumed.
Red cells coated with lytic antibodies are
then added to the mixture, if a specific
antigen–antibody interaction has taken place
no complement will be available to bring
about red cell lysis. If serum does not contain
specific antibodies, complement will not have
been fixed and will remain available for red
cell lysis in the second reaction (Fig. 21.6). A
number of controls must be included with each
test, as follows:

1 A complement control which measures the
  ability of the complement to lyse sensitized
  red cells.
2 The antigen control which confirms that
  the antigen has no complement-activating
  properties (anti-complementary activity).
3 The serum control which confirms that the
  test serum does not contain anti-complementary activity.
4 A standard serum of known titre must be
  included.
5 A negative control serum.

Complement fixation tests are technically
difficult to perform and are labour intensive.
They are very specific but are not as sensitive
as other methods. Each of the components of
the complement fixation test must be regularly
titred to minimize inter-assay variation.
Reference sera and unknown sera from other
laboratories should regularly be tested to
confirm the reproducibility of results between
one laboratory and another. The negative
control serum must also be included.

Immunofluorescence techniques

Immunofluorescence tests can be used in two
ways to detect specific antigen present in
patient specimens, the direct immunofluorescence test, or to detect specific antibody in
patient serum (indirect immunofluorescence
test). The basic principle of the immunofluorescence test is that fluorescent dyes such as
fluorescein produce an apple green fluorescence when illuminated by u.v. light. Antibodies
which have been conjugated with fluorescein
isothiocyanate can be used to detect the
antigen–antibody interaction (Fig. 21.7).

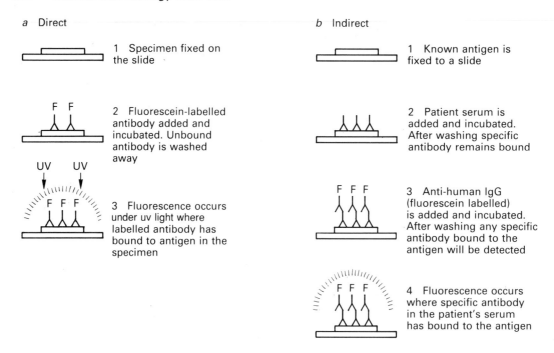

Figure 21.7 Diagram of the process of direct immunofluorescence (antigen detection) or indirect immunofluorescence (antibody detection)

Direct immunofluorescence tests

In the direct immunofluorescence technique the patient specimen (e.g. sputum or urethral pus) is placed on the microscopic slide fixed with methanol and dried. Specific fluorescein-labelled antibody is added and incubated at 37°C in a humidified chamber with control negative and positive specimens. After incubation, slides are washed thoroughly and examined under the u.v. microscope. If the fluorescein-labelled antibody has bound to the specimen an apple green fluorescence will be seen, implying the presence of the target antigen. Note: glycerol must be used as the fluid to prevent non-specific fluorescence which occurs with normal immersion oil.

Direct fluorescence tests are often used when culture is difficult, or is not available, e.g. in the detection of *Pneumocystis carinii*, *Gardia lamblia* and *Chlamydia trachomatis*.

Alternative fluorochromes can be used: rhodamine B can be conjugated to specific antibody and produces a red fluorescence in u.v. light. This is especially valuable when two antigens are sought. One antibody can be conjugated with fluorescein and one with rhodamine. If both antigens are present in the specimen apple green and red fluorescence will be detected.

Indirect fluorescence

In this technique a known antigen is fixed to a microscope slide. Dilutions of test and control sera are incubated and the slides washed. Antibody bound to antigen is detected by fluorescein-labelled anti-human immunoglobulin. In this assay the presence of fluorescence indicates specific antibody in the test serum. This technique is both specific and sensitive, and the reagents have a long shelf-life (in contrast to radioimmunoassay). Each test is time consuming to perform, however, and the observer is strictly limited in the number of tests that can be performed, not only because of the nature of the assay but also because of the difficulties of maintaining concentration in the examination of a large number of specimens.

This technique has found its application in the serological diagnosis of viral, parasitic infections and in a confirmatory test for syphilis (FTA). By changing the conjugated antibody to an anti-IgM, specific IgM can be detected and this technique is discussed in the diagnosis of syphilis and in the micro-immunofluorescence tests for *Chlamydia* (see p. 228).

Indirect fluorescent antibody tests are performed first at a screening dilution and all positive sera should be titred.

Radioimmunoassay (RIA)

Radioimmunoassay depends on the labelling of antibody or antigen with ^{125}I. When antibody and labelled antigen combine, a complex is formed. Bound and unbound antigen are separated by centrifugation and the complexed radioactivity is found in the centrifuged pellet where it can be counted by a gamma counter.

The concentration of antibody or antigen present in the unknown specimen is measured by referring to a standard curve.

Radioimmunoassay has many disadvantages for the routine microbiological laboratory. The equipment and reagents required are very expensive. The shelf-life of radioactive reagents is very short. In addition, extra precautions and monitoring are required when handling radiation and the disposal of radioactive reagents is strictly controlled.

RIA tests have similar sensitivity and specificity to ELISA, which is without these disadvantages. In view of this radioimmunoassay should be discouraged for routine use.

Enzyme-linked immunosorbent assay (ELISA)

Enzyme-linked immunosorbent assays (ELISAs) have transformed serological techniques. ELISAs depend on antibody–antigen being demonstrated by the action of an enzyme which has been covalently bound to the antibody or antigen. In these assays an antigen or antibody is attached to a solid phase support, of which a number have been described. The solid phase supports which have been used include beads, tubes or microtitre plates made of several different plastic materials, polystyrene, or polyvinyl chloride. This means that bound and free agents can be separated without the need for time-consuming centrifugation steps. For most routine purposes ELISA assays will be performed in microtitre plates or in small strips making up a portion of a plate.

The theoretical level of detection available by ELISA is one molecule, but in practice about 10 molecules is the effective limit. Enzyme assays are of two main types – homogeneous and heterogeneous. In homogeneous assays binding of antibody inactivates the enzyme thus eliminating the need to separate bound from unbound. This method has low detectability and is suitable for detection of small hapten-like molecules. It has found its principal use in antibiotic assay (see Chapter 20). Heterogeneous assays require separation of bound and unbound with washing stages and depend on the amplification provided by enzyme activity bound specifically to antigen.

Antigens

Antigens are most usually attached to the solid phase of the immunoassay for the detection of specific antibody, but can also be used when labelled in competitive ELISAs (Fig. 21.8). It is essential that antigens are of sufficient purity, and do not cross-react with antigens in other important organisms (e.g. *N. meningitidis* Group B capsular polysaccharide with that of *E. coli* K1). The antigen must be firmly attached to the solid phase, e.g. proteins adhere by electrostatic attraction. Some positively charged antigens can be made to adhere by coating the microtitre plates with poly-*L*-lysine and pneumococcal capsular polysaccharides have been bound to plates with specific rabbit immunoglobulin.

Antibodies

The antibody chosen for the various stages of the assay are of critical importance. Polyclonal and monoclonal antibodies have both found a role. The principal advantages of monoclonal antibodies are that they have a defined specificity, are pure and their homogeneous character means that it is easy to standardize

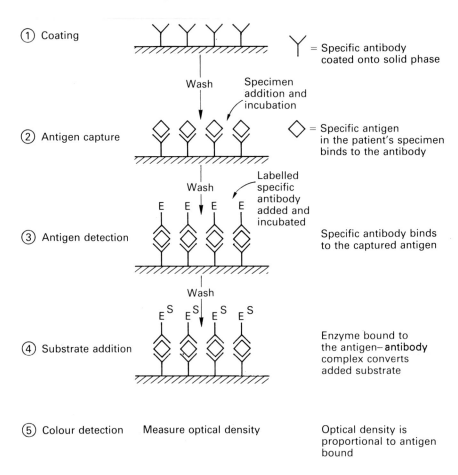

① Coating

Wash

Specimen addition and incubation

$\curlyvee$ = Specific antibody coated onto solid phase

② Antigen capture

Wash

Labelled specific antibody added and incubated

◇ = Specific antigen in the patient's specimen binds to the antibody

③ Antigen detection

E E E E

Wash

Specific antibody binds to the captured antigen

④ Substrate addition

E^S E^S E^S E^S

Wash

Enzyme bound to the antigen–**antibody** complex converts added substrate

⑤ Colour detection   Measure optical density

Optical density is proportional to antigen bound

Figure 21.8   Diagram of a double antibody–antigen capture ELISA method

reaction conditions. They are in general of lower affinity, however, and cannot distinguish between two antigens if they both contain the same epitope. In addition monoclonal antibodies may be very sensitive to freeze–thaw cycles, pH variation or bind poorly to microtitre plates. Antibodies should be specific with minimal cross-reaction with other relevant antigens.

Enzymes

Heterogeneous ELISAs depend on the amplification provided by enzymes. It is essential that the enzyme chosen should have a high activity, producing a readily measurable change in a substrate. It should be stable in normal laboratory conditions and readily obtainable in a pure form. A number of enzymes have proved valuable in ELISA assays and these include horse radish peroxidase, alkaline phosphatase, beta-galactosidase, urease and glucose oxidase.

Conjugation

The linkage of enzyme to antibody to antigen should result in a stable complex which retains full enzyme activity and unaltered antigen–antibody binding. Such conjugates can readily be obtained with the one- or two-step glutaraldehyde or periodate method.

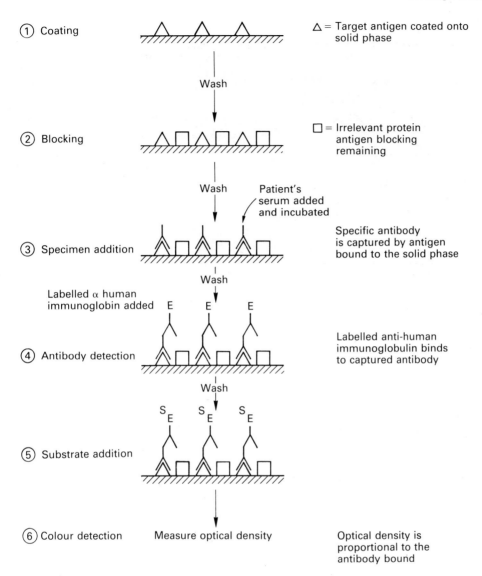

① Coating   △ = Target antigen coated onto solid phase

Wash

② Blocking   □ = Irrelevant protein antigen blocking remaining

Wash   Patient's serum added and incubated

③ Specimen addition   Specific antibody is captured by antigen bound to the solid phase

Wash

Labelled α human immunoglobin added   E   E   E

④ Antibody detection   Labelled anti-human immunoglobulin binds to captured antibody

Wash

S_E   S_E   S_E

⑤ Substrate addition

⑥ Colour detection   Measure optical density   Optical density is proportional to the antibody bound

Figure 21.9   Diagram of antibody capture enzyme-linked immunosorbent assay (ELISA) method

Substrates

The substrate provides the final window on the assay. Chromogenic substrates should be colourless before conversion, being converted into a strongly coloured compound by the action of the enzyme. The substrate should be readily soluble before and after enzyme activity.

Types of ELISA

Antibody capture

In this method the wells of a microtitre plate are coated with antigen. After washing, the test serum is added at an appropriate dilution and the plate washed again. The specific antibody present in the serum binds to the

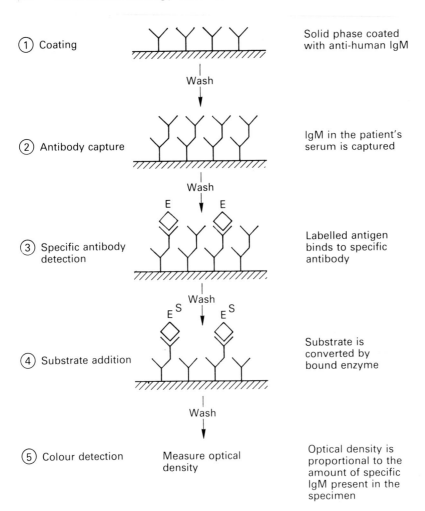

① Coating — Solid phase coated with anti-human IgM

Wash

② Antibody capture — IgM in the patient's serum is captured

Wash

③ Specific antibody detection — Labelled antigen binds to specific antibody

Wash

④ Substrate addition — Substrate is converted by bound enzyme

Wash

⑤ Colour detection — Measure optical density — Optical density is proportional to the amount of specific IgM present in the specimen

Figure 21.10   IgM antibody capture ELISA method

antigen and may be detected with an anti-human immunoglobulin conjugate/enzyme substrate system. The specificity of the anti-human immunoglobulin antibody conjugate can be altered to detect different isotypes and subclasses of immunoglobulin if needed (Fig. 21.9).

IgM method

It is difficult to detect IgM by altering the conjugate to an anti-IgM conjugate because of the large differential in concentration between IgG and IgM which may result in competition. IgM can be purified by sucrose density centrifugation, but ELISA antibody capture methods can simplify this process. Microtitre plates are coated with antibody to human IgM, IgM present in the serum sample is bound and specific IgM detected with labelled antigen (Fig. 21.10).

Double antibody sandwich

The double antibody sandwich is the conventional approach to antigen detection. The wells

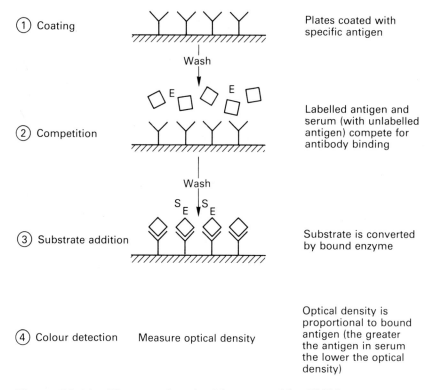

① Coating — Plates coated with specific antigen

Wash

② Competition — Labelled antigen and serum (with unlabelled antigen) compete for antibody binding

Wash

③ Substrate addition — Substrate is converted by bound enzyme

④ Colour detection — Measure optical density — Optical density is proportional to bound antigen (the greater the antigen in serum the lower the optical density)

Figure 21.11 Diagram of method for competitive ELISA

of a microtitre plate are coated with antibody specific to the antigen studied. After washing, the patient sample is added and antigen in the specimen is captured. The plates are washed again and enzyme-conjugated antibody specific for the antigen is added. Antigen captured in this assay is shown as a colour change and is quantified in comparison with a standard curve derived from a range of antigen concentrations (see Fig. 21.8).

Competitive antigen assay

In this assay the wells of microtitre plates are coated with antibody. An enzyme-labelled antigen is competed with the antigen which is to be quantified in the serum sample before the enzyme substrate is added. The difference between the colour change with labelled antigen alone and label and serum is proportional to the concentration of antigen in the serum (Fig. 21.11).

Defining a positive result

Like other serological investigations in which antibody concentration is measured, titres can be reported. This is most valuable in studies of antibody responses to vaccines or infectious agents. The means of recording titres is as follows: an arbitrary cut-off value for optical density (OD) is defined, e.g. 0.5. The titre is the lowest dilution which has a result greater than 0.5 OD.

Another way to define a positive result is to take a series of known normal specimens. The assay is run in the optimum manner and the mean and standard deviation of the control specimens is found. A positive sample is therefore defined as any sample with an OD greater than three standard deviations above this mean. In practice a serum with an OD near this value can be selected as a negative control and a positive result defined as any value higher than this control. Reference weak positive and strong positive sera should also be

Table 21.1   Examples of ELISA applications

Antigen detection
  Plasmodium falciparum
  Streptococcus pneumoniae
  Campylobacter in food
  Vero toxin (*E. coli*)
Antibody detection
  Syphilis
  Mycoplasma pneumoniae
  Toxoplasma gondii
  Brucella spp.

included. The reference sera can also be used to standardize the results obtained on different days. Variation in ELISA, as with any other assay, is inevitable and is due to variable binding to the plate and minor variations in reagents. These variations can be smoothed out by referring results to a reference positive.

In antigen assays the reporting of positive results is simplified by comparing specimen values against results obtained from a standard curve established with reference samples.

Applications of ELISAs

The features which make ELISAs an important technique for microbiology include the low cost, stability, and long shelf-life of the reagents. The simplicity of the technique and the ease with which large numbers of specimens can be processed make ELISA methods ideal for screening large numbers of specimens, e.g. syphilis in antenatal patients or malaria in blood donors. The ability to detect specific IgM or antigen enables a rapid diagnosis to be made in conditions where culture is difficult. A list of ELISA applications is found in Table 21.1.

Detection levels of various techniques

The level of detectability of each of these techniques varies due to the technical considerations already noted. With *S. pneumoniae* antigen detection as an example, CIE has a highly variable detection limit, and is less sensitive than latex agglutination and coagglutination.

Significance of positive results

Antigen detection methods have the virtue of being rapid, and are usually more sensitive than direct Gram stain. Antigen assays will remain positive during treatment and may be the only means of making a diagnosis if antibiotics have been administered before admission to hospital. The absolute concentration of antigen has been shown to be related to clinical outcome in pneumococcal meningitis, both in relation to survival and to neurological sequelae.

Bacteriological examination of water, food and air

Water

Introduction

Water-borne diseases are a major threat to health world-wide but are uncommon in developed countries because of the sophisticated water purification, distribution systems and sewage disposal in place. To ensure the safety of the water supply standards of water quality have been established by governments, the European Community and the World Health Organization, the current regulations should be consulted.

If water is inadequately treated bacteria, protozoa, and viruses may be transmitted to anyone drinking it. Pathogens may also gain access to the water supply after treatment in the distribution system, e.g. animals that may carry intestinal pathogens in their own gastro-intestinal tract may foul service reservoirs.

Standards

Potable water should not contain human pathogens but it is not feasible to use the presence of these organisms as an indicator of contamination because they are usually outnumbered by environmental and other faecal organisms and generally die out more rapidly. To overcome this difficulty indicator organisms are sought and their isolation is used to imply possible faecal contamination.

Coliforms

For this purpose a coliform is defined as a Gram-negative bacillus capable of growing on MacConkey's agar, which ferments lactose at 37°C in 24 hours and is oxidase negative. 'E. coli' are pragmatically defined as those organisms with similar reactions at 44°C which are indole and methyl red positive, and do not produce acetoin in the Vokes Proskaüer reaction or utilize citrate.

More recent UK Department of Health advice defines coliforms as members of a genus or species within the family Enterobacteriaceae, capable of growth at 37°C, and normally possessing beta-galactosidase. Faecal coliforms are thermotolerant coliform organisms which are capable of growth and of expressing their fermentative properties at 44°C.

As E. coli is the most numerous facultative organism in the gut and it can be detected at very low dilution, this makes it a sensitive indicator of faecal contamination.

Other indicator organisms

Enterococci are present at lower concentration in the gut, do not multiply in water, but survive for longer in the environment. Some consider that enterococci can be used to indicate the origin of faecal contamination. It can be used to clarify results when a high number of coliforms but no E. coli are found. The

Table 22.1 Guideline values for bacteriological quality of water

Organism	Units	Guideline value
A Piped water supplies		
A1 Treated water entering the distribution system		
faecal coliforms	number/100 ml	0
coliform organisms	number/100 ml	0
A2 Water in the distribution system		
faecal coliforms	number/100 ml	0
coliform organisms	number/100 ml	0
B Unpiped water supplies		
faecal coliforms	number/100 ml	0
coliform organisms	number/100 ml	0
C Bottled drinking water/emergency water supplies		
faecal coliforms	number/100 ml	0
coliform organisms	number/100 ml	0

presence of enterococci then confirms the faecal origin of the coliforms.

Clostridium perfringens is present in even lower concentrations in the gut than enterococci but are extremely hardy. They are present in most surface water as they are found in manured soil. Clostridia are more resistant to chlorine and they may not be inactivated by the concentration and contact time used. This is recognized by a standard for sulphite-reducing clostridia of not more than 5/100 ml. The presence of *C. perfringens* in treated water in the absence of coliforms known to have been present in source water indicates that treatment has been successful.

It is argued that the behaviour of clostridia is similar to that of the more resistant protozoan pathogens *Giardia* and *Cryptosporidium* and that it may be possible to use clostridia as an indicator for the protozoa.

The standards laid down by the WHO for drinking water at various stages of its supply are summarised in Table 22.1. No *E. coli* should be found/100 ml at any point in the distribution system, in bottled water or emergency water supplies. Numbers of coliform organisms are as set out in the Table. It should be noted that deviations from negative results should only be sporadic (<95% of samples) and not in consecutive samples. Similar requirements are made in the UK Water Act.

Water sampling should be frequent and regular. It should include measurement of chlorine in the sample and also take the engineering considerations into account. The frequency of bacteriological sampling at the treatment works depends on the volume of water supplied. The frequency of testing at the consumers' taps will increase in proportion to the size of the population served. Bacteriological testing will include coliform and faecal coliform counts together with total colony counts (Table 22.2).

Methods

Samples

The water supply may be sampled at any point through the distribution system including taps in customers' homes. In addition sampling of private untreated supplies, boreholes and wells may be undertaken.

Samples are usually obtained from strategic points in the system where taps for sampling may be fitted. Where taps in private houses or

Table 22.2 Frequency of sampling of water at consumers' taps

Population served	Minimum number of samples
Less than 5000	1 sample per month
5000–10 000	2 samples per month
10 001–20 000	4 samples per month
20 001–50 000	1 sample per 5000 per month

similar sources are sampled the taps should be those which are directly connected to the public main. The water should be run to waste for one minute and any external fitment should be removed. Metal stand pipes can be flamed.

Sterile containers must be used which contain sodium thiosulphate to neutralize chlorine. Samples should be kept cool in an insulated container, not exposed to the light and should be tested within six hours.

Detection of coliforms

There are two ways of detecting bacterial contamination of water in common use: the multiple tube presumptive coliform count and the membrane filtration method.

Presumptive coliform test

In this technique double strength or single strength indicator broth are dispensed into tubes of differing volumes. The volumes of the tubes is chosen by the likelihood of contamination. Thus when water of good quality is tested larger volumes are used: one 50 ml, five 10 ml of double strength medium. In contrast water of poor quality is inoculated into smaller volumes: one 50 ml, five 10 ml (double strength) and five 1 ml (single strength). The media are incubated at 37°C and inspected at 24 and 48 hours. Growth is demonstrated by a change in the indicator and gas production in Durham's tubes placed inside the tube. Acid and gas producing tubes are considered to contain presumptive coliforms. The number present in the original sample is calculated from tables of most probable numbers (MPN).

Presumptive positive isolates must be confirmed by the Eijkman test in which positive tubes are subcultured in duplicate into a medium which contains lactose and an inhibitor of clostridia which can produce a positive result in the presumptive coliform test. One tube is incubated at 37°C and the other at 44°C. Indole production is tested in parallel by subculture in tryptone water at 44°C. Coliforms will produce a positive result at 37°C but only *E. coli* at 44°C.

If coliforms are present but *E. coli* is not, the isolation of enterococci may suggest a faecal origin for the contamination. Positive tubes

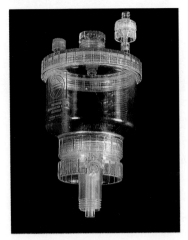

(a)

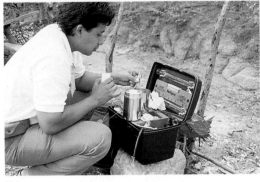

(b)

Figure 22.1 (*a*) Membrane filtration device. Water is drawn through the filter held in place in between the upper chamber and the outflow. (*b*) A portable water microbiology laboratory for application in developing countries based on membrane filtration. (The Del agua kit)

are subcultured into a medium such as glucose azide broth and incubated at 44°C. Tubes which show growth by a change in the colour of the bromocresol purple indicator are subcultured on bile aesculin azide agar.

Membrane filtration

In this method a measured volume of water is passed through a membrane filter with a sufficiently small pore size to retain the indicator organisms (Fig. 22.1). The filters are removed aseptically and placed on two pads of filter paper moistened with lauryl sulphate broth. Both are incubated for four hours at 30°C and one for 14 hours at 35°C for the presumptive count and one filter at 44°C for 14 hours for *E. coli*. The identification of *E. coli* is confirmed by subculture to lauryl sulphate tryptone broth and peptone water for indole testing at 44°C.

Detecting legionellas

Larger samples of water are required to detect *Legionella* spp. The water is filtered through a 0.22 µm filter and cut into pieces and placed into a volume of distilled water. The filter is shaken or vortex mixed to dislodge the organisms which are then concentrated by centrifugation. The deposit is inoculated on selective and unselective buffered charcoal yeast extract agar and also examined by a direct fluorescence technique.

Testing swimming pools

The most important test in the examination of swimming pools is the accurate measurement of the chlorine content. Bacteriological examination should be directed towards detecting staphylococci as these species are more resistant to chlorine and can survive on skin scales.

Milk

Introduction

There are several types of milk available for purchase by the public: pasteurized, sterilized and ultraheat treated milk. The quality and definitions of these products are laid down legally as are the tests to define their standard (see Further reading).

Milk testing

Several of the statutory tests are not bacteriological: the phosphatase test, and turbidity test. In addition a colony count test measures the total number of bacteria present in milk, and the number of coliforms and specific pathogens, in this case listeria, salmonella, and enterotoxigenic *S. aureus*.

Phosphatase test

This test measures a phosphatase found in cows' milk which should be denatured by the pasteurization process. The phosphatase liberates *p*-nitrophenol, which is yellow, from *p*-nitrophenol phosphate. The test is read with a colorimeter after two hours' incubation at 37°C. A control sample of milk heated to 100°C for at least three minutes is used as a negative control. The colour is compared with a Lovibond comparator disc and fully pasteurized milk should have less than 10 µg of *p*-nitrophenol.

Turbidity test

This is the test for sterilized milk in which the milk proteins become coagulable by ammonium sulphate if it has been properly treated. Ammonium sulphate is added to a sample of milk and the milk filtered. The filtrate is placed in a boiling water bath for five minutes. After cooling the tube is examined for turbidity. A control of milk which has been heated to 100°C for five minutes is tested in parallel. No turbidity should be seen in either test or control.

Colony count

For the colony count technique milk is pre-incubated at 6°C for five days or 21°C for 24 hours. Serial dilutions are made in 50 ml of maximum recovery broth and pour plates made. These are incubated at 30°C for 72 hours.

Coliforms are detected by taking 3 ml of milk and diluting it in 50 ml of violet red bile agar and incubating for 24 hours at 30°C. Coliforms are counted as all of the red colonies.

Standards of milk quality control differ in differing countries and the current edition of the regulations should be consulted.

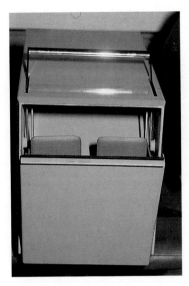

Figure 22.2 Stomacher is used to break up food before microbiological testing

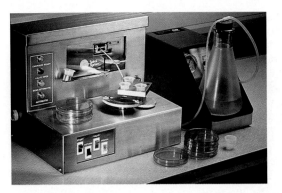

Figure 22.3 Spiral plater can be used to enumerate bacteria

Food

Introduction

A full description of food microbiology is beyond the scope of this book and further information should be sought from the references given in Further reading.

Microbiological examination of food is performed to establish standards of hygiene by total viable counts notable of Enterobacteriaceae, to establish the shelf-life of food by detecting food spoilage organisms, and to detect specific pathogens such as salmonellas implicated in an outbreak of food poisoning.

Samples

Food should be transported to the laboratory in its original containers or transferred aseptically to sterile containers. It should be held at 4°C until processed.

At least 10 g should be examined. Specimen processing is simple, if the food is liquid it can be mixed by inversion and dilutions made. If the food is solid it should be weighed aseptically and placed in sterile diluent and broken up by either a sterile homogenizer or a stomacher (Fig. 22.2). Dilutions are made and colony counts are performed.

Methods and media

Colony counts can be performed by a variety of methods. The standard plate count, pour plate, or the Miles and Misra technique can be used. A spiral plater can also be used successfully (Fig. 22.3).

It is usual to count all of the Enterobacteriaceae present in a sample not only the *E. coli*, as organisms such as *Klebsiella* spp. are more heat resistant than other organisms. The presence of enterococci should also be noted as the presence of these organisms may reflect failures in hygiene.

Media used for inoculation of food include MacConkey's agar, azide blood agar (for enterococci), neomycin blood agar (for clostridia). When food poisoning organisms are sought media specific for the infecting agent should be used. For salmonellas deoxycholate citrate agar and brilliant green MacConkey, selenite F enrichment can also be used to optimize the recovery of these organisms. Mannitol salt or mannitol salt lactose geltain can be used for isolation of staphylococci. *Bacillus cereus* can be isolated on a selective medium such as Holbrook and Anderson (see Table 22.1). Identification and typing is performed by the methods already described.

Air

Introduction

The bacterial quality of air is of importance to pharmaceutical and other manufacturing

Table 22.3 Examples of media used in the isolation of food poisoning organisms

Organism	Media
Salmonella spp.	DCA, Wilson and Blair
S. aureus	Mannitol salt, milk salt, phenolphthalein phosphate polymyxin
Clostridium perfringens	Robertson's cooked meat, neomycin blood agar
Vibrio parahaemolyticus	TCBS
Bacillus cereus	Glucose tryptone, chloral hydrate blood agar, *Bacillus cereus* selective

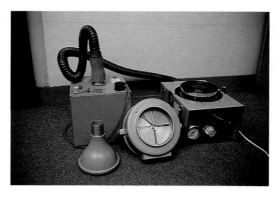

Figure 22.4 Casella slit sampler shown dismantled

industries. In the hospital environment air quality can also be important and testing required. The air supply to theatre suites should be monitored especially after building work has been performed. The bacterial count in air entering theatres through filters should be less than 3.5 colony forming units/m^3 and not more than one colony of *S. aureus* or *C. perfringens* in 35 m^3. Higher concentrations can be found nearer the operation site. Air quality is especially critical in those theatres where orthopaedic procedures are to be performed.

Immunocompromised patients are often highly susceptible to organisms in environmental air, notably *Aspergillus,* and many patients undergoing induction of remission for leukaemia or bone marrow transplantation are nursed in rooms with air which is HEPA filtered.

Methods

Settle plates

This is the simplest way of examining air quality. Nutrient plates are left exposed in a marked site for a given time. The plates are then incubated at 37°C overnight and for three days at 20°C for the detection of saprophytic bacteria, and for extended periods for moulds. All organisms isolated are identified by conventional methods.

The advantage of settle plates is the economy and simplicity of the method. The disadvantages are that only those bacteria carried on heavy particles which fall to the plate are detected and the results obtained are not quantitative.

Air samplers

The Casella air sampler draws air through a slit and deposits it on a blood agar plate in the machine. The plate rotates to distribute the impacted bacteria over the whole surface of the plate. The size of the slit allows the collection of particles of different sizes. An electric motor rotates the plate and draws a vacuum which draws in the air and the sampler is run until the required volume of air is collected. The plate is then removed and incubated as noted above.

The advantage of the Casella sampler is its ability to quantify the number of organisms in a given volume. The disadvantage is that it is a relatively cumbersome piece of equipment which to some extent limits the sites that can be sampled (Fig. 22.4).

Air centrifuge

The Reuter centrifical air sampler resembles a torch. Air is drawn into the top of the machine and is subjected to centrifugal acceleration so that it impacts on a plastic strip inside which is coated with agar. The strip is then removed for culture and identification of organisms.

The advantage of this device is its lightness and portability. As it is battery driven mains electricity is not required so that sampling can be performed in difficult areas of a building.

Further reading

General

Atlas RM. *Handbook of Microbiological Media*, Parks LC (ed). CRC Press: Boco Raton, 1993.

Ballows A, Hausler WJ, Herrman KL, Isenberg HD, Shadomey HJ *et al. Manual of Clinical Microbiology*, 5th edn. American Society of Microbiology. Washington, 1991.

Baron EJ, Finegold SM. *Bailey and Scott's Diagnostic Microbiology*, 8th edn. Mosby: St Louis, 1990.

Christie AB. *Infectious Diseases*, 4th edn. Churchill Livingstone: Edinburgh, 1991.

Isenberg HD (ed). *Clinical Microbiology Procedures Handbook*. American Society of Microbiology: Washington DC, 1992.

Lambert HP, O'Grady FW. *Antibiotic and Chemotherapy*, 6th edn. Churchill Livingstone: Edinburgh, 1992.

Mandell GL, Douglas RG, Bennett JE. *Principles and Practice of Infectious Diseases*, 3rd edn. Churchill Livingstone: New York, 1990.

Chapter 1: Introduction

Bridson EY. Media in Microbiology. *Reviews in Medical Microbiology* 1990; **1:** 1–9.

Difco Manual, 10th edn. Difco Laboratories: Detroit, Michigan, 1984.

Oxoid Manual, 6th edn, compiled Bridson EY. Alphaprint, Alton, Hants, 1990.

Snell JJS, Farrell ID, Roberts C (eds). *Quality Control: Principles and Practice in the Microbiology Laboratory*. Public Health Laboratory Service: London, 1991.

Chapter 2: Gram-positive cocci

Feldman RG, Fleer A. The immune response to Group B streptococcus. *Reviews in Medical Microbiology* 1992; **3:** 52–58.

Kehoe MA. New aspects of *Streptococcus pyogenes* pathogenicity. *Reviews in Medical Microbiology* 1991; **2:** 147–152.

Moellering RC. Emergence of Enterococcus as a significant pathogen. *Clinical Infectious Diseases* 1992; **14:** 2–13.

Ruoff KL. Recent taxonomic changes in the genus *Enterococcus. European Journal of Clinical Microbiology and Infectious Diseases* 1990; **9:** 75–79.

Stevens DL. Invasive Group A infections. *Clinical Infectious Diseases* 1992; **14:** 1173–1178.

Whitworth JM. Lancefield Group F and related streptococci. *Journal of Medical Microbiology* 1990; **33:** 135-151.

Chapter 3: Gram-positive bacilli

Alouf JE, Freer JH (eds). *Sourcebook of Bacterial Protein Toxins*. Academic Press: London, 1991.

Brooks R, Joynson DHM. Bacteriological diagnosis of diphtheria. ACP Broadsheet 125. *Journal of Clinical Pathology* 1990; **43:** 576–580.

Coyle MB, Lipsky BA. Corynebacteria in infectious diseases: clinical and laboratory aspects. *Clinical Microbiological Reviews* 1990; **3:** 227–246.

Drancourt M, Bonnet E, Gallais H *et al.* *Rhodococcus equi* infection in patients with AIDS. *Journal of Infection* 1992; **24:** 123–131.

Gorby GL, Peacock JE. *Erysipelothrix rhusiopathiae* endocarditis: microbiologic, epidemiologic, and clinical features of an occupational disease. *Reviews of Infectious Diseases* 1988; **10:** 317–325.

Kerr KG, Lacey RW. Isolation and identification of *Listeria monocytogenes*. ACP Broadsheet 129. *Journal of Clinical Pathology* 1991; **44:** 624–627.

Lamon JR, Postlethwaite R, McGowan AP. *Listeria monocytogenes* and its role in human infection. *Journal of Infection* 1988; **17:** 7–28.

McLaughlin J. The identification of Listeria species. *DMRQ Newsletter* 1988. 1–3.

Portnoy D, Chakraborty T, Goebe W, Cossart P. Molecular determinants of *Listeria monocytogenes* pathogenesis. *Infection and Immunity* 1992; **60:** 1263–1267.

Chapter 4: Mycobacterial infection

Brennan PJ. Structure of Mycobacteria: recent developments in defining cell wall carbohydrates and proteins. *Reviews of Infectious Diseases* 1988; **11:** 420–430.

Brisson-Noel A, Anzar C, Chureau C *et al.* Diagnosis of tuberculosis by DNA amplification in clinical practice evaluation. *Lancet* 1991; **ii:** 364–366.

Collins CH, Grange JM, Yates MD. *Organization and Practice in Tuberculosis Bacteriology.* Butterworths, London, 1985.

Cregan P, Yajko DM, Ng VL *et al.* Use of DNA probes to detect *Mycobacterium intracellulare* and 'X' mycobacteria among clinical isolates of *Mycobacterium avium* complex. *Journal of Infectious Diseases* 1992; **166:** 191–194.

Dannenberg AM. Immune mechanisms in the pathogenesis of pulmonary tuberculosis. *Reviews of Infectious Diseases* 1988; **11:** S369–378.

Health Services Advisory Committee. *Safe Working and the Prevention of Infection in Clinical Laboratories.* HMSO: London, 1991.

Heifets L. Qualitative and quantitative drug-susceptibility test in mycobacteriology. *American Review of Respiratory Diseases* 1988; **137:** 1217–1222.

Mitcheson DA, Allen BW, Manickavasagar D. Selective Kirchner medium in the culture of specimens other than sputum for mycobacterium. *Journal of Clinical Pathology* 1983; **36:** 1357–1361.

Chapter 5: Gram-negative cocci

Easmon CSF, Ison CA. *Neisseria gonorrhoeae*: a versatile pathogen. *Journal of Clinical Pathology* 1987; **40:** 1088–1097.

Granato PA, Franz MR. Evaluation of a prototype DNA probe test for the non-cultural diagnosis of gonorrhoea. *Journal of Clinical Microbiology* 1989; **27:** 632–635.

Mertsola J. Cytokines in the pathogenesis of bacterial meningitis. *Transactions of the Royal Society of Tropical Medicine and Hygiene* 1991; **85:** 17–18.

Moore PS. Meningococcal meningitis in sub-Saharan Africa: a model of the epidemic process. *Clinical and Infectious Diseases* 1992; **14:** 515–525.

Chapter 6: Gram-negative coccobacilli

Finch RG. Uncommon Haemophilus infections. *British Medical Journal* 1984; **289:** 941–942.

Gotuzzo E, Carillo C, Guerra J, Llosa L *et al.* An evaluation of diagnostic methods for brucellosis – the value of bone marrow culture. *Journal of Infectious Diseases* 1986; **153:** 122–125.

Heizmann W, Botzenhart K, Doller G. Brucellosis: serological methods compared. *Journal of Hygiene Cambridge* 1985; **95:** 639–653.

Moxon ER. The molecular basis of *H. influenzae* virulence. *Journal of the Royal College of Physicians of London* 1985; **19:** 174–178.

Parton R. Changing perspectives on pertussis and pertussis vaccination. *Reviews in Medical Microbiology* 1991; **2:** 121–128.

Rahman A, Mousa SA, Muhtaseb DS, Almudallal SM, Marafie K, Marafie AA *et al.* Osteoarticular complications of brucellosis: a study of 169 cases. *Reviews of Infectious Diseases* 1987; **9:** 531–543.

Young EJ. Human brucellosis. *Reviews of Infectious Diseases* 1983; **5:** 821–842.

Chapter 7: Gram-negative bacilli

Ewing WH. *Edward's and Ewing Identification of Enterobacteriaceae*, 4th edn. Elsevier Science Publishing: New York, 1986.

Dance DAB. Meliodosis. *Reviews in Medical Microbiology* 1990; **1:** 143–150.

Manthay CL, Vogel SN. The role of cytokines in host responses to endotoxin. *Reviews in Medical Microbiology* 1991; **3:** 72–79.

Qureshi N, Takayama K. Structure and Function of Lipid A. In *Molecular Basis of Bacterial Pathogenesis.* Iglewski BH, Clark VL (eds). Academic Press: London, 1990.

Chapter 8: Anaerobes

Duerdan BI, Draser BS (eds). *Anaerobes in Human Disease.* Edward Arnold: London, 1991.

Finegold SM, George WL (eds). *Anaerobic Infections in Humans.* Academic Press: London, 1989.

Hardie JM, Borriello SP (eds). *Anaerobes Today.* John Wiley: Chichester, 1988.

Willis AT, Phillips KD. *Anaerobic Infections.* Public Health Laboratory Service: London, 1988.

Chapter 9: Spiral bacteria

Barbour AG. Antigenic variation in relapsing fever *Borrelia* species. In *Molecular Basis of Bacterial Pathogenesis.* Iglewski BH, Clark VL (eds). Academic Press: London, 1990.

Penn CW. Pathogenicity and molecular biology of treponemes. *Reviews of Medical Microbiology* 1991; **2:** 68–75.

Chapter 10: Medical mycology

Barnes RA. Immunological diagnosis of fungal infections in the immunocompromised host. *Reviews in Medical Microbiology* 1990; **1:** 58–65.

British Society of Antimicrobial Chemotherapy Working Party. Laboratory monitoring of antifungal chemotherapy. *Lancet* 1991; **i:** 1577–1580.

Clayton Y, Midgely G. *Medical Mycology.* Gower: London, 1985.

Tang CM, Cohen J. Diagnosing fungal infections in immunocompromised hosts. *Journal of Clinical Pathology* 1992; **45:** 1–5.

Chapter 11: Parasitology

Beaver PC, Jung RC, Cupp EW. *Clinical Parasitology,* 9th edn. Lea and Febiger: Philadelphia, 1984.

Peters W, Gillies HM. *A Colour Atlas of Tropical Medicine and Parasitology,* 3rd edn. Wolfe: London, 1989.

Warren KS, Mahmoud AAF. *Tropical and Geographical Medicine,* 2nd edn. McGraw-Hill Books: New York, 1984.

Yamaguchi T. *A Colour Atlas of Parasitology.* Wolfe: Tokyo, 1981.

Chapter 12: Organization and quality assurance

Advisory Task Force on Standards to the Audit Steering Committee of the Royal College of Pathologists. Pathology department accreditation in the United Kingdom: a synopsis. *Journal of Clinical Pathology* 1991; **44:** 798–802.

Farrington M. Medical audit in the clinical microbiology laboratory in the United Kingdom. *Reviews in Medical Microbiology* 1992; **3:** 104–111.

Snell JJS, Hawkins JM. Quality assurance – achievements and intended directions. *Reviews in Medical Microbiology* 1992; **3:** 28–34.

Snell JJS, Farrell ID, Roberts C. *Quality control: Principles and Practice in the*

Microbiology Laboratory. Public Health Laboratory Service: London, 1991.

Chapter 13: Safety in the laboratory

Collins CH. *Laboratory-acquired Infections*, 2nd edn. Butterworths: London, 1988.
Control of Substances Hazardous to Health Regulations 1988. HMSO: London, 1988.
Health and Safety at Work Act 1974. HMSO: London, 1974.
Health Services Advisory Committee. *Safe Working and the Prevention of Infection in Clinical Laboratories.* HMSO: London, 1991.

Chapter 14: Collection of blood for culture

Bannister BA. Infection and the traveller. *Reviews in Medical Microbiology* 1990; **1:** 185–195.
Brown DFJ, Perry SF. Methods used in the United Kingdom for the culture of micro-organisms from blood. *Journal of Clinical Pathology* 1992; **45:** 468–474.
Freeman R. Blood cultures – principles, practice and pitfalls. *Reviews in Medical Microbiology* 1990; **1:** 92–100.

Chapter 15: Examination of specimens from the central nervous system

Bayston, Leung TSM, Wilkins BM, Hodges B *et al*. Bacteriological examination of removed cerebrospinal fluid shunts. *Journal of Clinical Pathology* 1983; **36:** 987–990.
Fallon RJ. *Microscopical Examination of Cerebrospinal Fluid.* ACP Broadsheet. British Medical Association: London.
Lambert PH (ed). *Infections of the Central Nervous System.* Edward Arnold: London, 1991.

Chapter 16: Infections of the respiratory tract

Barlett JG, Finegold SM. Bacteriology of expectorated sputum with quantitative culture and wash technique compared to transtracheal aspirates. *American Review of Respiratory Disease* 1978; **117:** 1019–1027.
Barret-Connor E. The non-value of sputum culture in the diagnosis of pneumococcal pneumonia. *American Review of Respiratory Disease* 1971; **103:** 845–848.
British Thoracic Society and Public Health Laboratory Service. Community-acquired pneumonia in adults in British hospitals in 1982–1983: a survey of aetiology, mortality, prognostic factors and outcome. *Quarterly Journal of Medicine* 1987; **62:** 195–220.
Kahn FW, Jones JM. Analysis of bronchoalveolar lavage specimens from immuno-compromised patients with a protocol applicable in the microbiology laboratory. *Journal of Clinical Microbiology* 1988; **26:** 1150–1155.
Murray PR. Microscopic and bacteriologic analysis of expectorated sputum. *Mayo Clinic Proceedings* 1975; **50:** 339–344.
Rein MF, Gwaltney JM, O'Brien JM *et al.* Accuracy of Gram stain in identifying pneumococci in sputum. *Journal of the American Medical Association* 1978; **239:** 2671–2673.

Chapter 17: Examination of faeces for bacterial pathogens

Blaser MJ. *Helicobacter pylori*: its role in disease. *Clinical Infectious Diseases* 1992; **15:** 386–393.
Duthia R, French GL. Comparison of methods for the diagnosis of typhoid fever. *Journal of Clinical Pathology* 1990; **43:** 863–865.
Furniss AL, Lee JV, Donovan TJ. *The Vibrios.* Public Health Laboratory Service Monogram 11. HMSO: London, 1979.
Gulig PA. Virulence plasmids of *Salmonella typhimurium* and other salmonella. *Microbial Pathogenesis* 1990; **8:** 3–11.

Helicobacter pylori (formerly *Campylobacter pyloris/pylori*) 1986–1989: a review. *Journal of Clinical Pathology* 1990; **43:** 353–356.

Pedler SJ, Orr KE. Examination of faeces for bacterial pathogens. *Journal of Clinical Pathology* 1990; **43:** 410–415.

Walker RI, Caldwell MB, Lee EC, Guerry P, Trust TJ, Ruiz-Palacios GM *et al.* Pathophysiology of *Campylobacter* enteritis. *Microbiological Reviews* 1986; **50:** 81–89.

Chapter 19: Investigation of specimens from the genital tract and diagnosis of sexually transmitted diseases

Albritton WL. Biology of *Haemophilus ducreyi. Microbiological Reviews* 1989; **53:** 377–389.

Hammann R. Newly recovered and delineated microbial species of the human genital tract. *Infection* 1989; **17:** 188–193.

Levett PN. Bacterial vaginosis. *Reviews in Medical Microbiology* 1992; **3:** 15–20.

Piot P, Van Dyck E, Goodfellow M, Falkow S *et al.* A taxonomic study of *Gardnerella vaginalis* (*Haemophilus vaginalis*). Gardner and Dukes 1955. *Journal of General Microbiology* 1980; **119:** 373–396.

Ridgway GL, Taylor-Robinson D. Current problems in microbiology: 1 Chlamydial infections: which laboratory test? *Journal of Clinical Pathology* 1991; **44:** 1–5.

Chapter 20: Antimicrobial susceptibility

Aymes SGB, Gemmell CG (eds). Antibiotic resistance in bacteria. *Journal of Medical Microbiology* 1992; **36:** 4–29.

British Society of Antimicrobial Chemotherapy (Working Party). Break-points in *in-vitro* antibiotic sensitivity testing. *Journal of Antimicrobial Chemotherapy* 1988; **21:** 701–710.

Davies J. Another look at antibiotic resistance. *Journal of General Microbiology* 1992; **138:** 1553–1559.

Reeves DS, Phillips I, Williams JD, Wise R. (eds). *Laboratory Methods in Antimicrobial Chemotherapy.* Churchill Livingstone: Edinburgh, 1978.

Chapter 21: Serological techniques

Hayden JD, Ho SA, Hawkey PM, Taylor GR, Quirke P *et al.* The promises and pitfalls of PCR. *Reviews in Medical Microbiology* 1992; **2:** 129–137.

Lambert PA. Immunodiagnosis of gram-positive infections. *Reviews in Medical Microbiology* 1990; **1:** 236–242.

Matthews RC, Burnie JP. Clinical applications of molecular biology to diagnostic microbiology. *Journal of Clinical Pathology* 1992; **45:** 465–467.

Voller A, Bidwell DE, Bartlett A. *The Enzyme-Linked Immunosorbent Assay (ELISA). A Guide with Abstracts of Microplate Applications.* Flowline Press: Guernsey, 1979.

Wreghitt TG, Morgan-Capner P. *ELISA in the Clinical Microbiology Laboratory.* Public Health Laboratory Service: London, 1990.

Chapter 22: Bacteriological examination of water, food and air

Collins CH, Lyne PM, Grange JM. *Collins and Lyne's Microbiological Methods,* 6th edn. Butterworths: London, 1989.

Humphreys H. Microbes in the air – when to count! (The role of air sampling in hospitals.) *Journal of Medical Microbiology* **37:** 81–82.

Lewis MJ. Water fit to drink? *Reviews in Medical Microbiology* 1991; **2:** 1–6.

World Health Organization. *Guidelines for Drinking-water Quality.* WHO: Geneva, 1984.

Index